Advance Care Planning in End of Life Care

Edited by

Keri Thomas

Ben Lobo

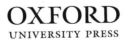
OXFORD

UNIVERSITY PRESS

OXFORD

UNIVERSITY PRESS

Great Clarendon Street, Oxford OX2 6DP
United Kingdom

Oxford University Press is a department of the University of Oxford.
It furthers the University's objective of excellence in research, scholarship,
and education by publishing worldwide. Oxford is a registered trade mark of
Oxford University Press in the UK and in certain other countries

British Library Cataloguing in Publication Data
Data available

Library of Congress Cataloging in Publication Data
Data available

ISBN 978-0-19-956163-6

Oxford University Press makes no representation, express or implied, that the
drug dosages in this book are correct. Readers must therefore always check
the product information and clinical procedures with the most up-to-date
published product information and data sheets provided by the manufacturers
and the most recent codes of conduct and safety regulations. The authors and
the publishers do not accept responsibility or legal liability for any errors in the
text or for the misuse or misapplication of material in this work. Except where
otherwise stated, drug dosages and recommendations are for the non-pregnant
adult who is not breast-feeding.

Foreword

One of the few certainties in life is the inevitability of death. Despite this, many people do not prepare for their own death and do not discuss their priorities or preferences for care as they approach the end of their lives, either with their families or with health and social care professionals. Professionals who care for people who are approaching the end of life may sometimes fail to recognize this or may lack the skills to initiate discussions with their patients about their priorities and preferences. Professionals may fear that raising such matters will cause distress. They may not appreciate that, if done well, discussions can enable patients and their families to prepare and can address fears and relieve anxiety. Discussion and planning can provide a patient with a much greater chance of dying in the place of their choice, with their preferences for care being respected.

The editors of *Advance Care Planning in End of Life Care* have brought together the insight and perspectives of a large number of leading experts in this field from the UK, Australia, Canada, and the USA. These include physicians, nurses, academics, health service managers, and those working for patient associations and charities. Importantly the authors include people working in hospitals, the community, care homes and hospices, and those caring for both young and older people. Each chapter is thoroughly referenced.

Interestingly, what emerges from the different contributors is a growing consensus about the benefits of having sensitive discussions with patients about their wishes for future care and recording patients' preferences. Most importantly the book provides excellent examples about how this can and has been achieved in a variety of settings.

The End of Life Care Strategy in England recognizes identification of people who are approaching the end of life and initiating discussions as the first step of an end of life care pathway. The strategy recognizes that lack of open discussion is one of the key barriers to the delivery of good end of life care.

I thoroughly recommend this book as a key resource to improve care at the end of life. I believe that many individual professionals will find it useful in their clinical practice.

Professor Sir Mike Richards, CBE, MD, FRCP
National Clinical Director for Cancer and End of Life Care
Department of Health
London, England

Preface

'The fear of death follows from the fear of life. A man who lives fully is prepared to die at any time.'
Mark Twain

'We will put patients at the heart of the NHS, through an information revolution and greater choice and control: shared decision making will become the norm: *no decision about me without me.*'
'Equity and Excellence: liberating the NHS', Department of Health, England Crown Copyright July 2010

Advance Care Planning as a key form of shared decision making is increasingly accepted around the world as an integral part of best practice in our care for people nearing the end of life. The purpose of this book is to help readers explore a wide range of issues and practicalities in Advance Care Planning (ACP) for all people, providing a clear framework of shared understanding, and facilitate good practice in a variety of settings and circumstances.

ACP is more widely used in some countries than others, with increasing integration of it as a key part of mainstream End of Life Care policies in the UK and elsewhere. We wish to present ACP in a wider context and draw on the considerable experience and expertise both from the UK and from other countries around the world. It is helpful to contextualize the professional, social, and cultural benefits and risks of ACP, and to be able to share expertise and experience in this important area within an international context. It is impressive that so many people in different countries are reaching the same conclusion at about the same time—that shared decision making through discussing and recording future possible needs and preferences with patients is important, is currently inadequately done, and is a vital means of improving end of life care.

This book takes a comprehensive look at the subject of ACP, frames the purpose, process, and outcomes and includes contributions from experts from around the world. In the different sections of the book, we explore the current evidence of use of ACP, the context and experience in the UK, the lessons learnt by others from the USA, Australia, and Canada, and provide some guidance on practicalities of delivering it in various settings. Although inevitably there may be some key messages that are repeated, each author takes a particular stance and focuses on a unique area, so that the consistency of the message may be affirmed in a variety of ways, and each chapter can be read independently or within the context of the whole. We hope that by promoting this systematic and transparent approach to ACP, more will be enabled to understand and implement ACP in their area, thereby enabling people to live well as they approach the end of life, and to die well in the place and manner of their choosing.

This book will be of great use for both the generalist and specialist professional in the provision of health and social care for people near the end of life, and those involved in commissioning or researching this area. It is comprehensive and far-reaching, presenting detailed evidence-based reviews, providing a number of summaries and reference materials, and enabling wider discussion of the implications of ACP. But it cannot be an exhaustive account, and where necessary readers are directed to other references and resources. We hope that the book will dispel some of the myths about the subject, and focus on meeting the needs of people facing the end of life in a broader and deeper context than previously covered, but we acknowledge the different opinions and variety of responses to this complex area and that there are rarely neat and precise scientific answers to some of these more complex questions.

The principles of ACP outlined here, underpinned by the highest professional standards and used in a spirit of respect and empathy, will help the integration and delivery of personalized, safe, and effective care to people nearing the end of life. Both of us as clinicians have particular experience within our fields of general practice, palliative care and geriatrics in caring for the frail, elderly, and people living with life-limiting conditions, but we include also the more specific areas that require a particular focus, such as people with disabilities, dementia, MND, children, in hospice care, and other areas. Since the majority of people who die in the UK are elderly patients with complex co-morbid non-cancer conditions, cared for by their usual healthcare provider, greater mainstreamed use of ACP in generalist settings of care homes, GP practices, and hospitals is greatly encouraged, supported by those with particular expertise. We mention but do not focus on such areas as euthanasia and Physician Assisted Suicide, as we wish to site ACP discussions within the broadly positive context of quality care and shared decision making relevant to all, to enable people to live well until they die. It is our experience that ACP discussions can help people to live better in that precious time before they die and to die well and as they had wished, when the time comes. As people and as professionals we will continue to strive towards the ambition of providing best care for our patients, fuelled by our sense of vocation, our shared experience, and our humanity. We hope this book makes a significant contribution to this national and international priority. We would also like to point to the growing international momentum of ACP across the world, as founder members of the International Society for Advance Care Planning and End of Life Care (www.acpsociety.org).

This book has been over two years in gestation, with much hard labour at the end. We would like to thank all the contributors to the book, our invaluable secretarial support from Emma Farquhar and Melanie Dakin (without whom undoubtedly we could not have completed the work) and our patient editors and publishers at OUP. We would also like to sincerely thank all other contributors to the book who have worked wonderfully well with us in bringing this to fruition.

Finally, we would like to thank our understanding and supportive families:

Keri—my husband, the 'ever-fixed Mark' (Shakespeare Sonnet 116) and wonderful five children Megan, Ben, Bethany, Sophie, and Imogen.

Ben—my wife Cheryl and Harriet my beautiful and brave daughter. This book is dedicated to them.

Contents

Section 3 **The UK experience of ACP: what's happening now?**

Contributors

Madeline Bass
Head of Education and
Clinical Lead,
St Nicholas Hospice Care,
Bury St Edmunds, Suffolk, UK

Sharon Baxter
Executive Director,
Canadian Hospice Palliative
Care Association; Secretariat for
the Quality End of Life Care,
Coalition of Canada, Canada

Jackie Beavan
Teaching Fellow in Clinical
Communication, University of
Birmingham, UK

Adrienne Betteley
Specialist Practitioner,
End of Life Care Programme Lead,
Merseyside and Cheshire
Cancer Network,
Preferred Priorities National Core
Team member, UK

Simon Chapman
Director of Policy and
Parliamentary Affairs,
The National Council for
Palliative Care, London, UK

Josephine Clayton
Associate Professor,
Staff Specialist and Head of
Department of Palliative Care,
Royal North Shore Hospital,
Sydney, Australia;
Associate Professor,
Faculty of Medicine,
University of Sydney;
Senior Research Member,
Centre for Medical Psychology and
Evidence-Based Decision-Making (CeMPeD),
University of Sydney,
Australia

Simon Conroy
Senior Lecturer/Geriatrician
University of Leicester School of Medicine,
UK

Karen M Detering
Respiratory Physician, Respecting Patient
Choices Program
Austin Hospital, Melbourne, Australia

Eric Fairbank
Director of Palliative care,
Southwest Health Care,
Victoria, Australia

Carolyn Fowler
Macmillan Lecturer Practitioner in
Palliative Care, East and North Herts
NHS Trust,
Education Lead for Cancer and Palliative
Care Mount Vernon Cancer Network

Rob George
Consultant Palliative Medicine Guy's
& St Thomas' NHSFT
Ethicist, Cicely Saunder's Institute,
Kings College London & King's Health
Partners, UK

Lynn Gibson
Manager of Northumberland Learning
Disability Physiotherapy Service,
Northumberland Tyne and Wear NHS
Foundation Trust

Tim Harlow
Consultant Palliative Medicine,
Hospiscare, Exeter, UK

Claire Henry
Programme Director,
National End of Life Care Programme,
London, UK

Jo Hockley
Nurse Consultant for Care Homes,
St Christopher's Hospice,
London, UK

Deborah Holman
Advancing Practice Nurse
End of Life Care,
Gold Standards Framework
Care Home Facilitator,
St Christopher's Hospice,
London, UK

Gillian Horne
Macmillan Research Fellow and
Director of Patient Care,
Rowcroft Hospice, Avenue Road,
Torquay

Sheila Joseph
Programme Manager
National End of Life Care Programme,
London, UK

Ben Lobo
Medical Director,
Consultant Physician and Community
Geriatrician,
Derbyshire Community Health Service
Derbyshire County

Joanne Lynn
Clinical Improvement Expert
Colorado Foundation for Medical Care
Chevy Chase, MD, USA

Heidi Macleod
Director of Care Development,
Motor Neurone Disease Association

Andrew Makin
Nursing Director, Registered
Nursing Home Association,
Independent Mental Capacity Advocate

Bruce Mason
Research Fellow,
Primary Palliative Care Research Group,
The University of Edinburgh, Scotland

Dorothy Matthews
Macmillan CNS Palliative Care
for People with Learing Disabilities,
Northumberland
Tyne and Wear NHS
Foundation Trust

Scott A Murray
Professor
St Columba's Hospice Chair of Primary
Palliative Care,
Primary Palliative Care Research Group,
The University of Edinburgh, Scotland
General Practitioner, Mackenzie Medical
Centre, Edinburgh

AnnMarie Nielsen
Canadian Hospice Palliative Care
Association; Secretariat for the
Quality End of Life Care;
Coalition of Canada, Canada

Simon Noble
Clinical Senior Lecturer,
Palliative Medicine Cardiff University,
Honorary Consultant Palliative Medicine,
Royal Gwent Hospital, Newport

David Oliver
Senior Lecturer in Elderly Care Medicine,
The University of Reading;
Consultant Physician at the Royal
Berkshire NHS Foundation Trust

Don Redding
Head of Policy and Communications,
Picker Institute, Europe

Claud Regnard
Consultant in Palliative Care Medicine,
St Oswald's Hospice, Newcastle Hospitals
NHS Trust and Northumbria University

Sir Mike Richards
Professor,
National Clinical Director for
Cancer and End of Life Care,
Department of Health, London

Sarah JF Russell
Doctoral Research Student,
Visiting Fellow University of Hertfordshire
Trainer, Education for Health, Warwick
Director of Education and Research,
Hospice of St Francis, Berkhamsted,
Hertfordshire

Nikki Sawkins
Specialist Practitioner,
National GSF Clinical Nurse Lead
for Care Homes,
Palliative Care Lead Nurse Waveney
Hospice Care

Jane Seymour
Sue Ryder Care Professor in Palliative and
End of Life Studies,
University of Nottingham
School of Nursing, Midwifery, and
Physiotherapy,
Queen's Medical Centre, Nottingham

W Silvester
Associate Professor, University of Melbourne;
Director, Respecting Patient Choices Program,
Medical Consultant, LifeGift Intensive Care
Specialist, Austin Hospital, Melbourne,
Australia

Dierdra Sives
Palliative Medicine Specialist,
Strathcarron Hospice, Denny,
Stirlingshire, Scotland

Les Storey
National Lead, Preferred Priorities for Care,
National End of Life Care Programme,
Advisor on Advance Care Planning Hospice,
New Zealand
Member of Older People Policy Group,
National Council for Palliative Care

Jennifer Stothard
Head of Commissioning,
Cancer and End of Life Care Services,
NHS Derbyshire County,
Derbyshire

Keri Thomas
Professor
National Clinical Lead for the
Gold Standards Framework Centre,
Hon Professor End of Life Care,
University of Birmingham,
Clinical Champion for End of
Life Care, Royal College of General
Practitioners,
Founder Omega,
The National Association for
End of Life Care

Angela Thompson
Palliative Care Lead Paediatrician
Coventry & Warwickshire,
Trustee of ACT,
Editor of International Journal of
PaedPalLit,
Executive member of Association of
Paediatric Palliative Medicine

Max Watson
Lecturer Palliative Medicine,
University of Ulster, Northern Ireland
Honorary Consultant Palliative Medicine
Northern Ireland Hospice,
Belfast and Princess Alice Hospice, Esher
Special Adviser the Hospice
friendly Hospitals Programme, Dublin

Anne M Wilkinson
Professor,
Western Australia Cancer
Council Chair in Palliative and
Supportive Care,
Western Australia Centre for Cancer
and Palliative Care Research
School of Nursing, Midwifery, and
Postgraduate Medicine
Faculty of Computing, Health and Science
Edith Cowan University
Joondalup, Western Australia

Abbreviations

ACP	Advance Care Planning		IMCA	Independent Mental Capacity Advocate
ACT	Association for Children's Palliative Care		LPA	lasting power of attorney
AD	Advance Directive		LPOA	Legal power of attorney
ADRT	advance decision to refuse treatment		LST	life sustaining treatment
AFMC	Association of Faculties of Medicine of Canada		MCA	Mental Capacity Act
			MND	motor neurone disease
ALS	Amyotrophic Lateral Sclerosis		MNDA	motor neurone disease association
CAD	court appointed deputy		NCPC	The National Council for Palliative Care
CHPCA	Canadian Hospice Palliative Care Association		NHMRC	National Health and Medical Research Council
CNS	community nurse specialist			
COPD	chronic obstructive pulmonary disease		NHS	national health service
CPR	cardiopulmonary resuscitation		NICU	neonatal intensive care unit
DSM	Diagnostic and Statistical Manual of Mental Disorders		OOH	out of hours
			OT	Occupational therapist
EFPPEC	Educating Future Physicians in Palliative and End-of-Life Care		PEG	percutaneous endoscopic gastrostomy
			PPC	preferred priorities of care
eLFH	e-learning for healthcare		PSDA	patient self determination act
EOL	end of life		QI	quality improvement
EoLC	end of life care		RCT	randomized control trial
GP	General Practitioner (family physician)		RPC	respecting patient choices
GSF	gold standards framework		SLA	service level agreements
HCA	health care assistants		SPC	specialist palliative care
IDT	interdisciplinary team			

Section 1

Introduction to Advance Care Planning: why do it?

Chapter 1

Overview and introduction to Advance Care Planning

Keri Thomas

'You matter because you are you, and you matter to the end of your life. We will do all we can not only to help you die peacefully, but also to live until you die.'
Dame Cicely Saunders, Founder of the Modern Hospice Movement

'The question is not whether we will die, but how we will live.'
Joan Borysenko

'End of life care—you can either do it right…or you can do it anyway.'
Sharon Baxter, Canada

This chapter includes:

- An introduction to Advance Care Planning (ACP)
- The purpose and principles of ACP in response to patient need
- Thoughts on the deeper significance of ACP conversations.
- Summary overview
- Suggestions for planning ACP discussions in different settings

---

Key Points

- Advance Care Planning discussions are important. They are a key means of improving end of life care and of enabling better planning and provision of care in line with the needs and preferences of patients and their carers.
- Advance Care Planning discussions are important conversations that can change practice, inform, and empower patients. ACP can be a process of discussions over time, need not be 'over medicalized' or too formalized, and could be undertaken by anyone involved in end of life care, although is best undertaken by experienced staff following some further training.
- The practice of Advance Care Planning affirms the use of advance statements, in which patients clarify their wishes, needs and preferences for the kind of care they would like to receive, and the means of leading a fuller life meanwhile. It can also include advance decisions or refusals of specific treatments including cardio-pulmonary rescuscitation, and the appointment of a person to act as a proxy surrogate e.g. Lasting Power of Attorney.

- The process of Advance Care Planning can be valuable in itself for all, but for many, it relates to the possible future development of incapacity i.e. clarifying wishes and preferences in anticipation of possible future decline.
- There can be a deeper significance of this discussion, in drawing closer to the person's sense of meaning core values and spirituality and in enhancing a sense of self- determination, control, preparedness and hope.
- A summary overview and practical suggestions are given for various settings and further areas signposted within the book.

An introduction to ACP

This book is essentially about having a conversation. It is a particularly important conversation between someone who faces a changing reality as they approach the end of their life, and someone who cares for them. It is usually part of an ongoing dialogue over time within a trusted relationship, or it might be an opportunistic one-off conversation, but either way it can be one of the most important conversations that is undertaken, with both 'life changing' and 'death changing' consequences. As such, at its simplest, it is a matter of seeking the views, choices, preferences, understanding and expectations of the person approaching the end of their life, along with their family and carers, with the aim of this informing and directing the care provided and the quality of life lived. Though essentially simple, within this lie multifaceted complexities that have an enormous impact on all involved in end of life care. This book is an exploration of this conversation and of some, not all, of the facets that underlie it.

As we as a society become increasingly keen on self determination, personalized care and control, ACP gives us a vehicle to express this at the most important of junctures, as we face the final stage of our lives. But there is more to this than meets the eye—the process is itself part of the reward. There are some that have reservations about the subject, and quite rightly warn us off a tick-box policy-driven formulaic response. But, how can listening, really listening, to people ever be wrong, and why might we find it so difficult? This conversation should never for forced, but those with responsibility for the care for our patients should be able to offer these discussions more openly and with the sensitivity to respond as needed. Many people express relief following these discussions, pleased that there is greater clarity on the way forward, that their feelings have been heard, their choices aired and noted. There is greater satisfaction with care following ACP discussions, with reduced anxiety from bereaved carers. (1)

So, with some natural caveats, and understanding the reservations of some clinicians, but encouraged by the common experience of others across the world, (see Chapters 12, and 17–22) this is a plea to colleagues. Let us be courageous and open up this conversation, listening to and acting upon the answers, so that our care can be aligned with the person's wishes and end of life care is the best we can possibly provide—the 'gold standard' that we aspire to. That, I hope, is the essence of Advance Care Planning.

'In coming to accept death, we can more fully embrace life.'

Frankl (1957) Man's Search for Meaning

Advance Care Planning has the potential to improve end of life care by enabling patients to discuss and record their future health and care wishes and also to appoint someone as an advocate or surrogate, thus increasing the likelihood of these wishes being known and respected at the end of life (2). This subject is important for those with the ability to make decisions now, to plan ahead and to live life as fully as possible until they die. It is also important to anticipate a time when they may not be able to make such decisions in future, and to plan for this eventuality. This aspect is stressed as a priority more by some than by others, and it refers to the legislation related to mental capacity and development of advocacy or best interest decisions, particularly in the context of the rising tide of dementia now facing us. This is therefore extremely important in the many cases in which people are unable to make clear decisions at a crucial stage in their lives, not just due to dementia, but also due to changes in levels of consciousness and the incapacity of severe illness.

In addition to this, it is widely thought that in fact the process of having this discussion is as important as the outcome. Advance Care Planning discussions provide the possibility of clarifying future directions and choices so that the issues can be raised, examined, and fully discussed; fears both trivial and huge can be clarified and addressed; and a more realistic and pragmatic approach can be taken to living out the final stage of life in the way that is important to that individual person.

Advance Care Planning discussions open up a space in which plans and reflections can be discussed, a place for contemplating future outcomes and eventualities within a safe environment in order to maximize life in the present. This is a 'liminal' space, a pause in the journey at which different routes and options can be explored and confirmed. This should be at the pace of the individual person and responded to appropriately, to be able to ensure that care is delivered in alignment with the person's requests and wishes. The conversation can be visualised rather like a waltz, with each person moving harmoniously in step with each other, responding to the movement and direction of the other, never treading on each other's toes or overwhelming them with more than they can cope with at the time. In this sense, the Advance Care Planning discussion can only be good.

If one was to assume that this was a simple and easy process, it would not take long to realize that despite sounding straightforward, it requires considerable skill and sensitivity due to the deep significance of the subject. We are talking about something as big as death, as terrifying as loss of all we hold dear, the most threatening subject known to the human race. It can't be quite that simple—there will always be complexities; sensitivities about how to approach and handle the subject; how to say the right words; how to respond to heartfelt longings, to allay fears; how to maintain hope despite the declining reality; how to handle back-lash or denial; how to respond appropriately to optimistic expectations—how to waltz effectively with our patients. This is the deep and powerful fact of death that we quite naturally go to lengths to avoid until we have to— and sometimes not even then. The so called 'death denying' instincts of us all are intrinsic in our make up, part of our survival DNA and we are right to tread carefully in this area and not demean their significance. Death of a loved one can be the most painful and devastating event that we ever face, so it is unsurprising that we naturally would avoid the discussion—whether as patients, carers, families or as professionals. Like other animals, our survival instincts are strong, and contemplating death is counter-intuitive. As TS Elliott put it, 'Humankind cannot stand very much reality', and for some, denial is a legitimate coping mechanism, which they do not wish to be shattered by another's well meaning honesty. Their family may regret this 'collusion of silence' but we must at all times respect the views of the person concerned, walking the sensitive tightrope of gently coaxing towards the opening up of a wider discussion if appropriate, whilst never forcing the conversation.

The underlying purpose and principles of ACP, in response to patient need

Advance care planning is defined as a process of discussion between a patient and professional carer, which may include family and friends. This dialogue has two main outcomes (see Fig. 1.1)—firstly

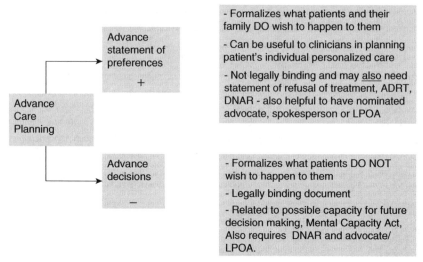

Fig. 1.1 Advance Care Planning—statement of preferences and advance decisions or refusals.

an 'advance statement', which describes the patient's positive preferences and aims for future care; and secondly an 'advance decision', which provides informed consent for refusal of specific treatment if the patient is not competent to make such a decision in the future. In addition, to both of these, a further output is the nomination of a proxy advocate for the person, in England known as the Lasting Power of Attorney. As with other countries (see Chapters 17,18, and 20–22), the focus of advance care planning is shifting from the second to the first, from eliciting refusal of treatment for a minority of patients to identifying the preferences for care of most patients. (Fig. 1.2)

So why should we discuss this difficult subject? We know within our current health and social care systems, that end of life care is inadequate and requires considerable improvement. Too often we are failing our patients through poorly coordinated, poorly communicated care. Unanticipated needs are often addressed through inappropriate crisis responses that do not meet the preferences of the individual. This is especially true of the frail elderly, many with cognitive impairment, who make up the majority of deaths and are the most vulnerable to over-medicalizing death and dying. A National Audit Office Report in England suggested that about half of residents from care homes who died in hospital could have died elsewhere, and that the frail elderly were the most vulnerable to over–hospitalization (2).

People's priorities for a good death have been described in many different ways, and in all of these a sense of being prepared, of not being a burden on others and of retaining some control are key elements (1–4).The usual understanding of the benefits of Advance Care Planning are respect for autonomy, preparation for possible future incapacity, and completion of formal directives. But in addition, patients see the benefits of Advance Care Planning to include preparation for end-of-life care and death, relieving anxiety, dealing with unfinished business, avoiding prolongation of dying, strengthening of personal relationships, relieving burdens placed on family, and the communication of future wishes (5) Some find the timing of the discussion a crucial factor in its success, and for some patients with cancer this can be particularly relevant, indicating that ACP for younger cancer patients might be a rather different issue than for the elderly in care homes or those with long term non-cancerous conditions (6).

There is a growing belief that we as health and social care providers have a responsibility to open up this dialogue in a sensitive and open way, because the benefits of doing so greatly outweigh the disadvantages and personal cost. Handled sensitively, such conversations are more likely to enhance life in the remaining time for these people, enabling them to grow through this staggeringly difficult challenge towards something greater than before, help to secure the kind of care that they feel is important to them, avert the kind of reactive over medicalized 'conveyer belt' of interventions and hospitalization that sometimes happens in our modern world, and enable people to grow in dignity and fulfilment of life as they face the final important stage.

Regarding preferred place of death, we know that about half do not die where they would choose (7). People whose preferences are discussed and recorded are more likely to attain them, than those for whom this issue has not been raised or noted. As dying at home is the preferred option of the majority, despite only about a third attaining it, this in itself has considerable economic implications in providing care closer to home and reducing excessive expensive hospitalization, something currently in the public eye. So ACP can be helpful in enabling us to make best use of scarce resources, and in aligning with patients' choices—a potential 'win win'.

The conversation can also trigger something very important within families, and help create the opportunity to say those things that otherwise may be left unspoken. People approaching death can find it easier than their families to discuss meaningful things, and yet such affirmations of a sense of pride, of approval, of shared memories, of forgiveness, of love can be with them in the memory for years to come. Ira Byock in his book, 'The Four things that Matter Most', suggests these four great affirmations are: I'm sorry, I forgive you, thank you, I love you (8). This brings about a sort of ending that may befit the life led. Initiation of such a discussion for the many is increasingly seen as being more valuable that specific refusal of treatment for the few.

Some who have been using Advance Directives as refusals of treatment for many years in the USA are sceptical about the benefit of focussing on the latter form of refusal decision exclusively. '… unexpected problems often arise to defeat ADs. Advance Care Planning should emphasize not the completion of directives but the emotional preparation of patients and families for future crises (9).' Many feel that things are shifting towards statements of wishes and preferences, being better prepared, and the conversation being more between the patient and family (see Chapter 17) (Fig. 1.2). In my experience in care homes, the early introduction of this discussion to families before admission to the home, eases the path and normalizes the process even before the later conversation with the clinician—as they say 'helping us to help you' or 'thinking ahead' so that they can provide best care in line with their hopes and expectations.

Traditional vs developing model of Advance Care Planning as used in USA	
Traditional model	**Developing model**
Purpose	Prepare for death
Prepare for incapacity	Achieved control in health system
	Relieve burden
	Strengthen relationships
Focus	
Written advance directive	Written advance directive only one aspect
Context	
Doctor/patient relationship	Patient/family

Fig. 1.2 Traditional versus developing model of Advanced Care Planning as used in the USA.

There are similar movements in other countries, and in the UK the focus has been on the completion of the statement of wishes for all people approaching the end of life, with the optional refusal of treatment for those to whom this applies. The discussion about resuscitation is for those relevant patients for whom resuscitation may possibly be of benefit, in an effort to prevent unwanted over medicalization of the dying process (see Chapter 10). For many in care homes, however, this will not be relevant as resuscitation would be futile (10), but this still needs to be recognized and communicated to others to prevent undignified, inappropriate resuscitation attempts.

There are growing movements in many countries which are focussing on improving end of life care by emphasizing the need to offer discussions which can lead to a positive statement of wishes and preferences for all appropriate patients. The emphasis on this is also growing in the UK with the use of the NHS End of Life Care Programme and an example of ACP, Preferred Priorities of Care, (see Chapter 11) and the GSF Thinking Ahead document (11), though we have a long way to go before ACP is fully integrated into current thinking and standardized practice. Although it's tough to do, important to do well, and can cause issues for some, it is too important to ignore; Advance Care Planning discussions are now here to stay.

Thoughts on the deeper significance of ACP conversations

For those of us working in this area it is intriguing that many patients express thankfulness for the jolt of some life-threatening experience or diagnosis, to reawaken their sense of values and priorities and enable them to live life to the full. Those who have gone through 'near-death' experiences say the same and live with a new perspective with less fear, more appreciation of the now, and a reawakened sense of what matters in life. In facing death, there is much we can learn about life.

Death focuses the mind as to what is important in life. If we were able to cope somehow with the reality of death, overcoming our fundamental death denying delusion, could we live in the context of our dying and would our lives be better for this? Many would say yes. If we admitted our mortality at a deep level, knowing that 'when' not 'if' we die, maybe then we could live life more fully, with more gentleness and forgiveness, with renewed perspective and priorities (12) (see Chapter 5).

Denying death is intrinsic in our make up—to live as if we live forever. But if we grow in awareness of the limitations of this life, it is the experience of many that we can live a fuller life now, more in line with our core values. If we can live lives more in the context of our dying, will this change the way we live? This is a big stretch for most of us, and yet those that have been stretched in this way have become 'bigger' people for it, with a wider horizon and a greater sense of the value of the present moment. The Greek symbol Omega derives from the great or 'mega' zero. 'Omega people' who live in the context of their dying tend to be people of joy, of profound presence, and of altered perspective, as found in many hospices and care homes across the land. This is the experience of many working in palliative care—that patients become our teachers and deeper lessons are there if we choose to see them. Likewise, we can discover this during these important ACP discussions, we can help people live fuller lives, of better quality, more in tune with their wishes and preferences in the time remaining to them, and help to bring their lives to a fitting and respectful conclusion.

Hope and expectations

'To me having information, it's critical. Even if it's bad news I want to know what it is so I can cope with it. I want to know what's going on, what I can set myself up for' (13)

Realistic information, sensitively provided, helps patients and their families to maintain a feeling of normality and allows them to adapt and develop new coping strategies. Such discussions engender hope. Such hope is not an aspiration for a cure, but for assuaging of fear, understanding the process of dying, and for reassurance that support will be given during a variety of eventualities. In a fascinating Canadian study of renal failure patients contemplating the use of ACP in fostering hope, Davison and Simpson describe the importance of these discussions in normalizing life and enhancing hope, even when to the outsider it seems that all hope is lost (13). Planning for death with our patients may be an uncomfortable concept but is likely to engender resilience and realistic hope in many rather than dispel it (14).

If we assume we will live for ever, it can be a shock to discover we do not—expectations of the baby boom generation may be particularly high and unrealistic. But most would agree that quality of life is more important than quantity, and there is a strong emphasis now on maintaining this quality of life for as long as possible 'bringing years to life and life to years'. Calman described quality of life in terms of the gap between patients' expectations and reality—the greater the gap suggesting the more distress and 'dis-ease' (15). Our role as healthcare providers may be to help reduce this gap, negotiate realistic changes in expectation, by discussing likely trajectories and prognoses through Advance Care Planning, and providing concurrent improvements in reality, with good symptom control and support services, thereby improving quality of life in the final months and weeks. (See Box 1.1 for an overview of ACP in the UK.)

'We should aim for a life well lived and a death worth dying for'

Terry Pratchett. The Times; Jan 2010

Suggestions for planning ACP in different settings

Within each setting and context the appropriate plans for introduction of Advance Care Planning discussions as part of mainstream practice and policy must be made. More details of these are in the relevant sections of this book. A systematic structure such as use of the Gold Standards

---

Box 1.1 Overview of Advance Care Planning in England (16,17)

What is ACP? (16,17)

ACP is a process of discussion between an individual and their care provider, and this may also include family and friends

There are two different types:

An Advance Statement—a statement reflecting an individual's preferences and aspirations, that can help identify how the person would like to be cared for. Though not legally binding, it is likely to be taken into account

An Advance Decision—the decision must relate to a specific treatment and specific circumstances. It will only come into effect when the individual has lost capacity to give or refuse consent. (Used to be called Advance Directive/Living will)

Why is ACP important?

- Used extensively across the world
- A cornerstone in improving end of life care
- Encourages pre-planning of care
- Enables better provision of service, related to patient needs
- Empowers and enables patients and family
- May increases quality of life, sense of control, preserve normality and hope
- Increasingly required by patients and their families

Box 1.1 Overview of Advance Care Planning in England *(continued)*

Why do it? Advantages

- Respects the person's human rights
- Most people are happy to discuss advance care planning
- This may improve patient satisfaction, and bereaved carer satisfaction
- Encourages full discussion about end of life decisions
- Doctors are more likely to give appropriate treatment
- Helps difficult decision-making
- Family/friends do not have to take difficult decisions
- Better planning and provision of care and services to meet needs and preferences
- More likely to die in preferred place of care if this is stated, especially home death.
- May help prevent inappropriate admissions, death and resuscitations, with economic implications
- Helps to begin realistic dialogue and encourage resilience and realistic planning
- Can be a catalyst for deeper discussions, reflection on meaning and priorities, and spiritual considerations
- Can help deepen relationships through enhanced communication and reduce feeling of being a burden
- Can enable a sense of retaining control, self determination and empowerment
- Helps determine future goals and provide insight

Why not do it? Disadvantages and Difficulties

- Difficulty in initiating discussion
- Sensitive sometimes difficult discussion requires good judgement
- Can appear to back fire if poorly undertaken
- Anticipating the future and how an individual responds to such circumstances is complex
- Frequently updating any advanced decisions
- Availability of documentation
- Ensuring the advanced decisions can be interpreted within a healthcare setting
- Right to demand certain treatments
- Left to junior staff to initiate discussion
- Busying over routine clinical issues
- 'Death Anxiety' of staff
- Making time
- Sensitivities and sadness
- May require extra communication skills

Barriers

- Client/individual
- Family availability unaware of need
- Healthcare professionals— inexperience lack of knowledge, discomfort, lack of time, doctors uncertainty of appropriateness
- System factors—lack of communication, legislation etc
- Public awareness

Box 1.1 Overview of Advance Care Planning in England *(continued)*

How—Tips for a successful ACP discussion (see excellent RCP Guidelines) (17)

- A step-by-step approach should be used.
- It is a process, not a single event—discussions on more than one occasion (over days, weeks, months) and in most circumstances usually not on a single visit
- The person needs to be ready for the discussion—it cannot be forced
- Patients can refuse, defer, review, wish only for verbal discussion or wish to discuss other issues
- It takes time and effort and should not be done as a checklist, but in comfortable, unhurried surroundings
- An ACP tool to guide the discussion may help
- Clear information must be given; clarify, check, and reflect with the patient (see Chapter 23)

The discussion is characterized by truthfulness, respect, time, compassion, and empathy

- Look out for cues that they wish to end the discussion, summarize and check understanding with the patient, and plan for a review
- The discussion should be documented if the patient so wishes
- Not all people will be able to document their wishes, but may well be able to nominate their preferred decision maker and discuss their long-term values, as these come to mind more readily than anticipating abstract situations

How—policy and tools

- Greater public awareness e.g. 'Dying Matters' Let's Talk campaign
- Staff may need special support and communication skills training
- May need leaflets or guidance materials to give to families before the discussion
- Region-wide ACP documents to be used and agreement as to when they should be used
- Information transfer—health and social care providers including out of hours, emergency services, and ambulance, especially related to preferred place of care and DNAR status
- Make both Advance statements and ADRTs accessible as needed

When—Triggers

Specific examples

- Following a new diagnosis of life limiting condition
- In conjunction with prognostic indicators
- Multiple hospital admissions
- Admission to a care home
- Expressed need of patient or family

General examples

- Life changing event e.g. death of spouse or close friend or relative
- Making or changing a will

Who

- Patient and family—supporting patients and their families to discuss this early e.g. using an introductory leaflet e.g. Planning Your Future Care (18)
- The usual healthcare provider who has a long standing relationship e.g. GP, community nurse, or healthcare provider
- Secondary care—specialist consultant hospital ward staff, etc
- Palliative care specialist
- Sometimes trained non-clinical facilitator

Box 1.1 Overview of Advance Care Planning in England *(continued)*

What is a Lasting Power of Attorney (LPOA)?

See Chapter 8

A LPOA is a person (an 'attorney') to take decisions on their behalf if they subsequently lose capacity. This can extend to personal welfare matters as well as property and affairs (previously called Enduring Power of Attorney in England). This person may be appointed to make specific health and welfare decisions on their behalf, should they lose capacity

Resuscitation discussions

Do Not Attempt resuscitation (DNAR), not for CPR and Allow Natural Death (AND) are specific forms of refusal of treatment. They may not be relevant in every case. Many areas are developing a standard DNAR form and process. This is not the same as ACP policy.

Framework (GSF) can help improve the organisation, triggers, and uptake of the ACP through-out the team (19, 20). GSF is a systematic common-sense approach to formalizing best practice, so that quality end of life care becomes standard for every patient. It helps clinicians identify patients in the last year of life, assess their needs, symptoms and preferences, and plan care on that basis; enabling patients to live and die where they choose. GSF embodies an approach that centres on the needs of patients and their families and encourages inter-professional teams to work together. GSF focuses on enabling 'generalists' or the usual frontline healthcare provider to provide best care for all patients nearing the end of life. It is widely used in the UK, through specific programmes in primary care, for care homes, and in hospitals. In this context, the ACP discussions are more likely to occur using the coordinated approach of GSF; e.g. as a trigger ena-bling every resident in the care home to be offered an ACP discussion, for all patients on the GPs GSF/palliative care register, and all appropriate hospital patients to be offered ACP discussions. In summary, ACP can be offered in many settings (see Boxes 1.2 and 1.3).

Box 1.2 A summary of ACP in different settings

- ◆ All settings
  - Following consultation, agree a policy, plan and means of communication across the whole setting
  - Involve family, carers and the usual healthcare providers
  - Back policy up with systematic education, especially of doctors who may take longer to be persuaded of the benefits of ACP (1)
  - Audit the proportion dying in their preferred place of care e.g. using GSF After Death Analysis (ADA) (19) and use as feedback against target
  - Note and communicate DNAR status where appropriate (not the same as ACP)
- ◆ ACP in Primary Care Teams (see Box 1.3 and Chapter 13)
  - All patients on the QOF palliative care/GSF register should be offered an advance care planning discussion i.e. those identified to be in the final 6–12 months of life
  - This register should include non-cancer patients and an assessment of the proportion of all practice deaths on the register should be made (see Next Stage GSF website (19))

Box 1.2 A summary of ACP in different settings *(continued)*

- Preferred place of care should be sought sensitively, recorded, and communicated to others involved in their care, e.g. out of hours providers, ambulance staff (perhaps through the use of the handover form)
- At the team meeting the patient's ACP and known preferences including place of care should be discussed and efforts made to attain this where possible, being aware that decisions can change due to changing circumstances such as carer breakdown

◆ ACP in Care Homes (see Chapter 12)
- Every resident should be offered an ACP discussion following admission to a care home
- Care homes could produce their own leaflet describing ACP for visiting relatives to help initiate the discussion before coming to the home and once settled in, as in the GSF Care Homes Training Programme
- For those with reduced capacity or dementia, a best interest discussion with relatives can be completed and, over time, indications of preference can become clear (see dementia ACP Box 12.4)
- The ACP becomes pivotal in planning more 'personalized' care around the resident and their relatives

◆ ACP in Hospitals (see Chapter 20)
- Develop coordinated ACP policy within hospital
- Note ACPs already available for hospital inpatients or outpatients
- Note patients approaching the end of life and ACP discussion offered, often by a specified trained person able to hold ACP discussions
- Follow guidance such as Respecting Patient Choices (1)

◆ ACP in hospices (see Chapter 14)
- Develop coordinated policy for all patients to be offered ACP discussions
- Ensure high levels of staff support and training
- Ensure communication to others in the community and secondary care during admission and at discharge

◆ ACP in wider healthcare organisations (see Chapter 18)
- Develop coordinated system wide policy for ACP. This is in addition to that for resuscitation decisions (DNAR)
- Develop 'campaign' in line with greater public awareness
- Ensure good information transfer including emergency services and coordination centres e.g. handover forms, 'message in a bottle' etc
- Where there is use of a locality register, patient passport, patient held record, or use of cross boundary GSF ensure information follows patient

Box 1.3 ACP suggested five point plan for GPs (14)

1. **Identify** patients nearing the end of their life (within the final 6–12 months) and include them on the palliative care/GSF register (14 GSFwebsite identify link
   a. Use of Surprise question or GSF Prognostic Guidance) (19)
   b. Multiple admissions to hospital
   c. Admission to a nursing home
   d. Other factors such as death of a spouse
2. **Discuss management plan** of care with the primary care team using the palliative care/GSF Register
3. **Advance Care Planning discussion** with the patient and family/carers; using an agreed tool and communicated to others. (Advance Statement). May have Lasting Power of Attorney (LPOA)
4. **Advance Decision** and Advance Decision to Refuse Treatment (ADRT)—used if the possibility of future incapacity to refuse a specific treatment is being questioned; written with the help of hospital/hospice specialists and lawyers—in line with the guidance in the Mental Capacity Act: this may include a Do Not Attempt Resuscitation (DNAR) form or Lasting Power of Attorney (LPOA)
5. **Provide services and review**—Use the advance statement to enable provision of the required services where possible, and review regularly with patient and carers/family.

Finally, one of the key aims of Advance Care Planning discussions is to help people be better prepared for the future, to 'hope for the best but prepare for the worst', but in doing so, to support more realistic glimpses of possible scenarios. It therefore has a benefit far greater than is at first apparent, in supporting deeper communication, better transfer of information, greater quality of life and enabling the person and their family or carers to live life more fully in the way they wish to live. Advance Care Planning, skilfully undertaken, integrated into standard practice, respectfully delivering care aligned with the person's wishes, can be literally a life enhancing experience, and plays a major role in enabling best end of life care for all.

This book includes many examples of good practice in Advance Care Planning in different settings and scenarios from around the world, and though it does not cover every possible area, it paints a picture of a time when Advance Care Planning might become the norm, and might routinely inform all areas of care. This might therefore act as an encouragement and a resource for all striving to implement ACP within their area of care, and enable more to be able to live well and die well in the place and the manner of their choosing.

References

1 Detering KM, Hancock AD, Reade MC, Silvester W (2010). The impact of advance care planning on end of life care in elderly patients: randomised controlled trial. *BMJ*, **340**:c1345.
2 National Audit Office Report in En of Life Care Nov 08 www.nao.org.uk
3 Smith R A good death 'Age Concern Debate of the Age' *BMJ*, **320**:129–30.

4   Steinhauser KE, Clipp EC, McNeilly M, Christakis NA, McIntyre LM, and Tulsky JA (2000). In search of a good death: observations of patients, families, and providers. *Annals of Internal Medicine*, **132**(10): 825–32.

5   Department of Health End of Life Care Strategy July 2008 London www.dh.gov.uk/en/Healthcare/ IntegratedCare/Endoflifecare/DH_299

6   Barnes K, Jones L, Tookman A and King M (2007). Acceptability of an advance care planning interview schedule: a focus group study Palliative Medicine, **21**:23–28

7   Gomes B and Higginson IJ (2006). Factors influencing death at home in terminally ill patients with cancer: systematic review. *BMJ*, **332**:515–21.

8   The Four things that matter most Ira Byock Simon & Schuster 2003

9   Perkins HS (2007). Controlling Death: The False Promise of Advance Directives experience of dying. *Annals of Internal Medicine*, **147**:51–57. www.annals.org

10 Conroy SP, Luxton T, Dingwall R, Harwood RH, and Gladman JRF (2006). Cardiopulmonary resuscitation in continuing care settings: time for a rethink? *BMJ*, **332**:479–82 (25 February)

11 GSF Advance care Planning www.goldstandardsframework.nhs.uk

12 http://www.5wishesbook.com/video.php

13 Davison SN and Simpson C (2006). Hope and advance care planning in patients with end stage renal disease: qualitative interview study, *BMJ*, **333**:886

14 Murray SA, Sheikh A, and Thomas K (2006). Advance care planning in primary care *Uncomfortable, but likely to engender hope rather than dispel it,* Editorial *BMJ*, **333**:868–914

15 Calman KC (1984). Quality of life in cancer patients—an hypothesis. *Journal of Medical Ethics*, **10**:124–7.

16 Advance Care Planning A guide for health and social care staff Aug 2008 NHS End of Life Care Programme www.endoflifecareforadults.nhs.uk/publications/pubacpguide

17 Advance Care Planning—Concise Guidance to Good practice no 12 Royal College of Physicians Feb 2009 www.bookshop.rcplondon.ac.uk

18 Planning your Future Care www.endoflifecareforadults.nhs.uk

19 http://www.goldstandardsframework.nhs.uk/TheGSFToolkit/ToolsandTemplates

20 Thomas K (2003). Caring for the dying at home. Companions on a journey. Oxford. Radcliffe Medical Press.

Chapter 2

Advance Care Planning for the end of life: an overview

Jane Seymour and Gillian Horne

This chapter includes:

- ◆ Brief introductions
- ◆ Outline of development of ACP
- ◆ Selective summary of ACP research
- ◆ Discussion of the social and cultural challenges with ACP
- ◆ Practice and policy developments to promote ACP in England
- ◆ Focus on the perspectives of patients and the public on ACP and related issues

---

Key points:

- ◆ ACP developed in the latter half of the twentieth century alongside concerns about the risks of futile and inappropriate use of life prolonging medical technologies
- ◆ ACP has been promoted as a means of setting on record the views, values, and specific treatment choices of those living with serious, progressive conditions that are likely to cause incapacity or loss of the ability to communicate wishes to others in the future
- ◆ Various initiatives in law, policy, and healthcare systems across the Western world are actively and strongly promoting practice based as well as strategic initiatives to support implementation of ACP
- ◆ There has been recognition that a whole-systems approach to Advance Care Planning is necessary to bring about change in end of life care
- ◆ Community based complex interventions have been developed which go beyond the objective of completing an advance directive (AD) form and embrace process issues. Some interventions appear to have enabled greater congruence between treatment at end of life and expressed preferences, in addition to a greater use of palliative care services
- ◆ A new perspective has begun to emerge in which emphasis is placed less on leaving an instruction to guide medical care and more on the potential for Advance Care Planning discussions to help patients and their families prepare for death, review their immediate goals and hopes for the future, and strengthen their relationships (see Chapter 17)
- ◆ There are gaps in the research literature about how best to initiate ACP and its timing.

Introduction

The urgent need for initiatives aimed at addressing barriers to improving the quality of palliative and end of life care was highlighted by a report released in the UK during 2007 which analysed complaints to the Healthcare Commission: the NHS watchdog in England (1). The report analysed 16000 complaints made between July 2004 and July 2006, finding that more than half (54%) of complaints from bereaved family members about hospital treatment were about end of life care and, of these, most centred on failures perceived in relation to communication and degree of 'preparedness' for the death. Over the last decade or so, research evidence suggests a similar picture has emerged from many other developed countries. Among the largest and most frequently cited is the US SUPPORT study, which found that among a large sample of patients recognized as at high risk of dying, 50% had a 'do not attempt resuscitation' order written in the last two days of life and more than one third spent their last days in ICU (2).

In the not too distant past, serious illness led to death quite quickly. Dying was encapsulated into a few weeks or days and there were fairly clear norms of social and clinical behaviour surrounding the person who was dying and their companions. Now, with the rise of what has been called the 'indistinct zone' (3) of chronic illness and the concentration of death in older age, life has fundamentally changed: we tend to live for a long time with illnesses that are eventually fatal and die perhaps when no one expects us to. New questions have emerged to which we have not yet found the answers to either personally, socially, or institutionally:

1 When?

    The first question is about prognostication and timing: how do we know when our focus should shift from trying to prolong life to trying to provide comfort as life comes to an end and, when a prognosis is given, whom does this benefit?

2 Who decides?

    The second turns around decision making: what principles should guide the decisions that may be required at the bedside of a dying person, whose dying risks being prolonged by the inappropriate use of medical technology or who needs rapid relief from pain?

3 Who acts?

    The third question relates to authority and responsibility: who should take the lead in managing end of life care? The clinician? The patient? The patient's family?

4 Whose values?

    The last question relates to the interpretation of concepts and values: what does it mean to die with dignity? How can we achieve this when we know that this term means so many different things to different people?

Advance Care Planning (ACP), usually defined as a process of discussion between an individual, their family, and care providers, has been widely promoted as one means of addressing these multiple questions and first appeared as an umbrella term describing a range of interventions and associated outcomes in the literature in the early 1990s (4). ACP has been promoted as a means of setting on record the views, values, and specific treatment choices of those living with serious, progressive conditions that are likely to cause incapacity or loss of the ability to communicate wishes to others in the future. The goals of Advance Care Planning have been identified as:

◆ Ensuring that clinical care is in keeping with the patient's informed decisions and preferences when the patient has become incapable of decision making; improving the health care decision making process by facilitating shared decision making

♦ Improving patients' well being by reducing the frequency of either under or over treatment. (4,5).
Advance Care Planning commonly results in one or more outcomes, all of which are well described in the literature (5,6). In summary, these are:

1 The setting out of **general values and views** about care and treatment. In England, these are known as 'statements of wishes and preferences', and are promoted as a useful record to guide future care (7).

2 An instructional directive: often known as a 'living will' or advance directive (AD), which sets on record positive or negative **views about specific life prolonging treatments** such as cardiopulmonary resuscitation (CPR) or ventilation, in defined circumstances. Those that set out an advance refusal, now have legal force in most countries when assessed as valid and applicable. In England, these are called **'advance decisions to refuse treatment'** (ADRTs) under the provisions of the Mental Capacity Act (8). Both generic and disease specific directives are described in the literature (9).

3 **The nomination of a proxy**: often known as an 'attorney', who then has the authority to represent the patient once they have lost capacity in relation to decisions surrounding their medical treatment. In England, the introduction of provisions for 'lasting powers of attorney' under the Mental Capacity Act of 2005 (8) is one example.

Various initiatives in law, policy, and healthcare systems are actively and strongly promoting practice based as well as strategic initiatives to support implementation of ACP, although the exact form of implementation and the terms used differs across states and countries (10).

Brief history

The rising popularity of ACP arguably reflects trends in late modern palliative care towards emphasizing the value of 'open awareness' around death and dying, and a wider societal concern with the promotion of personal autonomy (11), as well as the containment of health care costs and amelioration of the consequences of what many perceive as the 'run away train' of medical technology. The cultural stance and response of the USA to these factors has arguably been a major influence across the Western world. The concept of a 'living will' was initially proposed in 1969 in the USA (8), and was subsequently embedded in US legislation which followed two high profile cases of the 1970s and 80s (see Chapter 17). These involved the withdrawal of life support from young women left in persistent vegetative states—Karen Quinlan, was 21 when she had a cardiac arrest related to substance abuse; Nancy Cruzan was 32 when she was involved in a near fatal car accident. In Cruzan's case, it was seven years before her parents were successful in persuading the courts to authorize the removal of the artificial feeding keeping her alive (12). The passage of the Patient Self-Determination Act in the USA during the 1990s—hot on the heels of the conclusion to the Cruzan case—made it mandatory for all patients admitted to a health care institution or enrolled with a health care agency to be given written information about their rights on decision making and the right to prepare an advance statement relating to their future medical care (13). As a result of legislative processes in the US, the emphasis there has been until recently on the completion of instructional directives or the nomination of proxies using the principle of 'precedent' or prospective autonomy (14,15). In the last ten years, this emphasis has begun to change as evidence emerges of what is important to patients and families. A new model has emerged in which emphasis is placed on the potential for ACP discussions to help patients and their families prepare for death, review their immediate goals and hopes for the future and strengthen their relationships (16) (see Chapter 17). The move towards a 'self care' model of Advance Care Planning for example—'Lets talk' (17) (appendix 1) additionally provides a means for individuals to access information and on-line tools to make their own decisions about future medical care.

Developments similar to those occurring in the USA have taken place in Canada, Australia, and Northern Europe since 1990, often in association with high profile cases. However, it is probably true to say that it is only in the last few years that there has been any serious debate among practitioners, researchers, and policy makers about whether and how ACP should be implemented, and what are its risks and benefits in clinical care. The frequency of use of ACP records varies markedly across the world, with very low take up reported in most countries except some areas in North America (5). For example, one study in New South Wales, Australia, has shown that less than one per cent of people have a record in their notes of any discussion about Advance Care Planning (18), despite initiatives in other parts of the country (see Chapters 20 and 21). However, there appears to be a groundswell of opinion in favour of the idea of ACP and some evidence of efforts to engage at a practice level with ACP discussions, even if these are not formally recorded. In the UK, NHS initiatives such as the Preferred Priorities of Care (19), Gold Standards Framework (20), and Liverpool Care Pathway for the Dying Patient (21) may all be seen as challenging organizations and practitioners to engage with users of services about aspects of ACP, particularly as they relate to place of care. The potential for ACP to contribute to better end of life care outcomes for patients has been significantly emphasized in the End of Life Strategy for England (22) and the associated national review of NHS services (23).

Outcomes of ACP: the evidence base

Several studies have identified benefits which result from ACP, although there is conflicting evidence. An association between having a advance directive and dying outside the acute hospital has been observed, although there is little understanding of how the directive or the processes of Advance Care Planning leading to its completion may have contributed to decisions around place of care (24–26). Perhaps, as a logical sequel of the expectation that having an AD may result in less 'high tech' and hospital inpatient care, there have been some hotly contested claims that ACP could result in reduced health care costs (27). For example, Fries et al. state '… advance directives, such as a living will or durable power of attorney, that emphasize humane and dignified care at the end of life can reduce costs as well as ensure desired care' (28).

There is some evidence that ACP may increase individuals' autonomy in terms of sense of control (29,30). Some interventions, particularly where they go beyond the objective of completing an AD form and embrace process issues, appear to have enabled greater congruence between treatment at end of life and expressed preferences (23,30–32). The most well known of these is the 'Respecting your Choices' programme (33) implemented by Bernard Hammes and his team in Wisconsin, USA and now taken up in several other states and countries, including Australia and Canada (see for example *www.polst.org*). This involves a multi faceted educational programme with skilled facilitators whose job it is to help patients document a range of goals, wishes, and plans for the future. It has the following objectives:

- To help people understand what options and decisions might be faced, help them reflect on those decisions, work through the issues and then both make decisions and communicate these decisions to each other and ultimately to the health professionals
- To enable systems to track and make use of documents and preferences
- To make sure retrieval from the medical record was possible
- To influence care so that advance directives would be carefully considered in decision making (31).

A similar programme called 'Let me Decide' implemented in Canada in nursing homes and hospitals, has shown similar results to those emanating from the latter programme (32). A further example is the 'Choices' intervention (Comprehensive Home Based Options for Informed Consent for End Stage Services) which, for 208 patients with advanced chronic illness, has been shown to result in more time spent at home, more palliative care, and less time in hospitals (34). In the specialist intensive care literature similar results have been found. Interventions involving intensive communications training and a systems focus towards change were found to increase options for palliative care as opposed to aggressive intensive support (for a review, see reference 35, p89).

Where the focus has been mainly on completion of an AD form, with little supplemental work to change attitudes or influence the quality of communication, the evidence has been much less positive (35,36). In the most famous of the many studies, SUPPORT, it was found that an intervention based around the completion of AD forms which were then made available to patient's physicians, had no impact on the style of communication between doctor and patient, on the incidence or timing of DNAR orders, or on the knowledge that doctors reported they had about patients' preferences (2). It has been recognized latterly that an important limitation of traditional ADs is that they tend to relate to scenarios which are either too vague (if I am close to death) or too specific (if I am in a persistent vegetative state) to be useful (37).

ACP facilitating a process of shared decision making

In the last few years, a number of studies using qualitative methods to interview patients and their care-givers have been published which shed light on the particular contribution Advance Care Planning can make to the quality of life of patients living with an illness that will eventually be fatal. These draw attention to the importance of the process rather than outcomes of ACP, illustrating how it may offer a vehicle for communication and choice about end of life care through facilitating mutual understanding between parties involved and enhancing openness and discussion of concerns. Among these, is one study from Canada (38) reporting interviews with patients with renal failure who were either about to, or had recently commenced, dialysis. The patients reported that they found that the ACP discussion could be an important opportunity to articulate their hopes for the future and to reflect on how to make sense of, and make plans for the impact of, their illness on their daily life, and on their family:

> Hope was central to the process of advance care planning for these patients in that their hopes helped to determine their future goals of care and provided insight into the perceived benefits of facilitated advance care planning and their willingness to engage in end of life discussions. Patients' hopes, therefore, became the cornerstone of facilitated advance care planning by providing a focus for end of life discussions (38, p887).

In one of our own studies, which examined the views of a diverse sample of 32 older people (39), advance statements were seen primarily in terms of the potential they have for providing a guide for family members, especially where a person may have only one or two surviving relatives. A particular issue was how advance statements might help to ensure that the 'burden' of decision making placed upon adult children was lessened. For example, during discussion of artificial feeding in one group, a participant spontaneously referred to the potential for a 'living will' to protect his family from '… the hassle of trying to make minds up' (39). In this study, the older people who took part had moral concerns about their family obligations which ranged far beyond any narrow concern with autonomy (40). Similar findings were found by Singer et al. (41), in a study of the views of 48 patients receiving renal dialysis in Canada who had been given the opportunity to complete an advance statement. Early findings from another of our studies (42) that sought the views and experiences of people with lung cancer about discussing future care reveal that concerns for family are more important than individual needs for future care.

Philosophical, social, and cultural challenges

The fundamental constraint on advance directives is that they derive their ethical and legal justifications from the principle of individual autonomy. Advance directives exist primarily to protect patients' rights to refuse medical interventions at the end of life. Many patients do not seek this protection or define their right to influence treatment decisions differently from advance directives. The current autonomy based procedures and policies shaping end of life decision making do not match the needs of many patients and their families, including many older adults and those from different racial and cultural backgrounds (43, p872)

The examples of qualitative research briefly reviewed above suggest that the traditional autonomy focused framework of Advance Care Planning and emphasis on the completion of instructional directives about specific treatments is out of step with the perspectives and needs of patients, and suggests that new, broader initiatives that start by trying to discover the personal goals and values of patients may be more helpful. Further evidence challenging the traditional focus of ACP on autonomy comes from a range of studies among minority ethnic communities which show that concepts of 'truth telling' and 'autonomy' vary culturally, both between countries and between cultural groups living in different countries. For example, in work with older Chinese people who had been resident for many years in England, it was found that by far a bigger concern was the maintenance of good spirits in the face of life threatening illness. Entry to a hospice, classically an arena where one would expect there to be opportunities to engage with ACP, was regarded negatively because it contradicted assumptions about the right way to die (44). Such perceptions are not limited to non westerners, but an integral part of some European cultures. For example, Dr Nunez Olarte, writing in 2000 about his personal views of the applicability of Advance Care Planning in Spain, observed that:

Autonomy does not mean assaulting patients with truth, or assaulting them with informed consent, or assaulting them with advance directives (45, p50)

Even in the USA there are differing opinions about whether people should be 'forced' to have discussions about their future medical care (2,46) recognizing that some people may choose to discuss their preferences with their family or others, rather than their physician (47).

As well as these cultural challenges to the traditional bases of ACP, another problem relates to the assumption that patient's views about treatment or position on decision making styles will be reasonably stable over time. However, it has been observed that at least one third of people change their minds over a comparatively short timescale (48). This may be due to the phenomenon of 'response shift' in which patients facing rapidly changing health care states 'downsize' their perceptions of what is a reasonable quality of life and may change their views and perspectives on medical decision making quite fundamentally (49). Furthermore, some evidence is beginning to emerge from research in the UK (42,50), which suggests that, for some very ill patients the recollection of the disclosure of 'bad news' so overshadows them subsequently, that they find it exceedingly difficult to engage with ACP, preferring instead to 'carry on as normal', live in the present, and 'hope for the best'.

The frailty of extreme old age, as well as critical life experiences shaped by war, may induce a similar response among older adults, and explain findings which suggest that some older people are resistant to discussing the future and prefer to 'take one day at a time' or delegate decision making to others (51).

Two case studies

One woman, who had been married for 60 years, described how she was the main carer for her husband, who was very ill. She said that she was devoted to her husband and hoped, quite selflessly, that she would be the one to be left on her own eventually. Nevertheless, she had a dread of ultimately being on her own—being agoraphobic added to her concerns—and she didn't want to inconvenience her family. She said that they were both dreading anything happening to either of them and were 'just living a day at a time'. She prayed for ideal solution—that they would die together or within a very short time of each other (52).

Andy, a 73 year old man with lung cancer and an abdominal aneurysm, talked about living 'one day at a time' and not thinking about the future. He'd been told his prognosis was only six to twelve months, but he wanted to get on and live as normal a life as possible. His wife, Amy, was quiet when Andy spoke about living for 'now'. Several times Amy said she wanted to know more about what would be available when the time came, but Andy said he didn't want to talk about that (42).

Such findings are often further compounded by the fears induced by a realistic perception that there are few services or resources which older people can access to help them as they face the last period of their lives: this perspective emerges in work with older members of the public about end of life care (52). In addition to age, a person's gender or family responsibilities may also influence decisions about whether to engage in ACP. It has been suggested that ACP is a social as well as a medically focused undertaking (53).

A final challenge relates to the contexts in which attempts may be made to introduce Advance Care Planning. This has been clearly shown in the UK, where efforts to introduce initiatives to support the Mental Capacity Act (7), which for the first time makes legal provision for the completion of advance decisions to refuse treatment, were widely reported in the media as a 'back door to euthanasia' (54), probably because of parallel debates about the legalisation of assisted dying that were taking place at the same time. This seems to have affected the way in which members of the public in England perceive ACP, with some worrying that the completion of advance directives may lead to medical actions which are akin to 'pulling the plug' or out of step with the 'real intent' of the person in question (52).

Changing practice and policy

Realistic information, sensitively provided, helps patients and their families to maintain a feeling of normality and allows them to develop new coping strategies. Such discussions engender hope. Such hope is not for a cure but for understanding the process of dying and for reassurance that support will be given during a variety of eventualities (55, p869).

Where does this leave us as we try to make sense of what is the right thing in clinical practice? How is it possible, within the many constraints imposed by our health care systems, to attend to the many different perspectives patients and their families have, and be mindful of the rich complexity of cultural and ethnic heritages that underpin these?

There is a distinct gap in the literature about how best to raise, conduct, and record Advance Care Planning discussions, what questions should be employed to guide such discussions, or how they should be recorded. There is increasing evidence from the USA of the success or failure of some initiatives (see Chapter 18). There has also been uncertainty about the timing of ACP discussions, or by whom they should be led. However, a systematic review which has resulted in valuable guidelines for practice (5) makes it clear that any Advance Care Planning intervention needs to take a broader approach than merely trying to increase the completion of advance directives. Approaches need to be developed in which primacy is given to the patient's and, where they have one, their family's point of view. This will involve a sensitive assessment of whether or not they are ready to engage in thinking about the future, and then helping them to talk and communicate with each other, as well as with their professional care givers. This might involve the articulation of fears about death and dying, but this is certainly not automatic, neither should this be forced. Talking about what might seem more mundane issues, but which may have a critical impact on daily life, might be more important for some. Equally, it is likely that only a minority of people will have strong and specific views about particular medical treatments. However, with help, most will be able to set out a number of areas or goals of importance in their lives; or will have views about how their future care should be organized as their health deteriorates to best fit in with their family life and preserve their sense of identity, dignity, and control. It will be important to acknowledge uncertainty, since no amount of discussion or horizon scanning can predict how things will unfold, and it may add to distress to try to do this (56). It will also be important to acknowledge that patients and their families may not perceive many 'real' choices, and that indeed the health services available may not be able to deliver reliably some things that are 'chosen', such as death at home for example (57).

There may be concerns about the time and resources required from health and social care professionals and their needs for training (10), if ACP as we have sketched out here, is to be effectively introduced into every day practice. Any initiatives that are developed must take account of these and work with professionals to build on their existing practice, rather than expecting them to engage in anything they may see as fundamentally new and alien.

Preliminary work in the UK in relation to developing an aide memoire for nurses to use with patients with lung cancer, drawing inspiration from studies by Linda Briggs in the US (58), suggests that it is possible to help clinicians develop their practice such that they feel more comfortable and confident about opening up an ACP discussion with seriously ill patients, but much more work is required to further develop this (59). Many of the principles involved are ones which will be familiar to those from specialist palliative care: skills of listening and reflecting, of summarizing, and of unconditional regard for the point of view of the patient and their family. Work under the auspices of the National End of Life Care Programme (9) has identified a number of possible triggers to help clinicians to assess whether the timing of an ACP discussion is appropriate. Box 2.1 provides some pointers for good practice in Advance Care Planning.

Developing approaches to ACP that are feasible to use in the busy pressurized world of practice, that are sensitive to the needs, fears, and varied perspectives of patients and their families, and which actually make a difference in terms of providing better end of life care depends on much more than the preparation and training of health care professionals. It requires a sea change in attitudes to discussing and anticipating end of life care among the public, and a commitment among politicians and policy makers to developing systems of health and social care so that those who face the end of life can trust that adequate help and support will be provided to them and their families. In particular, the persistent inequalities which mean that people with palliative care needs have sharply different opportunities to engage in preparation and planning for death need to be addressed. It has been recognized that systems of care provision that are poorly adapted to the realities of demographic change mean that many older people living in Europe with complex care needs are simply just not 'in the loop' of assessment, delivery of health and social care, and proactive planning for long term and end of life care (60).

Summary and conclusions

Advance Care Planning has moved from being a process which aims to elicit specific instructions about medical treatment at the end of life, to being recognized as an opportunity to help patients and their families to prepare, in their own terms, for the changes wrought by serious progressive illness and work with them to plan nursing, social, and medical care so that it better fits their needs, hopes, and aspirations. In thinking about the use of Advance Care Planning, we would do well to remember that being and becoming ill engenders a paradox in which it is likely that we both welcome an opportunity to 'take control' and reject it, because of feelings of fear and uncertainty, and a basic human need to feel safe and cared for during illness (61). Making an Advance Care Plan is not something that we may all wish or feel able to do. As we face illness, what were once clear preferences may become blurred and uncertain, we may want others to make decisions on our behalf, and we may not be able to talk easily about the end. It is also difficult for clinicians to raise Advance Care Planning conversations and to know how to manage them. Many feel similar discomforts and anxieties to their patients, with some having made attempts to initiate a discussion that was not welcomed, resulting in a breakdown of trust within the patient-clinician relationship. Moreover, it is clear that raising awareness of Advance Care Planning and associated issues before illness is necessary; which means grasping the nettle of developing approaches to public education about a sensitive topic for use in schools and in the wider community.

Finally, in order for Advance Care Planning to be successful, it needs to be embedded in systems of care designed to provide comprehensive support to those facing the end of life, in recognition that serious illness and dying are worthy of the same care and attention that we give to birth, acute illness, and injury.

Box 2.1 Good practice guide

- Consider if the person has hit a trigger point in life and may be thinking about the future in the context of, for example: bereavement, recent diagnosis, change in treatment, hospitalization, retirement, change in marital status, nursing home admission, or disclosure of a prognosis.
- Recognize cues from the patient and/or family indicating that they wish to talk about the future.
- Don't force a conversation about end of life care; rather be led by the person themselves. Be open to revisit the conversation in the future if new cues are given by the patient.
- Offer opportunities to talk about a patient's concerns or wishes for the future, either with yourself or another member of the health/social care team whom they trust.
- A person may express a preference for a family member or another significant person to be provided with information on their behalf about future care and choices available. This should be respected.
- Document the person's expressed preferences or wishes and gain their consent to share these with other members of the health and social care team.
- Offer people guidance about additional resources to provide information about their condition or situation. This may be particularly important if they express an interest in making an advance decision to refuse treatment.

Acknowledgement

This chapter is based on the text of a plenary lecture delivered in Budapest to the European Association of Palliative Care. We are grateful to the Association for their invitation to prepare the latter, and to Macmillan Cancer Support for the funding of Gillian Horne's PhD study.

References

1 Healthcare Commission (2007). Spotlight on Complaints. Available at: http://www. healthcarecommission.org.uk/_db/_documents/spotlight_on_complaints.pdf (Accessed 15 May 2007).

2 SUPPORT Project Principal Investigators (1995). A controlled trial to improve care of seriously ill hospitalized patients: the study to understand prognoses and preferences for outcomes and risks of treatment (SUPPORT). *JAMA*, **174**:1591–8.

3 Lynn J (2005). Living long in fragile health: The new demographics shape end of life care. In: Improving end of life care: Why has it been so difficult? *Hastings Center Report*, **35**(6):S14–S18.

4 Teno JM, Nelson HL, and Lynn J (1994). Advance care planning: priorities for ethical and empirical research. *Hastings Center Report*, **24**:S32–36.

5 Conroy S, Fade P, Fraser A, and Schiff R (2009). Advance care planning: concise evidence based guidelines. *Clinical Medicine*, **9**(1):76–79.

6 Horne G, Seymour J, and Payne S (2009). Advance care planning: evidence and implications for practice. *End of Life Care*, **3**(1):58–64.

7 Henry C and Seymour JE (2007). *Advance Care Planning: a guide for heath and social care professionals*. National End of Life Care Programme, Leicester. (Revised 2008)

8 Department of Constitutional Affairs (2005). *Mental Capacity Act*. HMSO, London.

9 Singer PA (1994). Disease specific advance directives. *Lancet*, **244**(8922):594–6.

10 Dunbrack J (2006). Advance care planning: the Glossary project. Health Canada. Available at: http://www.hc-sc.gc.ca/hcs-sss/alt_formats/hpb-dgps/pdf/pubs/2006-proj-glos/2006-proj-gloss_e.pdf (Accessed 15 May 2007).

11 Sanders C, Rogers A, Gately C, and Kennedy A (2008). Planning for end of life care within lay-led chronic illness self-management training: the significance of 'death awareness' and biographical context in participant accounts. *Social Science and Medicine*, **66**:982–93.

12 Brown BA (2003). The history of advance directives: a literature review. *Journal of Gerontological Nursing*, **29**(9):4–14.

13 Ulrich LP (2001). *The Patient Self-Determination Act: Meeting the Challenges in Patient Care*, Georgetown University Press, Washington.

14 Rich BA (2002). The ethics of surrogate decision-making. *Western Journal of Medicine*, **176**(2):127–29.

15 Dworkin R (1993). Life's *dominion. An argument about abortion and euthanasia*. Harper Collins, London.

16 Martin DK, Emmanuel LL, and Singer PA (2000). Planning for the end of life, *Lancet*, **356**:1672–76.

17 Fraser Health Authority (2007). Planning in advance for your future health care choices. http://www. fraserhealth.ca/News/NewsReleases/Documents/ACP-Ebook160309.pdf. (Accessed 16 April 2009).

18 Chiarella M (2007). *Practicalities of advance care planning: an international perspective*. Paper presented to St Barnabas' Hospice, Lincoln, UK. April.

19 The Lancashire and South Cumbria Cancer Network http://www.cancerlancashire.org.uk/ppc.html

20 The National Goldstandards Framework Centre http://www.goldstandardsframework.nhs.uk

21 The Liverpool Care Pathway for the Dying Patient, MPCIL http://www.mcpcil.org.uk/liverpool_care_pathway

22 Department of Health (2008). *End of Life Care Strategy—Promoting High Quality Care for all Adults at the End of Life*. The Stationery Office, London.

23 Darzi, Professor the Lord Darzi of Denham KBE (2008). *High Quality Care for All: NHS Next Stage Review Final Report.* The Stationery Office, London.

24 Ratner E, Norlander L, and McSteen K (2001). Death at home following a targeted advance care planning process at home: the kitchen table discussion. *Journal of the American Geriatrics Society,* **49**:778–81.

25 Degenholtz H, Rhee Y, and Arnold R. (2004). Brief communication: the relationship between having a living will and dying in place. *Annals of Internal Medicine,* **141**:113–7.

26 Caplan GA et al. (2006). Advance care planning and hospital in the nursing home. *Age and Ageing,* **35**(6):581–85.

27 Connolly C (2005). Experts Dispute Remark That Living Wills Save Money. *Washington Post,* A09.

28 Fries JF, Everett Koop C, Sokolov J, Beadle CE, and Wright D (1998). Beyond Health Promotion: Reducing Need and Demand for Medical Care. Health care reforms to improve health while reducing costs. *Health Affairs,* **17**(2):70–84.

29 Hanson LC, Danis M, Garrett J (1997). What is wrong with end-of-life care? Opinions of bereaved family members. *Journal of the American Geriatrics Society,* **45**(11):1339–44.

30 Morrison RS, Chichin E, Carter J, Burack O, Lantz M, and Meier DE (1995). The effect of a social work intervention to enhance advance care planning documentation in the nursing home. *Journal of the American Geriatrics Society,* **53**(2):290–94.

31 Hammes B and Rooney B (1998). Death and end-of-life planning in one Midwestern community. *Archives of Internal Medicine,* **158**:383–90.

32 Molloy DW, Guyatt GH, Russo R, Goeree R, O'Brien BJ, Bedard M, et al. (2000). Systematic Implementation of an Advance Directive Program in Nursing Homes: A Randomized Controlled Trial. *JAMA,* **283**(102):1437–44.

33 Innovations in End-of-life care at http://www2.edc.org/lastacts/archives/archivesJan99/featureinn.asp

34 Stuart B, D'Onofrio CN, Boatman S, and Feigelman G. (2003). CHOICES: promoting early access to end of life care through home based transition management. *Journal of Palliative Medicine,* **6**(4): 671–83.

35 Lorenz KA and Lynn J (2004). *End of life care and outcomes.* Agency for Healthcare Research and Quality, US Department of Health and Human Services.

36 Fagerlin A, Ditto PH, Hawkins NA, Schneider CE, and Smucker WD (2002). The use of advance directives in end-of-life decision making: Problems and possibilities. *American Behavioural Scientist,* **46**(2):268–83.

37 Hickman SE, Hammes BJ, Tolle SW, and Moss AH (2004). A visible alternative to traditional living wills. *Hasting's Center Report,* **35**(5):4–5.

38 Davison S and Simpson C (2006). Hope and advance care planning in patients with end stage renal disease. *BMJ,* **333**(7574):886–90.

39 Seymour J, Gott M, Bellamy G, Ahmedzai SH, and Clark D (2004). Planning for the end of life: the views of older people about advance care statements. *Social Science & Medicine,* **59**(1):57–68.

40 Beauchamp TL and Childress JF (2001). *Principles of Biomedical Ethics,* 5th Ed.Oxford University Press, New York.

41 Singer PA, Martin DK, Lavery JV, Thiel EC, Kelner M, and Mendelssohn DC (1998). Reconceptualizing Advance Care Planning From the Patient's Perspective. *Arch Intern Med,* **158**(8):879–84.

42 Horne, G, Seymour JE, and Payne S (2005-10). *Advance care planning for patients with lung cancer.* Macmillan PhD Research Fellowship, University of Nottingham, Nottingham.

43 Winzelberg, GS, Hanson, LJ, and Tulksy, J (2005). Beyond autonomy. Diversifying end of life decision approaches to serve patients and families. *Journal of the American Geriatric Society,* **53**:1046–50.

44 Seymour, JE, Payne, S., Chapman, A., and Holloway, M (2007). Hospice or Home? Expectations about end of life care among older white and Chinese people living in the UK. *Sociology of Health and Illness,* **29**(6):872–90.

45 Nunez Olarte, J (2000). Cultural Attitudes Toward Death and Dying in Spain. In: Solomon, MZ, Romer, AL, Heller, KS (eds) *Innovations in End of Life Care. Practical Strategies and International Perspectives*. Mary Ann Liebert Inc. Publishers, New York.

46 Coppola KM, Bookwala J, Ditto PH, Lockhart LK, Danks JH, and Smucker WD (1999). Elderly adults' preferences for life sustaining treatments: the role of impairment, prognosis and pain. *Death Studies*, **23**(7):617–34.

47 Larson D and Tobin D, (2000). End-of-Life Conversations: Evolving Practice and Theory. *JAMA*, **284**(12):1573–78.

48 Hines S, Glover J, Holley J, Babrow A, Badzek L, and Moss A (1999). Dialysis Patients' Preferences for Family-based Advance Care Planning. *Annals of Internal Medicine*, **130**(10):825–28.

49 Seamark, DA, Seamark CJ, and Halpin DMG (2007). Palliative care in chronic obstructive pulmonary disease. *Journal of the Royal Society of Medicine*, **100**(5):225–33.

50 Clayson, H (2007). *The experience of mesothelioma in northern England*. Unpublished MD thesis, University of Sheffield, Sheffield.

51 Carrese JA, Mullaney JL, Faden RR, and Finucane TE (2002). Planning for death but not serious future illness: qualitative study of housebound elderly patients. *BMJ*, **325**(125):127.

52 Clarke A and Seymour J (on behalf of the Peer Education Project Group) (2006). *Opening the door for older people to explore end of life issues*, Help the Aged, London.

53 Black K (2007). Advance care planning throughout the end-of-life: focusing the lens for social work practice. *Journal of Social Work in End-of-Life and Palliative Care*, **3**:39–58.

54 The Daily Telegraph (2004). MPs defeat bid to block 'back door' euthanasia http://www.telegraph.co.uk/news/1478975/MPs-defeat-bid-to-block-back-door-euthanasia.html (Accessed 20 April 2009).

55 Murray S. (2006). Advance care planning in primary care. *BMJ*, **333**:868–69.

56 Drought TS and Koenig B (2002).'Choice' in end of life decision making: researching fact or fiction? *The Gerontologist*, **42**:114–28. Sp Iss III.

57 Tonnelli MR (1996). Pulling the plug on living wills: a critical analysis of advance directives. *Chest*, **110**(3):816–22.

58 Briggs L (2003). Shifting the focus of advance care planning: using an in-depth interview to build and strengthen relationships. *Journal of Palliative Medicine*, **7**(2):341–49.

59 Horne G, Seymour J, and Shepherd K (2006). Advance care planning for patients with inoperable lung cancer. *International Journal of Palliative Nursing*, **12**(4):172–79.

60 Seymour JE, Witherspoon R, Gott M, Ross H and Payne S (2006). *End of life care: promoting comfort, choice and well being among older people facing death*. Policy Press, Bristol.

61 Seymour JE (2007). Quality of life to the end: commentary. *Communication and Medicine*, **4**(1):117–8.

Chapter 3

Listening to the patient's voice

Heidi Macleod, David Oliver, and Don Redding

We wanted to commission a specific chapter that looked into the detail of the patient and carer experience. We are pleased that the MND Association, patients, and partner organizations took up this challenge. Although the editors recognize there are many other equally challenging conditions we believe that the spectrum of issues relating to this type of progressive neurological disease represents excellent examples and opportunities for learning.

Introduction: a perspective of the MND Association

Advance Care Planning is something that everyone ought to think about after all, life is a fatal condition! However, few people even want to contemplate their fate so it is something that doesn't get discussed until a terminal illness like Motor Neurone Disease (MND) is diagnosed. MND is without any effective treatment and it relentlessly robs those with it of the ability to use their limbs, speak, swallow, and finally breathe. The prognosis is poor; half of those diagnosed dying within 14 months. For people with MND it is especially important to plan ahead, as there is a high chance at some stage of being unable to communicate their wishes and decisions usually resulting in the loss of capacity. The reality of Advance Care Planning for MND patients varies. Some patient's psychological reaction results in a process of denial or worse still nihilism which restricts or precludes this approach. For others, the speed of progression means their plans never catch up as the people at the heart of the matter lurch from event to event, crisis to crisis. Sadly there are still patients and carers that are not properly supported by professionals and such planning opportunities pass them by.

The Motor Neurone Disease Association (MNDA) know what matters and help through a number of ways to pay attention to the detail that is essential to effective care and support when people face this aggressive neurological condition. Individuals perceive quality of life differently and just being alive equates with significant distress to themselves and those close to them. There is a spectrum of response in people with this disease, from those people who fight to stay alive at all cost to those who actively seek and achieve (sometimes assisted) suicide. ACP offers a framework to the individual to personalize their approach helping to meet sometimes diverse needs and expectations. Planning ahead increases the likelihood of supportive measures being implemented in time, reducing the risk of distress, and helping to avoid crises. The ACP might also include legally binding decisions e.g. an advance decision to refuse treatment. In the process of making an ACP people decide what is important in their life. This can generate other problems too, sometimes exaggerating unresolved interpersonal/family issues. The MNDA recognize the need for effective support for the people and professionals at the heart of care. MNDA provide specialist advisers that support and help educate key workers and care providers.

Planning enables individuals to focus on their own priorities, but remember that in a society where we promote choice we must respect their autonomy and allow people to change their mind.

The patient's voice: told through stories

Story one

When I was first diagnosed with MND I was so frightened about how the end would be for me I considered assisted suicide. I discussed it with my close friends who have given me the most amazing support no matter what decision I came to. After a few months my head cleared of the haze I had been in and I realized my initial plan was one made out of desperate fear. My faith has always been very important to me and therefore I could only have a natural end of my life.

I decided against the percutaneous endoscopic gastrostomy (PEG) as I had made the decision not to have any invasive procedures. Also as a single person, I would need to rely on friends and family to assist me when travelling and decided that I could not ask them to be responsible for the care of a PEG. I had already considered non invasive ventilation (NIV) having read the MNDA information pack and also information from the internet by the time I started having headaches, feeling sleepy and unable to concentrate (symptoms of poor respiratory function). A friend, whose husband had died from MND, suggested I should ask my consultant if I could try the NIV. The overnight change in me was amazing, but I decided that I would only use it at night and when the symptoms returned in the day, then I would stop using the machine.

As a single person without children and living on my own I had to plan ahead and realized I would need outside help. I worked as a team with my physio, speech and occupational therapist, and district nurse. Initially I was adamant that I would stay in my home till the end. My physio was a tremendous support; she didn't hide the reality of the next stage and what I would need. She supported my wish to stay in my home, she brought in the OT immediately who set up a life line, a key safe to enable people to gain entry in an emergency, and made changes around my flat to make it safer. I had wonderful support from my GP and social worker. A carer came twice a day, but after 6 months it became very clear to me and 'my team' that I was not safe on my own and I agreed to move into a residential home.

The Advance Directive (Advance Decision to Refuse Treatment) was instigated by myself following discussion with my sister. Having told her that I prefer to have a shorter life with quality, she replied that she would keep me alive as long as she could regardless of my suffering. The MNDA sent me information to help me make my decision. I asked a very close friend, if she would be my Power of Attorney and we then had a meeting with my solicitor to make it legal. I did not discuss this with my family at the time, it was about my right to decide on my end of life. My Advance Decision is that when I feel that I cannot cope with either the pain, am unable to eat naturally, or have lost total quality of life, I will stop using my NIV, refuse antibiotics for chest infection and will only have morphine or other medication to make me comfortable.

I trust my friend that whilst she wants me to live for ever, she will totally respect my wishes. That is why I believe Power of Attorney would be better with her and not with a member of my family who for example may be in line to inherit from my will. Once the documents were in place I informed my close family, friends, GP, consultant, residential home, and district nurse of my decision. The document allows me to change my mind at any time. I have donated my brain and spine to be used for research after my death. All my adult life I have let it be known that if I were to have a serious illness I would not have prolonged treatment so the decisions I have made relating to MND have not really changed.

With the team who planned my care and the advance decision in place, I can't think of any area that I would have changed. I do realize how lucky I have been with the support I have been given from MND Association and my team. I don't know how much would have changed had I been married with children although I did discuss all my decisions with my closest friend. At the end of the day it has to be what I want and need; it may be the first time in a person's life where they can and possibly have to be, selfish.

Story two

As someone with a form of MND that is slower in progression, ACP and Advance Decisions are things that I haven't yet fully addressed. This does not mean that I haven't thought about the issues that are likely to confront me, but it is a recognition that I have time on my side to get it right!

For me, quality of life is more important than quantity. Death itself is not something to fear, but with this disease, the process of getting there is worrying. Independence is hugely important to me and increasing disability and reliance on others for care does not get any easier to deal with. ACP is important to me in indicating what I am and am not prepared to accept, and gives me significant peace of mind, because at least when I can no longer indicate my wishes, the burden of the decision is lifted off the shoulders of my family. My family are supportive, but it is not easy for them to discuss issues which they don't want to confront and that currently seem quite distant. I think to get ACP right for oneself needs objective discussion and the family find that hard to do. It is much better to talk it through with a professional in the field and to clarify how best to approach the many issues. It doesn't mean that the family shouldn't be involved, but it is sometimes hard to discuss honestly what it acceptable to oneself without upsetting them. MND involves so many disciplines of health care professionals that it is a big advantage to have a plan that can be worked to by everyone and minimize confusion. My slower disease means that a care plan drawn up whilst communication is no problem, relieves the fear of what might happen when it is.

ACP gives the opportunity to address all the difficult issues and get care plans mapped out for the time when I might no longer be able to communicate my wishes. Whether it is planning for dependent care or invasive support, it is helpful for all concerned. For some people, it might mean pulling out all the stops to keep life going, whatever the degree of dependence on ventilators and relentless locking in with one's body. For me, it enables the line to be drawn at a point of my choosing. Plotting the end of my disease gives comfort that my wishes will be respected and that I don't need to fear unwanted interventions. Of course, that is where an Advance Directive comes into play and it is so important to have in place. It avoids crisis situations and ideally, prevents the family from having to resort to sudden, life-affecting, emotional decisions. A relief to me, and I hope to them, at a difficult time.

Story three

'I'm deaf!... Well I've got a STUTTER!'

A seminal moment, in my teens, trying to hear a customer over a busy chemist's counter, getting more and more flustered because I couldn't hear what they were saying. This response to my indignant utterance made the tension vanish. At the time, it was just an amusing anecdote and a touching moment of connection with my poor customer who was, no doubt, struggling with her own sense of frustration and embarrassment. It is essential to remember not only do we struggle to hear the patient voice, but they struggle to communicate with us.

Effective communication is the key to any relationship and especially in the provision of personalized health and social care. Communication is the core element to Advance Care Planning and all the policies and strategies about 'End of Life'. It underpins the very NHS constitution. Communication is enhanced using effective tools encouraging us to hear better, actively listening and understanding more about the person in front of us. 'You matter because you are you, and you matter until the very last moment of your life' as Dame Cicely Saunders so deftly puts it. Furthermore, it is not enough to simply hear and listen to the patient and carer voice, but to act on it in order to help people live as well as possible for as long as possible.

The National Council for Palliative Care (NCPC) advocates both listening to, and hearing the patient voice, from individual interactions, to planning, commissioning, delivering, and evaluating care. They acknowledge the expertise of both patients and carers not only in their own condition and experience of services, but also in life experience and skills. We encourage the extension of the patient/professional dialogue into all areas of health and social care. This contribution will therefore, focus on hearing the patient voice at an organizational and strategic level.

In this context, I encourage you to think about how to hear the patient voice when planning your approach to end of life care and in particular Advance Care Planning and when planning and delivering communication skills training.

How do we do it? In general, working in partnership with patients and carers in end of life care is publicly encouraged but privately feared. The practicalities of being too ill to talk, coupled with the sensitivity of end of life issues leads us to the question: 'Is it right to ask people to be involved?' Our view is that it is wrong not to. How to do this, however, is another matter.

Here are a few, practical tips to consider in your practice and organization:

1 Not everyone is too ill to talk

2 Don't make it harder for yourself: we tie ourselves up in knots trying to be sensitive about this delicate issue of end of life. Not everyone feels so sensitive about it. Let people decide for themselves whether it's too difficult for them to talk about end of life issues. Don't censor their voice by failing to give them an opportunity to talk. Also—don't only ask carers. They do have a valid perspective but it does not always reflect the patient's view.

3 Start small: You don't have to change the world overnight. Have a go!

4 Think big: look at your organization. How can you consistently work in partnership with patients and carers in all activities?

5 Accept help: work with patients and carers to formulate your approach. We won't instinctively know how to involve patients and carers effectively and meaningfully. They can tell us what helps them to communicate effectively. Metaphorically speaking, they can tell us if they have a stutter! We can then adapt our involvement processes to accommodate.

6 Create a culture of communication: listen and show that you are listening. Give people lots of opportunities to tell you what they think and in many ways

7 Think outside the box: people nearing the end of life are likely to be tired, and may struggle with mobility so meetings are unlikely to be a reliable way of hearing their voices. Provide flexible ways of getting input. Go out to them. Think creatively. (*www.ncpc.org.uk/users/share_your_story*)

8 Resources are key. Allow financial resources to support travel and carer expenses, and allow staff time to get alongside patients and carers, providing support, training and building good rapport. Service users need support and training and it is also vital to tell them what has happened as a result of their involvement.

9 Share your experiences: share your learning as you go along so that we can all improve. *www. ncpc.org.uk/users/share*

10 Many patients and carers want to turn a bad experience into a good one, leave a legacy for others, or take control of their life at a time where they have very little control. Give them this opportunity.

11 Imperceptible beauty: the impact of involving patients and carers may not be dramatic, high profile changes of policy direction (although they may be). It may simply be that the individual interactions with professionals subtly and powerfully transform their perceptions. In other words—foster empathy. Empathy is the foundation of good care. Without this, we would not have a health service. Don't underestimate its value. Look for changes like this when evaluating the impact of involvement on your organization.

The message is simple: let patients and carers help us to fashion better listening strategies so that we can hear that still, small but powerful voice.

A carer's view

End of life issues are a very sensitive and discussions can be a painful area as they focus on the impending trauma of loss for all involved. An open acknowledgment and having issues resolved in advance, relieves much of the emotional and practical pressure at a hugely stressful time. Not doing so creates barriers of pretence which make planning unrealistic and a satisfying outcome very difficult to achieve. Final wishes carry great significance later so it is important to get it right for everyone.

The ability to discuss a terminal diagnosis and its implications between partners or significant others, will vary between individuals; some finding it relatively easy and some almost impossible. Discussing practicalities with a caring professional can open the door to the sharing of emotional issues, a really important aspect of living well to the end.

The best care may involve many professional disciplines. So where to start? A need may be flagged up by the patient or carer, often to the GP. This can be an opportunity to begin to talk about future needs and for a formal, written plan to evolve. A home visit is ideal. A sensitive GP or nurse will raise the need for planning if none has been forthcoming. Discussion of preferences and needs should take place as soon as possible to allay worries and ensure all services are anticipated then put in place quickly rather than wait for a crisis and be rushed into hospital. This also builds up confidence & trust.

Team work is of the essence. A book with contact numbers for all involved is a lifeline for the carer and a means of communication for professionals. There may be many disciplines or agencies involved. The nursing and social care plan should be clearly written and kept at home, so that any professional/carer can see what should be done, especially in a crisis. This might include the choice of whether to be transferred to a hospice or hospital.

It is also vital to ensure that personal affairs are in order, especially financial matters. A revised will may be needed. Access to a financial advisor and estate planner may be necessary as well as funeral services, so preferences can be made and problems resolved.

If unnecessary or unwanted interventions/treatments are to be avoided, it is essential that an Advance Decision is made and shared especially with the GP and community team, as they are usually the first port of call. This Decision may contain issues such as the use of antibiotics, PEG feeding, non-invasive or invasive ventilation, life support, and resuscitation. If this is in place it will give confidence that end of life decisions will be known and they will be respected removing any guess work. The main carer, often the next-of-kin, will not be expected to make any almost unbearable decisions with which they will have to live with.

A carer's view (continued)

In my case, I was very fortunate that my husband and I had discussed all the above issues, with the help of professionals who were able to spell out some of the pros and cons of different interventions and situations. When broncho-pneumonia struck, out of the blue, there was no question of antibiotics or hospital because my husband had clearly refused these. With wonderful support from our GP and team of nurses, John was kept comfortable and pain free, with the minimum of 'fuss' at home. After many years nursing the elderly, I can honestly say that John's last hours were amongst the most peaceful I have ever witnessed. This was due largely to the skill and compassion of the team, but underpinning it all was the knowledge that John's wishes were being fulfilled. Advance Care Planning and my husband's Advance Decision had made it clear what he wanted and for that I am so very, very thankful and it helped the team to do its job and feel tremendous satisfaction.

All this is a very tall order. It requires the highest level of professional skill, commitment, caring, and cooperation. Many people would say they fear the process of dying rather than death itself. With good planning and practice a 'good death' can be achieved. This is the best possible platform for the ensuing bereavement process.

The professional: expert in listening

I would like to emphasize the importance of listening by starting this piece with a case study.

Case study: Use of advanced decision to refuse treatment (ADRT)

G was a 66 year old retired handyman and lived with his wife. At the end of an operation on his knee he was unable to breathe sufficiently well by himself and he was transferred to the Intensive Care Unit, a tracheostomy was formed and he was continued on 24 hour ventilation. It appeared he had been breathless over the previous year and investigations subsequently confirmed a diagnosis of motor neurone disease (MND), in G's case it is a rare presentation of newly diagnosed MND after a planned operation.

G was eventually transferred to a hospice near his home. He continued to need continuous support of his breathing but he was able to swallow, speak, and move reasonably normally. He was keen to return home and after a great deal of discussion a care plan for home was agreed.

G also wanted to discuss his future care. Over a series of meetings the diagnosis and probable progression of MND was discussed. He was very keen to remain at home and not to be readmitted to hospital or hospice unless absolutely necessary. He realized that if there were problems with ventilation at home he would probably die before any help, such as an ambulance, could come to him. The clinicians involved in his care discussed the use of ADRT. He, with the support of his family, decided that if he became very ill, having reached the point when he could no longer swallow safely, could not move his arms or legs, or could not speak clearly or communicate his wishes, he would wish to not receive life prolonging treatment and to have ventilation withdrawn. He wanted the right care to keep him comfortable. An ADRT was completed—stating that he did not wish cardiopulmonary resuscitation, antibiotic treatment, artificial hydration, and he did wish ventilation to cease in the circumstances he decided.

G was able to return home and enjoyed a good quality of life at home for several months. He slowly deteriorated. His chest problems got worse and the ventilator was switched off at his request. He received medication to lessen his symptoms of breathlessness and he died peacefully as few minutes later, with his wife and the nurse with him.

The ADRT allowed G to make clear decisions while he had capacity to do so, and these were then respected. His wife felt that his wishes and aims in life had been respected and he was able to die as he wished – at home with his family with him.

Some people and professionals are good at listening but most people need help in learning communication skills. Often good clinical practice is supported by the use of tools and techniques that have been refined and evaluated.

Use of patient preference questionnaires

It is important to involve all patients in the significant decisions about their care. This can be complex and challenging particularly in the palliative care of people with progressive disease, irrespective of diagnosis. The patient, and those close to them, can be particularly anxious about their condition and find decision making an extra demand. These decisions can be made more challenging if postponed and left until a crisis arises. Moreover, specific physical and cognitive change may occur with disease progression such that the patient might loose capacity to make decisions in the future.

At the Wisdom Hospice a Patient Preference Questionnaire has been incorporated within the routine assessment of patients when they are seen by members of the multidisciplinary team— whether this assessment occurs in hospital, at home, or in the hospice ward. The questionnaire is based on examples used in elderly care and palliative cares settings (1,2). The aim is to allow the patient to express their wishes and preferences on the care they receive and to ascertain the way they would like to make decisions and involve others, including their professional carers and family. The questions considered are:

◆ Preference for knowing information about the illness

◆ How they have found previous information they have received

◆ Permission to talk to family members if they ask about the illness

◆ Knowledge of anyone in the family to whom information should not be given

◆ Preference for a family member or friend to be with the person to hear results, or discuss or make important decisions

◆ Any preferences for or against specific treatments

◆ Details of any written wishes for care or treatment.

The discussions may lead onto further exploration of specific issues, such as consideration of Lasting Power of Attorney or an Advance Decision to Refuse Treatment or Do Not Attempt Resuscitation. The discussion also provides very helpful information for the clinicians if decisions have to be made later in the best interests of the patient who has lost capacity.

The completion of the questionnaire is not a single event but a process and the questionnaire can be updated over time. The patient's views may change over time and with the progression of the disease. The multidisciplinary team is aware of the need to ensure that the views and preferences of the patient are continually but sensitively reviewed as part of the ongoing assessment.

The use of the Patient Preference Questionnaire allows a deeper understanding of the views of the patient and is helpful in encouraging wider discussion, with professionals and family, on areas of care that may be complex and difficult to discuss.

The expert organization

Shared decision-making: where are we at?

In the NHS in England, official interest in and support for shared decision-making between patients and professionals is growing, professional orientation and skills are slowly improving, but as yet there is no evidence that this is having any impact on patients' engagement in their own

care and treatment. Paradoxically, England is further along the policy curve than other advanced industrialized countries, but further behind on measures of engagement.

Policy recognition

The loudest recent statement comes from the newly minted NHS Constitution (3) which includes three relevant 'rights' for patients:

- to be involved in discussions and decisions about your healthcare, and to be given information to enable you to do this
- to be given information about your proposed treatment in advance, including any significant risks and any alternative treatments which may be available, and the risks involved in doing nothing
- to accept or refuse treatment what is offered to you.

Professional standards

Importantly, there is increasing recognition that sharing decisions is part of the mainstream standards for health professionals. The General Medical Council states that one of the duties for all doctors is to 'work in partnership with patients', which comprises:

- listen to patients and respond to their concerns and preferences
- give patients the information they want or need in a way they can understand
- respect patients' rights to reach decisions with you about their treatment and care
- support patients in caring for themselves to improve and maintain their health (4).

The Nursing and Midwifery Council's Code lists similar elements under the heading of 'collaborate with those in your care', although the requirement to 'uphold people's rights to be fully involved in decisions about their care' falls under the 'informed consent' heading (5).

Clinical guidance

These top-line standards are increasingly flowing into additional specific guidance. For example the GMC's guidance on securing consent locates it clearly within the wider context of shared decision-making (not vice versa) (6). Recent NICE guidelines on medicines adherence, developed with the Royal College of General Practitioners, is equally emphatic that both evidence and best practice show that patients are more likely to adhere to courses of medication where these have been the subject of a shared decision with their doctor (7).

System regulation

System regulation is gearing up to move in the same direction as professional regulation. The Standards for Better Health only included the need for patients to be 'supported to make choices and shared decisions' as an optional, 'developmental' standard which the Healthcare Commission did not include in its annual health check (8). But its successor, the Care Quality Commission, even before assuming its duties on 1 April 2009, announced its vision of 'high quality health and social care which… helps individuals, families, and carers make informed decisions about their care'.

At the time of writing the regulations for health and social care providers, which replace Standards for Better Health and against which the CQC will regulate, had still not been published; but the consultation draft suggested that 'involving people in making informed decisions about their care and treatment' will be a bottom line standard.

Reality

National patient surveys have a common core question asking whether, during a recent episode of care, patients 'were involved in decisions about your care and treatment as much as you wanted to be'; to which the answer can be 'yes, definitely'; 'yes, to some extent'; or 'no'.

In every patient survey, regardless of care setting or condition, at least one third and up to one half of patients do not answer 'yes, definitely'. From recent surveys we can see that those not involved in decisions as much as they wanted to be included (9):

◆ 30% of primary care patients (2008)

◆ 30% of women in maternity care during labour and birth (2007)

◆ 38% of emergency department patients (2008)

◆ 49% of hospital inpatients (2007)

With regard to primary care, it should be noted that the most common decision here is the prescription of a new medicine—a decision in which 40% of patients did not feel as involved as much as they wanted to be.

International comparison and trends over time

Patient experience measures are not yet comparable internationally. However, the Picker Institute made a comparison of indicators of patient engagement drawn from Commonwealth Fund data for 2004 and 2005 and covering the UK, Australia, Canada, New Zealand, Germany and the US. This found that fewer UK patients than in the other countries said their doctors usually involved them in treatment decisions (10). Although this study needs updating it is unlikely that much has changed. The Picker Institute's analysis of trends over time in the English national patient surveys from 2002 to 2007 found no improvement over time (11).

The implementation gap

There is no clear explanation yet as to why the degree of patient engagement in decisions is not improving. One hypothesis is that there is improvement in levels of engagement, but that this is balanced by rising patients' expectations of involvement

A second hypothesis is that although the high level professional bodies are now backing shared decision-making, this message has not got through to practitioners (and/or that practitioners are resisting it because of professional attitudes and behaviours instilled through old educational models).

A third is that professionals may increasingly be getting the message, but think that they are practising shared decision-making already. It is notable that professionals and patients often have very different perspectives about what constitutes, for example, good information provision.

A fourth (not mutually exclusive) hypothesis is that we have to some degree been misled by the assumption that better information and communication will ipso facto deliver shared decision-making.

As communication skills training has permeated medical education, and as Department of health (England and Wales) policy has increasingly emphasized information for choice, it appears that patients are reporting better information, explanations and communication from their professionals. Yet patients' involvement in decisions does not increase. It may be that we now need to look at what additional skills and competencies—such as active listening, eliciting views, values and preferences, and sharing authority—our professionals may require as part of their toolkit for partnering patients.

Shared decision-making

Shared decision-making is a process in which patients are involved as active partners with the clinician in clarifying acceptable medical options and choosing a preferred course of clinical care (12).

What is involved?

Choosing an appropriate treatment with full patient involvement can be a complex process (13). It involves a number of steps:

- Recognize and clarify the problem
- Identify potential solutions
- Discuss options and uncertainties
- Provide information about potential benefits, harms and uncertainties of each option
- Check understanding and reactions
- Agree a course of action
- Implement the chosen treatment
- Arrange follow-up
- Evaluate the outcome.

When is it appropriate?

Shared decision-making is appropriate in any situation when there is more than one reasonable course of action and no one option is self-evidently best for everyone.

This situation is very common since there are often many different ways to treat a health problem, each of which may lead to a different set of outcomes. In these cases the patient's attitude to the likely benefits and risks should be a key factor in the decision. The principles of shared decision-making ought to be observed whenever clinicians have to obtain informed consent or communicate risks.

Two experts

Shared decision-making relies on two sources of expertise:

- The health professional is an expert on the effectiveness, probable benefits, and potential harms of treatment options
- The patient is an expert on herself, her social circumstances, attitudes to illness and risk, values and preferences.

Both parties must be willing to share information and accept responsibility for joint decision-making. The clinician must provide patients with information about the diagnosis and treatment options. The patient must tell the clinician about their preferences.

Summary

This chapter has tried to convey the importance and sometimes complexity of 'listening to the patient's voice'. We have listened to many perspectives and the authors hope that this has led to a deeper understanding of the ideas, concerns, and expectations of the people involved. In order to make sure that Advance Care Planning for the end of life is personalized, effective and safe we must never forget to:

Listen (using every energy)

Learn (to achieve a deeper understanding)

Lead (to deliver care that puts people at the heart, because it matters)

Further resources

NCPC: *Listening to Users; Listening to the Experts.*
Available from www.ncpc.org.uk/users/resources

References

1 Sayers GM, Barratt D, Gothard C, Onnie C, Perera S, and Schulman D (2001). The value of taking an 'ethics history'. *J Med Ethics*, **27**:114–117.

2 Murtagh FE and Thorns A (2005). Taking an 'ethics history'. *J R Soc Med*, **98**:442–443.

3 The NHS Constitution, DH, London, 2009: http://www.dh.gov.uk/en/Publicationsandstatistics/Publications/PublicationsPolicyAndGuidance/DH_093419

4 Good Medical Practice, GMC, 2006: http://www.gmc-uk.org/guidance/good_medical_practice/duties_of_a_doctor.asp

5 The Code: Standards of conduct, performance and ethics for nurses and midwives, NMC, 2008: http://www.nmc-uk.org/aSection.aspx?SectionID=45

6 Consent: patients and doctors making decisions together, GMC, 2008: http://www.gmc-uk.org/guidance/ethical_guidance/consent_guidance/index.asp

7 CG76 Medicines Adherence, NICE clinical guideline, 2009: http://www.nice.org.uk/Guidance/CG76

8 Standards for better health, London: Department of Health, 2004

9 The key findings reports from these surveys are available at http://www.nhssurveys.org/publications

10 Coulter A (2006). Engaging patients in their healthcare: how is the UK doing relative to other countries? Oxford, Picker Institute Europe.

11 Richards N and Coulter A (2007). Is the NHS becoming more patient-centred? Oxford, Picker Institute Europe.

12 Sheridan SL, Harris RP, and Woolf SH (2004). Shared decision making about screening and chemoprevention: A suggested approach from the U.S. Preventive Services Task Force. *Am J Prev Med*, **26**:56–66.

13 Elwyn G and Charles C (2001). Shared decision making: the principles and the competences. In Edwards A, Elwyn G, (eds) *Evidence-based patient choice*, 118–43. Oxford: Oxford University Press.

Chapter 4

Advance Care Planning for older people

Simon Conroy

Key points
- ◆ The oldest old are a rapidly growing section of society, in whom conditions affecting capacity are prevalent
- ◆ Advance Care Planning may be helpful in allowing frail older people to exert greater control over their care
- ◆ Case managers are ideally placed to help initiate Advance Care Planning, preferably in primary care in anticipation of future events which may impair capacity
- ◆ Professionals involved in helping people draft Advance Care Plans should be aware of their own area of competence and ask for help when necessary.

Context

Older people are growing rapidly as a proportion of the UK population as a whole; since the 1970s the population aged over 65 has grown by 31%, from 7.4 to 9.7 million, whilst the population aged under 16 declined by 19%, from 14.2 to 11.5 million. Up to 23% of the UK population will be aged 65 or older by 2031. The oldest old, usually considered to be those aged 85 years or more, are growing especially quickly and numbered 1.6 million in 2006.

Whilst increased longevity is something to be celebrated—a marker of a successful society, the shift in population dynamics has major implications, not least in the provision of health and social care. Despite many advances in medicine and efforts to promote healthy ageing, many older people develop chronic diseases or long term conditions, which impact on their quality of life.

There is a growing impetus for people with long term conditions to take more control over their health care. This is reflected in the growth of self-management, for example in diabetes, where individuals are increasingly managing their diabetes with only minimal input from health care professionals. The promotion of autonomy—exercising one's own choices about treatment, is also reflected in other areas, such as end of life care. Whereas in the past it was commonplace for doctors and other health care professionals to protect patients from bad news, such as a diagnosis of cancer (paternalism), there is now a growing openness about such issues, although it is not for everyone.

How is ACP relevant for older people?

Advance Care Planning (ACP) is especially relevant for frail older people, as a group with a high prevalence of long-term conditions and an increased risk of loss of capacity, for example because of dementia or stroke.

The rationale behind ACP is that it provides information to health care professionals about a person's wishes and preferences when individuals no longer have the capacity to do so and are unable to express themselves. ACP is also one possible means by which people can exert greater control over their treatment, often, but not exclusively relating to end of life care issues. ACP is a process of discussion about future care between an individual and their care providers, irrespective of discipline (1).

The goals of ACP include:

- ensuring that clinical care is in keeping with a patient's preferences when the patient has become incapable of decision making (loss of capacity)
- improving the health care decision making process by facilitating shared decision making
- improving patient well being by reducing the frequency of either under or over treatment.

ACP discussions may lead to an advance statement (a statement of wishes and preferences), an advance decision to refuse treatment (ADRT—a specific refusal of treatment(s) in a predefined potential future situation) or the appointment of a personal welfare Lasting Power of Attorney (LPA). All or any of these can help inform care providers on the individual's best interests should the individual lose capacity. Equally there may be no specific output, though the discussion itself may hold intrinsic value. Some individuals will not want to engage in ACP discussions, and it is important not to pressurize these individuals in to unwanted discussion.

Where and when should ACP discussions take place?

The majority of individuals are comfortable discussing ACP in primary (general practice) and outpatient care settings, when their condition is stable (2–5) in anticipation of future ill-health (6,7). In this context discussions are usually initiated by professionals who have an established relationship with the individual. The relationship of trust is an important facet in creating the right environment for such a delicate discussion to take place. But there are some obvious tensions, for example, GPs have limited time for what can be sensitive and complex discussions. Some have suggested involving case managers in the initial phase of discussion, which is covered in more detail later in this chapter.

ACP discussions often occur at the time of hospitalization or around the time of diagnosis of a life threatening illness (8), but some patients with terminal disease (8) or serious illness requiring hospitalization (9) may not feel ready or able to engage in such discussions. Whilst early studies focused on in-patients and trying to involve them in ACP, there was limited engagement and little overall impact. Reasons for this are probably related to the absence of an established relationship, the fact that such patients are often sick and perhaps not in the best frame of mind for ACP discussions. Furthermore, patients in hospital often change their minds about treatments that they would and would not want, related to their on-going treatment and hopefully, recovery.

Before initiating ACP discussions, professionals should ensure that reversible factors impacting on decision-making, such as delirium, sensory impairment, being pain-free, fed, not too tired, etc are all addressed. This may be better achieved when not a hospital in-patient, and also relieves any perception that the health service has provided 'undue influence'. ACP discussions take time; they may evolve over a period of hours, days, or weeks. They cannot be rushed. Some people change their minds about their plans, so it is useful to review maters on a regular basis. It is not clear how often matters should be reviewed, but some people have suggested every 12 months, or after any major life event. For frail older people issues such as a major change in physical function, or admission to a care home may be the factors that influence a change in thinking.

Case managers and ACP

Given that an established trusting relationship is a necessary condition for successful ACP discussions, case managers are in an ideal role to help facilitate the discussions. Case managers are becoming more and more common place in modern health care, and are typically nurses who have specialized in a certain field. For example, heart failure nurses 'case manage' patients with heart failure. Their duties involve managing the medical condition, such as advising on drug doses and monitoring, but can also include providing social and moral support to patients. Other examples include respiratory nurses for patients with lung disease, or community matrons for frail older patients. The common feature of the patient groups is that they all have long term conditions. Case managers are not exclusively nurses, and can come from any background, but the key components are a long term relationship with the individual and some specialist knowledge relevant to the individual's condition. Good communication skills are a *sine qua non*. ACP discussions with patients with long term conditions (6,10–12) or as part of a broad end of life care management programme (13–15) can increase patient satisfaction, though evidence that ACP has any impact on other health service related issues, such as hospital admission rates, is lacking.

Case study

Mildred is an 84 year old lady who lives alone. Her husband died some years previously. Though she manages independently most of the time, she has recently been diagnosed with heart failure. Janet, her community heart failure nurse has been in to see her on several occasions to help get Mildred's treatment organized. They get to know each other well and enjoy sharing stories. Mildred confides in Janet about her fear of losing her independence. Janet takes the opportunity to ask Mildred more detail about her fears. Mildred outlines some of the things which she values, such as being able to get down to the shops, and meeting up with her friends for coffee mornings. Mildred mentions that one of her friends was recently admitted to hospital and how awful the experience was for her. Janet asks Mildred how she would feel about being admitted to hospital; although Mildred would not be keen, she accepts that 'if you have to go, you have to go'. Janet asks if Mildred would like to document her wishes and preferences, but Mildred states that she would prefer not to at this stage. Janet leaves the discussion there.

This is a good example of ACP–a naturally occurring conversation, with the offer of formalizing wishes and preferences, but no pressure to do so when Mildred declined.

Is ACP not just a way of saving the NHS some money?

The original proponents of ACP in the United States did think that it would save the health service money whilst improving patient care—something of a holy grail. But like the mythical holy grail, this belief turned out to be illusory. According to studies, ACP does not reliably reduce health care costs (13,16), except when used systematically in the care home setting (17). Any cost reduction associated with ACP is probably related to avoiding 'terminal hospitalization'(18), i.e. because people choose to die at home rather than in hospital, or because people with an ADRT are less likely to receive life-sustaining therapy when hospitalized. The bigger point to be made here is that death is an expensive process, irrespective of where and when a person dies. It is said that people consume the majority of their individual health care budget at the end of life—whether they die at 18 or 80 years old (19).

Are you the right person to be initiating ACP discussions?

Assuming that there is a natural rapport with the patient/individual, and that the context is right, anyone with sensitive communication skills might initiate an ACP discussion. For example, a

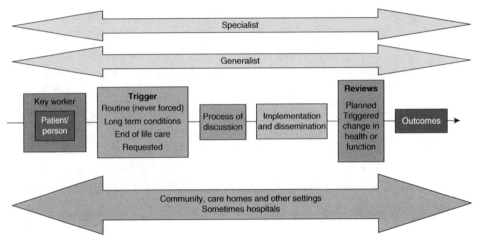

Fig. 4.1 A model for Advance Care Planning.

carer in a nursing home might be well placed to start a discussion and get people thinking ahead about the future.

High quality conversation skills are essential to allow ACP to take place, as well as dedicated time. Discussions take time and effort and cannot be completed as a simple checklist exercise; they usually need to take place on more than one occasion (over days, weeks or months) and should not be completed on a single visit in most circumstances. A variety of training courses are available.

The more detailed the discussion becomes, the more knowledge and skills the professional leading the discussion will need to have. So whilst the nursing home carer might be exactly the right person to get the discussion started, they may not be the correct person to discuss specific aspects of treatment, and so referral to a nurse or the general practitioner may be required. In some cases, specialist advice will be needed—for example, discussing the intricacies of artificial nutrition, or the likely success or failure of cardiac resuscitation. Such a model of generic and specialist input into the ACP process is summarized in Figure 4.1.

When carrying out discussions, professionals should be aware that older people especially, may be concerned about the burden of their own illness on their family and the impact that may make on their choices.

What should be discussed?

The content of the discussion will depend on individual circumstances and there is no set format. The discussion will need to be general and open ended in the first instance, and the questions used in the Preferred Place of Care document can be helpful in that regard. Other forms have been suggested to act as a template for such discussions, such as the Hammersmith Expression of Healthcare Preferences (20).

Case study continued

Mildred is reviewed at the hospital following a recent heart scan; Janet is able to accompany her. The consultant explained that the heart scan showed an enlarged heart. The consultant started talking about a defibrillator (like a pacemaker). Mildred was not keen and wanted to think about it further. Later on, Janet and Mildred were able to explore Mildred's concerns about the defibrillator, in which discussion Mildred recounted the experience of her husband's death. He died from a heart attack and underwent cardiac resuscitation in their home; Mildred was understandably very traumatised by the event. She is very clear with Janet that she would not want to be resuscitated. Janet is not sure how to handle the discussion at this point, but suggests that Mildred might discuss it when she goes back to see the consultant. A few weeks later, Mildred, again supported by Janet, is able to discuss the defibrillator and resuscitation with the cardiologist. In the end, Mildred decided that she wanted neither. Janet again raises the possibility of completing a document to this effect, and for the specific issue of cardiac arrest, Mildred agreed.

This is a good example of how a specific issue might trigger a review of a previous ACP discussion.

Summary

ACP may not be for everyone, but it is potentially a very useful tool for opening up discussions about difficult subjects. A sensitive approach, based on an established relationship is more likely to be effective. For older people, case managers initiating discussions in primary care, may be especially helpful in this regard.

Further resources

- The Royal College of Physicians has published guidelines for ACP. http://www.rcplondon. ac.uk/clinical-standards/organisation/Guidelines/concise-guidelines/Pages/RCP_ ConciseGuideline_AdvancedCarePlanning.aspx The court of protection can help advise on and resolve difficult problems: http://www.publicguardian.gov.uk/about/court-of-protection.htm

- Any professional making decisions on behalf of a person without capacity is required by law to have regard to the Mental Capacity Act Code of Practice: http://www.publicguardian.gov. uk/docs/code-of-practice-041007.pdf

- Office of Public Guardian: www.publicguardian.gov.uk

References

1 NHS End of Life Care Programme (2008). Advance Care Planning: A Guide for Health and Social Care Staff. DH Gateway, London,. http://eolc.cbcl.co.uk/eolc/files/F2023-EoLC-ACP_guide_for_staff-Aug2008.pdf (Accessed 22 June 2010).

2 Fried TR, Rosenberg RR, and Lipsitz LA (1995). Older community-dwelling adults' attitudes toward and practices of health promotion and advance planning activities. *Journal of the American Geriatrics Society*, **43**(6):645–9.

3 Johnston SC, Pfeifer MP, and McNutt R (1995). The discussion about advance directives: Patient and physician opinions regarding when and how it should be conducted. *Archives of Internal Medicine*, **155**(10):1025–30.

4 Torroella Carney M and Morrison RS (1997). Advance directives: when, why, and how to start talking. *Geriatrics*, **52**(4):65–73.

5 Edinger W and Smucker DR (1992). Outpatients' attitudes regarding advance directives. *Journal of Family Practice*, **35**(6):650–3.

6 Kass-Bartelmes BL and Hughes R (2004). Advance care planning: preferences for care at the end of life. *Journal of Pain & Palliative Care Pharmacotherapy*, **18**(1):87–109.

7 Hughes DL and Singer PA (1992). Family physicians' attitudes toward advance directives. *CMAJ: Canadian Medical Association Journal*, **146**(11):1937–44.

8 Barnes K, Jones L, Tookman A, et al. (2007). Acceptability of an advance care planning interview schedule: a focus group study. *Palliative Medicine*, **21**(1):23–8.

9 Hofmann JC, Wenger NS, Davis RB, et al. (1997). Patient preferences for communication with physicians about end-of-life decisions. SUPPORT Investigators. Study to Understand Prognoses and Preference for Outcomes and Risks of Treatment. *Annals of Internal Medicine*, **127**(1):1–12.

10 Tierney WM, Dexter PR, Gramelspacher GP, et al. (2001). The effect of discussions about advance directives on patients' satisfaction with primary care. *Journal of General Internal Medicine*, 16(1):32–40.

11 Molloy DW, Bedard M, Guyatt GH, et al. (1997). Attitudes training issues and barriers for community nurses implementing an advance directive program. *Perspectives*, 21(1):2–8.

12 Finucane TE SJ, Powers RL and D'Alessandri RM (1988). Planning with Elderly Outpatients for Contingencies of Severe Illness: A Survey and Clinical Trial. *Journal of General Internal Medicine*, 3(4):322–5.

13 Engelhardt JB, McClive-Reed KP, Toseland RW, et al. (2006). Effects of a Program for Coordinated Care of Advanced Illness on patients, surrogates, and healthcare costs: A randomized trial. *American Journal of Managed Care*, 12(2):93–100.

14 Rabow MW, Dibble SL, Pantilat SZ, et al. (2004). The Comprehensive Care Team: A Controlled Trial of Outpatient Palliative Medicine Consultation. *Archives of Internal Medicine*, 164(1)83–91.

15 Horne G, Seymour J, and Shepherd K (2006). Advance care planning for patients with inoperable lung cancer. *International Journal of Palliative Nursing*, 12(4):172–8.

16 Taylor JS, Heyland DK, and Taylor SJ (1999). How advance directives affect hospital resource use. Systematic review of the literature. *Canadian Family Physician*, 45:2408–13.

17 Molloy D, Guyatt GH, Russo R, et al. (2000). Systematic implementation of an advance directive program in nursing homes: A randomized controlled trial. *JAMA: Journal of the American Medical Association*, 283(11):1437–44.

18 Emanuel EJ (1996). Cost savings at the end of life. What do the data show? *JAMA: Journal of the American Medical Association*, 275(24):1907–14.

19 Peter Zweifel SFMM (1999). Ageing of population and health care expenditure: a red herring? *Health Economics*, 8(6):485–96.

20 Schiff R LM, Shaw M, Rajkumar C, and Bulpitt CJ (2005). Tool For The Expression Of Healthcare Preferences (EHP). *Age & Ageing*, (34):ii24–26.doi:10.1093/ageing/afn235

Chapter 5

Spiritual aspects of Advance Care Planning

Max Watson

'I am ready to meet my Maker. Whether my Maker is prepared for the great ordeal of meeting me is another matter.'
Winston Churchill

This chapter includes:

- Linking spirituality and Advanced Care Planning
- Fear and Advance Care Planning
- Religious views and Advance Care Planning
- Denial and Advance Care Planning
- Personal control and Advance Care Planning
- The spiritual work of Advance Care Planning
- Adaptation and Advance Care Planning
- Ritual, sacrament, and Advanced Care Planning

Key Points

- Dying is not primarily a medical event.
- The process of thinking about end of life issues can significantly impact on an individual's attitudes, values, and belief systems. The end (conclusion) of life leads us to think about the end (purpose) of life. It is a time of changing perspectives, important reflections on the past, and a stronger sense of what is most important in people's lives.
- Dying patients can challenge the cultural illusion that life is going to last forever. This can be hard for families and professionals to accept and challenges their own fears around mortality.
- An Advance Care Plan (ACP) can provide some comfort through bestowing a sense of control at a time in life when otherwise opportunities to influence events might not pertain. Care can be tailored to personal needs and preferences and this can be important for patients, their families, and healthcare professionals.
- ACP discussions can help in adapting to a new reality for patients and their families. This can bring about a sense of 'realistic hope' and increased resilience leading to better quality of remaining life. It can also trigger discussions with others at a deeper level, voicing unspoken but important truths at this significant time, which can live on in the memory of the bereaved.
- The importance and wisdom of religious rituals and religious symbolism cannot be ignored even in the most secular of contexts as they bring comfort to many.

Linking spirituality and Advanced Care Planning

Death is not primarily a medical event. Death is a personal, relational, and spiritual event, yet the majority of professional effort is concerned with the medical aspects of the end of life, often to the neglect of the more pertinent issues facing the dying and their families. Over many years and especially in the last two centuries, we have tended towards making the natural dying process a clinical event, in a similar way to the medicalization of giving birth.

'It's not that I am afraid of dying. I just don't want to be there at the time.'

Woody Allen

Manifestations of the death denying nature of society include:

- The use of euphemisms to describe death
- The hiding of death or references to death from children
- The 'sanitization' of dying in hospitals and the funeral industry
- The closing of coffins at funerals
- Loss of death and bereavement rituals and practices.

It is worth speculating as to how this unbalance became so common in clinical practice. Is it because health care professionals have been affected by the same death denying culture that affects the rest of western society? Perhaps clinical professionals use their ability to 'do' something clinically as a means of avoiding dealing with other issues and the essential demand of end of life care to 'be' with the dying.

Modern medical science describes with increasing accuracy the biological processes of dying, but is usually silent about what dying and death actually is for the individual person.

If health care professionals share the same attitudes towards death and dying as the rest of society, it is no surprise when it comes to Advance Care Planning that there could be some hesitancy in initiating planning discussions. Discussing death and dignity is inherently 'counter-cultural' and against our societal instincts.

Much attention has been given to the legal and medical implications of Advanced Care Planning and how patients can exercise choice when they no longer have the capacity to do so. Less attention has been paid to how the process of thinking about your own end of life plans impacts on your emotional, familial, psychological, and spiritual life. Consciously thinking about, and planning around your own end of life has a particularity about it which affects most people. Frequently it may cause people to reflect on existential issues and raises questions which may never have been truly faced before. Such a process can challenge our values and have an impact on the way we view the world.

Advance Care Planning has a profoundly spiritual and existential dimension that needs to be acknowledged and supported, regardless of the religious or non religious background of those involved. For those professionals conducting such discussions it is important to appreciate this or they risk missing out on important existential cues given by the patient and the opportunity to support them in the final stage of life.

The end (conclusion) of life forces us to think on what is the end (purpose) of life.

Fear and Advance Care Planning

The sociologist Ernest Becker in his book *The Denial of Death* (2) suggests that the fear of death is a pervasive force which permeates mankind's subconscious. He contends that many of man's heroic, religious, and secular dramas derive from an attempt to overcome death in some way and escape or deny its reality:

> The idea of death, the fear of it, haunts the human animal like nothing else; it is a mainspring of human activity—designed largely to avoid the fatality of death, to overcome it by denying in some way that it is the final destiny of man.

Becker's work has been built on by others who decided to assess whether his thesis could be proved. In some fascinating experiments they showed that thinking about death, even if only for a very short time, has the capacity to make people change previously held attitudes and preferences often in favour of more traditional, dualistic, and authoritarian approaches, or regress to paradigms from their formative years.

How thinking about death changes us (1)

A group of students was asked to fill out a questionnaire. The control group filled out a range of questions about their life experience including a section about their experience of pain, such as a fracture or an operation. The other group of students were asked to answer exactly the same questions but the questions of pain were replaced with questions about death. Where would you like to die? How would you like to die? etc.

On completion of the questionnaire the students were ushered into a classroom where they had to wait for the certificate of completion. Sitting in the room already were some students. These students were clearly identifiable as being from different racial groups and religions. The control group of students sat down in seats in a completely random fashion. The students who had been made to think about death significantly gravitated towards sitting beside others of their own cultural/ religious background.

Such experiments carried out across the world have shown that thinking about death even for only a short time can change voting preferences, as well as your sympathy for more extreme elements within your own tradition. In short, death thoughts for many people can trigger fears and uncertainties at a subconscious level of such strength that they change personal preferences and can promote conservatism.

The process of Advanced Care Planning is primarily concerned with ensuring that life is lived for as long as possible in the way that is preferred. It is about helping people adapt to a new reality that life is limited and has to be lived out in the context of dying. By their nature these discussions promote facing up to mortality, and as such could cause a significant impact. The process itself can change people's values if mortality is not something he or she has pondered. Indeed, often people who begin the process of Advance Care Planning end up choosing options which would not have been thought of as obvious for them at the outset. The very process of planning has changed their way of thinking.

Religious views of Advance Care Planning

The truth of this has long been appreciated in spiritual traditions and teaching. Rather than being morbid, or using fear of death to persuade people to change their ways, these practices have been used for thousands of years to help people face reality with a degree of detachment so they are better able to balance their lives in the present and live in the context of their own mortality.

> 'The brothers should contemplate their death eac1h day so that they can be freed from the cloying impact of the cares of the world.'

> St. John of the Cross Carmelite friar and priest

'The way you live and the way you die are one.'

Montague

'Contemplate the dead and the difference between your body and theirs that you may better live in this world.'

Buddha

'What you are now, we once were; what we are now, you shall be.'

Plaque in the Capuchean ossary in Rome

And he said: 'You would know the secret of death. But how shall you find it unless you seek it in the heart of life? The owl whose night-bound eyes are blind unto the day cannot unveil the mystery of light.'

Khalil Gibran, The Prophet: On Death

' . . . when we finally know we are dying, and all other sentient beings are dying with us, we start to have a burning, almost heartbreaking sense of the fragility and preciousness of each moment and each being, and from this can grow a deep, clear, limitless compassion for all beings.'

Sogyal Rinpoche

'Real spirituality is all about what you do with your pain—you either transmit it or transform it!'

Richard Rohr

Hundreds of years before Becker the major religions of the world were encouraging their followers to overcome fears of death through facing them and thus being freed from their shadow.

Death awareness and death inevitability have been a more accepted feature of most civilizations until relatively recently. The surfeit of death denial which is a feature of western hubris is actually in stark contrast to what has gone on before. Other societies at different times, be it through the building of a pyramid in Egypt or through the purchase of a Co-op funeral in Manchester have been more pragmatic about death and dying.

Denial and Advance Care Planning

Death, and all that is associated with it, including Advance Care Planning, undermines western society's confidence for it clearly implies that modern man is unable to fix everything. From within the cultural bubble that life is going to last forever it can be very hard for an individual to burst the taboo and expose the lie by expressing wishes in relation to their end of life. By so doing they are giving birth to the discomfort of mortality for everyone involved. Our natural and almost automatic response to such expressions is to stifle them, or deem the individuals concerned as being morbid, pessimistic or depressed.

'Mum don't be talking like that, you are going to be fine . . .'

In order to overcome this reticence individuals may have to metaphorically shout to have their voice heard which can make them seem emotionally unbalanced, thus confirming the initial label of instability.

Case Study

MG, a widow of 84 years with advanced chronic obstructive pulmonary disease (COPD), type two diabetes, and angina had been admitted to hospital three times in as many months with chest infections. She had witnessed several people who appeared healthier than her dying on the ward, yet whenever she asked the nurse or doctor about her death she was told not to bother herself thinking like that. The dissonance between what she was seeing and feeling with her own eyes and body and what she was being told by the professionals confused and upset her. She confided in her priest, 'Nobody is telling me the truth, and it makes me feel very frightened and alone'.

Some of this dissonance is due to many of the caring professionals being younger than the patients they are looking after, younger in years and also in terms of life experience, and maybe in spiritual maturity.

It would be wrong to expect these professionals to not share some of the youth values of the society in which they were trained and work. These same professionals and their peers are targeted by youth centred advertising, youth centred music, youth centred media and youth centred entertainments. There is little room on their television schedules for soap operas set in nursing homes or music dealing with old age concerns. Mick Jagger can now draw his old age pension, but our youth centred perspective turns a blind eye to images denoting his old age.

This youth focus leaves our society, with less knowledge and respect than earlier generations for the wisdom that comes through experience and age; wisdom which other cultures and times have prized and valued highly. This can make cross generational communication difficult, particularly in such a sensitive area as Advance Care Planning for it requires a degree of empathy and understanding.

Personal control and Advance Care Planning

A common concern of many near the end of life is retaining a need for control and self determination. Seven of the 12 factors for a good death in the Age Concern debate of the age, related to retaining control—control of place, of people present, and other factors (3). At a time when life appears out of control, this can be very important, especially within our more secular society.

'I do not want anybody else to be making my choices for me.'

For such an individual personal autonomy and choice may be understood as essential expressions of their very personhood. An Advance Care Plan in this context can provide existential comfort through bestowing control at a time in which they are in fact losing control at a very deep level. To individuals for whom control has been very important, the prospect of losing control can cause a very real and deep distress (existential/spiritual pain) because control is so linked to who they think themselves to be. If personhood is understood to be the sum and collation of thoughts, preferences and decisions, the loss of this capacity can feel like a loss of their very 'self', or even a loss of everything that is worthwhile in life. This fear, which such a huge loss can signify, is surely one of the motivators for the passion of those wishing to introduce laws on physician assisted suicide in the UK.

The motivations of the individual completing an Advance Care Plan often influence the nature of the directive. Where control is crucial the plan may become a very detailed document requiring regular updates, additions, and increasing detail to ensure that it is as accurate as possible and conforms with the latest thinking of the individual. The plan itself can become the means by which the individual maintains and expresses their identity. This can increase levels of anxiety among professionals who realize that the prospects of fulfilling such detailed objectives will be difficult to fulfil in the context of real, end of life clinical experience.

The spiritual work of Advance Care Planning

For those who are from a religious or spiritual tradition or who have a yearning for the same, an Advance Care Plan may include expression of religious or spiritual activities or aspirations that patients would like to complete. Examples of these activities might include a trip to Rome, Mecca or Benares or a particular sacramental act. It might also include the fulfilment of dreams such as swimming with dolphins, seeing an Australian sunset, or climbing the Himalayas.

Less dramatic expressions of spiritual aspects of Advance Care Plans might include a desire to reconnect with a previous community, to fulfil particular religious observances, or reconcile a previous difference or conflict, or simply to spend time visiting a favourite place maybe in the countryside or near the sea. Such activities can bring comfort both to patients as well as relatives, and provide a context in which previous family tensions can be reduced, and in which meaning and spiritual assurance grow.

There can be a strong draw to go home, to die in the village of their birth, as is witnessed by many from the UK Asian community going back to Asia—the so called 'Salmon instinct'. It is not unusual for end of life thoughts to raise the importance of spiritual issues for patients and heighten the search for meaning in life. For the professional listening to such thoughts it is necessary to appreciate their importance and to try to avoid prescribing physical treatments for spiritual discomforts. Conversely it is important not to be so sure that a patient's pains are spiritual that their physical needs are neglected!

An Advance Care Plan provides opportunity for reflection and taking stock on one's life. Not only does it give the chance to plan for the future it also encourages the individual to reflect on the past. Advance Care Planning without reflecting on the past is building a house without foundations. It can be done but the plans are unlikely to be robust or authentic.

In relation to the reflective component of an Advance Care Plan there may be personal issues of hurt which come to mind coupled with a desire for reconciliation and resolution of unfinished business. This drive within us exists at a very powerful level as anybody who has worked in a hospice has witnessed.

Case study

Shortly after Joe was diagnosed with lung cancer he made a promise to his daughter that he would escort her down the aisle on her wedding day. The disease was rapid and Joe's condition deteriorated and within months was spending most of the day in bed. He refused to let his daughter bring the wedding day forward, despite his deterioration. When he was admitted to hospice the family gave up hope that he would keep his promise. But Joe didn't die. He remained focused on his goal and despite all the physical indicators he fulfilled his promise and accompanied his daughter, all be it in a wheel chair down the aisle, and then died two days later.

This is a very common human emotion and relates to an innate desire to complete things where possible, and no more so than in terms of resolving relationship difficulties. The process of ACP can trigger deep emotions and enable important discussions to take place that will live on in the memory of the bereaved.

In his book *The Four Things That Matter Most* Ira Byock (4) suggests that there is a universal generic quality to the nature of this emotional work which is common to many people facing the end of their life. He suggests there is a common need to sort relationships out before it is two late.

'Please forgive me', 'I forgive you', 'thank you', and 'I love you' are the outward verbal expressions which Byock gives to these important relational tasks. Tasks which may also be part of an individual's personal Advance Care Plan.

The need for sharing and receiving forgiveness for mistakes that have been made or experienced, for pain given, and pain received is common. As death approaches there is a natural desire to resolve conflict, to pay restitution, and to leave the slate clean as much as possible. Such sentiments in our secular world may be viewed with suspicion, but those working regularly in end of life care both with religious and non religious patients will attest to the power and importance of forgiveness in bringing a sense of peace and restitution in the final stages. Forgiveness is a central part of the faith of many but also deeply healing in psychological terms, removing self-loathing and anger, and bringing about 'wholeness' at a time when a physical cure is not possible.

When tasks of forgiveness and reconciliation have been completed it can have a profound impact on the nature of the last days of a person's life confirming a phrase often quoted from Dame Cicely Saunders,

'The last part of life has an importance out of all proportion to its length'

Planning for reconciliation is of course, impossible but planning to ensure that there is at least opportunity for such work is important. This work is not just for the patient but also for the individuals who will have to live with the consequences of reconciliation or lack of reconciliation long term.

Bound up in the pain of physical disease is the pain of loss and the pain of suffering. Making sense of this suffering is the journey of a lifetime.

Adaptation and Advance Care Planning

The discussion of issues related to living out the final stage of life, brings us face to face with the taboo that is death. Gradually there may be an adaptation to this new reality, a coming to terms with the fact that death will happen, so planning for it is perhaps the best we can do in terms of reducing its impact and control. This growing realization may well come to the dying person before it dawns on their family and loved ones—especially with older people as they face the inevitable with perhaps a degree of expectation and relief.

Case study

A mother, 82 years old, and her 50 year old daughter were having a discussion about Advance Care Planning with a nurse in the care home, as a routing part of their ongoing care. The old lady expressed the wish to die in her favourite Victorian lace nightdress, and wished the nurse to write this down specifically. The daughter was horrified and blurted out 'it would be a waste—why on earth do you want that'. Her mother said quite calmly that she wished to wear that nightdress to look nice for her family to see her after she had died. There was a frisson in the room as the realization dawned on the daughter that her mother was calmly facing her death, whilst she was still fighting it.

Ritual, sacrament, and Advanced Care Planning

'Now faith is the assurance that what we hope for will come about and the certainty that what we cannot see exists.'

Hebrews 11 verse 1, The Bible

'Sacraments are the outward and visible sign of an inward invisible truth'

Common Prayer Book

For those who are religious, faith and religious practices may have a profound effect on how they view their dying and on how they plan for their future. Such people may receive great comfort and reassurance from the support of their religious community through sacraments, pastoral visits, prayer and affirmations of their religions beliefs and hopes. Secular health care delivery systems may struggle with creating space where such religious observance can take place but religious support for the dying is too important to many people to be excluded from health care. The influence of organized religion in Advance Care Planning has an impact that extends beyond those who society would readily identify as being 'religious'. This is because:

◆ The confirmation of mortality that accompanies worsening health may reconnect people with religious experiences and memories from their past

◆ Many of the texts, icons and teachings of the major religions relate to themes and issues which the dying can readily relate to, and draw comfort from

◆ In the search for meaning at the end of life it is not unusual to look beyond the self to religious references and understandings which help provide answers to the challenging questions that mortality poses

◆ 'There are no atheists in fox holes,' first coined during the Second World War, points to the fact that people often turn to God in times of extreme stress when they feel powerless

◆ There is a significant population who find difficulty identifying with or supporting particular religious communities, but who still have strong personal religious beliefs.

Asking patients about what is important to them is vital, and this is usually the first step in holding an ACP discussion.

If it is appropriate to introduce religious sacraments and symbols in the most appropriate way these may have a significant impact on how the patient and their family both view the future and plan for the future. A skilled pastoral care approach will discern the best level of religious ritual that is authentic and comfort-bringing for the individual and the family involved.

Such activities may include some of the following.

◆ Prayer, meditation, and reading of sacred texts

◆ Worship services

◆ Blessings

◆ Religion-specific sacraments and use of holy objects

◆ Weddings and sacred unions

◆ Observance of holy days

◆ Guided meditation for pain reduction and relaxation

◆ Music, sacred or familiar to the patient/family

◆ Life review and creation of a legacy document or recording for family

◆ Guided meditation for inner guidance or connection to God or a Higher Power.

The beliefs and values of patients and families need to be identified and respected in as much as the health care team can ethically and reasonably accommodate them. Such practices should not be assumed just because patients belong to a particular religion, or to no religion but should always be asked about. For example, grieving 'non religious' families may receive seemingly incongruous comfort by knowledge that after-death rituals and practices have been adhered to in accord with religious rites, though they may also be deeply offended by such practices. The only way to find out is to ask and never assume.

The level of religious ritual which is appropriate for each individual and family from their own culture and faith will vary according to the particular situation; the search for authenticity in religious expression and a non judgmental and accepting attitude from the professionals involved can be transformational. Even the most hardened sceptic has found comfort and support from specific rituals and prayers in facing and planning for the future. In this multi-cultural world we live in there is a need to refer to an authoritative source for advice on the different rituals linked to different religions. These may vary considerably in different localities, so seeking guidance from the patient, family, and local faith leaders is important (5).

As well as religious rituals, other rituals may be helpful for patients. It can be important for staff to create a sense of ritual security around the dying where, despite the approach of death, there is the support to allow people to feel accepted and given the space and time to complete the tasks of dying—the completion of their Advance Care Plan. As C Saunders notes in *The Management of Terminal Malignant Disease*:

> The real presence of another person is a place of security. I recall remarking to two psychiatrists that when patients are in a climate of safety they will come to realize what is happening in their own way and not be afraid. One said: 'How can you speak of a climate of safety when death is the most unsafe thing that can happen?' To which the other replied: 'I think you are using the wrong word. I think it should be "security". A child separated from his mother may be quite safe—but he feels very insecure. A child in his mother's arms during an air raid may be very unsafe indeed—but he feels quite secure. (6)

Ultimately how the individual copes with their pending death and the process of facing up to the responsibility of this time through Advance Care Planning is hard to predict.

Speaking of his experiences in the concentration camps in world war two Victor Frankl wrote (7):

> Even though conditions such as lack of sleep, insufficient food and various mental stresses may suggest that inmates were bound to react in certain ways, in the final analysis it becomes clear that the sort of person the prisoner became was the result of an inner decision and not the result of camp influence alone.

The capacity to function in the face of mortality relates in part to the quality of resilience which the individual retains. Some aspects of resilience are connected with genetics, some with upbringing, and the remainder are strengthened or weakened through life events (8). In helping people complete Advance Care Plans it is often humbling to observe just how resilient some people are to life and all that it has brought them, in contrast to how lacking in resilience others may appear.

Our role as midwives in the birth of Advance Care Plans is not to praise or condemn, but as fellow travellers to help deliver the most authentic declaration of the future aspirations of the individual as possible, in the knowledge that one day we too may need the services of just such a 'soul friend'.

Further resources

Pyszczynski T, Solomon S, Greenberg J, Maxfield M, Cohen F. Fatal attraction: the effects of mortality salience on evaluations of charismatic, task-oriented, and relationship-oriented leaders. *Psychol Sci.* 2004;15(12):846–51.

Simon L, Greenberg J, Harmon-Jones E, Solomon S, Pyszczynski T, Arndt J, et al. Terror management and cognitive-experiential self-theory: Evidence that terror management occurs. *Journal of Personality and Social Psychology*. 1997;72(5):1132–46.

References

1 Solomon S, Solomon S, Greenberg J, and Pyszczynski T (1991). A Terror management theory of social behavior: The psychological functions of self-esteem and cultural worldviews. In Zanna M, (ed.) *Advances in experimental social psychology*, **24**, 93–159. Academic Press.

2 Becker E (1973). *The Denial of Death*. New York: Simon & Schuster.

3 The future of health and care of older people: the best is yet to come (1999). London: Age Concern.

4 Byock I (2004). *The Four Things That Matter Most: A book about living*. New York: Free Press.

5 Emmanuel L and Neuberger J (2004). *Caring for Dying People of Different Faiths*, Oxford: Radcliffe Medical Press.

6 Saunders C (1984). *The Management of Terminal Malignant Disease* (2nd edn). London: Edward Arnold.

7 Frankl V (1963). *Man's Search for Meaning: An Introduction to Logotherapy*. New York: Washington Square Press.

8 Watson M (2007). Resilience and the psychobiological base. In: Monroe B, Oliviere D, (eds) *Resilience in Palliative Care - Achievement In Adversity*, 29–38. Oxford: OUP.

Chapter 6

Advance Care Planning: politically correct, but ethically sound?

Rob George and Tim Harlow

'When a man lies dying he does not die from his illness alone but from his whole life.'
Charles Peguy 1875-1914, Basic Verities 1943

This chapter includes:
- Introduction
- The fundamental question: Why are decisions necessary at all?
- Background
- Laying the foundations
- Defining and understanding Terms
- What are goods and harms?
- Building the theory
- Are we the same person as time passes or minds change?
- Practical implications
- Conclusion

Key Points
- ACP is valuable as it helps people reflect on and prepare for the end of their life
- The politics, ethics, and philosophy of ACP can be simple or complicated depending on the need and want of the decision maker and the life they have and do lead
- ACP is not a precise science and it offers both potential benefit as well as risk to the future self because autonomy is not future proof and comes at a price
- Despite the laudable efforts of the Legislature to codify people's advance decision making at the end of life; clarity for the many can never remove the uncertainties for the few.

Introduction

In a society such as the UK, which prizes the individual's autonomy, and has a natural scepticism of central authority, the idea of Advance Care Planning (ACP)—that one's personal wishes must be respected, and in some cases followed as a matter of law—seems, self evidently, to be a Good Thing. The attention that is now being paid to End of Life Care (EoLC), exemplified by government initiatives, is widely welcomed and genuine attempts to increase personal choice are found throughout the National Health Service (NHS) and in other sectors, yet it is well known that despite around two thirds of people probably wishing to die at home less than a third actually do so (1). This disparity can act as a potent driver for initiatives to increase ACP for EoLC and even to use the realization of such wishes for place of death to be markers of success. Palliative care places the individual needing care at the centre of its ethos—as Cicely Saunders said, 'You matter because you are you'. Being able to plan, or at least indicate in a real and potentially enforceable way, ones wishes beyond a time when one is able to formulate or communicate them, seems a natural and reasonable extension of this principle.

Any attempt therefore to criticise ACP seems at first sight to devalue these accepted principles of autonomy, of improving EoLC and of valuing the individual. However, in Advance Care Plans we are not just dealing with someone's preferences over taking sugar: ACP may include Advance Decisions to Refuse Treatments (ADRT) that prolong life, enhance quality, or reduce suffering. These are profound and deep issues so it is a matter of moral rigour and a social responsibility that such matters survive explicit scrutiny. It is all too easy to roll over in a fit of political correctness without considering as best we may what unintended adverse consequences are opened up by introducing and legislating for such processes.

Although the motive and intent of ACP cannot be doubted there must be a critical appraisal to see if ACP delivers the right outcomes in improving EoLC as far as is realistically possible. Ethics are only helpful if they guide us in real life decisions.

This chapter gives a very brief view of the underlying theory and philosophy that forms the fundamental moral justification for decision making, either in advance for oneself or on behalf of another, and how this applies to people with failing or fluctuating capacity; and then reflects on the practical implications that any problems and objections throw up.

The fundamental question: why are decisions necessary at all?

Generally, living entails decisions, some so commonplace or banal as to appear barely decisions at all, yet the control they give to influence one's environment is an integral part of what it means to be human. During the series of losses that dying may entail, this affirmation of a person's human- ity and individual significance by acts, no matter how small, is an inherently worthwhile end in itself.

Specifically circumstances that might require decisions will be heavily influenced by their exact nature and the information prevailing at the time, such as whether to accept palliative chemo- therapy or admission to a hospice. They may also be fundamentally important components of the quality of life and death of the person who has to make them. Such decisions, therefore, ought all to be determined by the individual as the subject of the intervention.

In any system there is more than one way of doing things. In UK there is respect for individual- ity and the personalization of EoLC care, whereas other societies with a potentially totalitarian system might relegate this or not recognize it at all. Our system is founded upon individual human freedoms. An individual who is deemed to have capacity to enact their freedoms is legally entitled to do so. The idea of others taking decisions away from us unjustifiably is a modern anathema in its fullest sense. We would all say that this is why we need the option, in case of fluc- tuating capacity, to plan our care in advance and so does society. Hence ACP will help guide the decisions that we know or expect to be taken when we near the end of our life and may no longer be able to take them for ourselves:

♦ This is justified because it promotes autonomy—a socially approved goal;

♦ The knowledge that our wishes will be respected by such ACP can be a comfort and help to all concerned and brings reality to bear upon what is happening—a social good;

♦ Care becomes more efficient and practical plans can be made, such as providing a hospital bed and other equipment at home—a social utility;

♦ The existence of ACP can provide a measure against which EoLC can be audited. In the example of places of death (*supra*) a reduction in hospital deaths might be a measure of success in EoLC and may make better use of resources—an economic utility.

These, then, are the common and plausible *prima facie* justifications for ACP, yet we must be clear that morality and practicality is highly complex and some surprises are in store.

Laying the foundations

First, there are key theoretical considerations that place question marks over the very conception of ACP. For example, and most basically, can autonomy as formulated in the liberal tradition ever exist? Can or should we ever be able to determine proscriptively what a future self might want or need, and indeed can we know in advance even who that future self will be? These are interconnected and fundamental to the premises upon which ACP is based and so they must be firm.

We will begin with some notes on terms and then outline various conceptions of autonomy, the implications these have for formulating our interests into the future and, in particular, when our capacity is too unstable or simply cannot engage in making known our views and judgements. Interwoven with this is the problem of personal identity and how this changes over time – the idea of a distinct, future self. What moral authority may we have over that future and as yet unknowable person and can we, therefore, ever make safe, binding decisions for them in advance? The philosophical literature on these questions is substantial and technical. Our summary is therefore necessarily brief and simple. You are encouraged to pursue the questions and objections that will arise. The referencing is confined to reviews and commentaries that will lead you into the source literature and detailed theoretical discourse. We acknowledge key thinkers by name, but leave the explicit references to the commentaries for ease and brevity. Finally we comment on any outstanding practicalities before concluding that ACP/ADRT is probably a good way forward, but not for the reasons most think.

Defining and understanding terms

'The beginning of wisdom is to call things by their proper names.'

Old Chinese proverb

Capacity and competence

Capacity is defined for legal purposes in the 2005 Mental Capacity Act (MCA) as the ability to understand, retain, and weigh information and then to communicate ones decision. The process is also decision-specific rather than general. This offers an apparently solid foundation for testing decision making. Consequently, the justification for planning in advance is the possibility that one may become incapable of making important decisions about one's care in that future. The problem, of course, is that a legal definition still does not, indeed cannot, give a factual and detailed measure of evaluative terms like understanding or weighing; they themselves are matters of individual evaluation and judgement along the way (what the MCA does to address this is that we must always presume in favour of a person being capable). Therefore, we must start by being clear as to what we mean by and how we might judge capacity and competence, so that we may have confidence in knowing when an ACP becomes active.

Whilst pedantic, it is critical to appreciate that no one has stable capacity. Tiredness, stress, excessive responsibility, too much work all impair one's faculties to process and weigh information and to make sound judgements. We call it 'not thinking straight'. Some would call this competence, to distinguish someone whose base capacity is undisturbed, but transient circumstances render them briefly incompetent to engage a task. Equally our patients' symptoms, and pain in particular, can impede both their capacity and competence either directly or through the distress that such things cause (2). Depression may do the same. To make things even trickier, there is also growing evidence of cognitive impairment in dying patients that often goes unrecognized, and meets the DSM-IV criteria for dementia (3). For some clarity and nuancing, then, we suggest the term capacity for the specific legal task in hand, and competence when decision-making seems impaired whilst overall background capacity is preserved.

In summary, the tests in the MCA are not tests in the factual, medical sense, but codified opinions: the term 'test' gives them a substance to which they are not really entitled. There is no hard delineation or box called capacity, especially in cases of dementia or other slowly progressive conditions where disease trajectories vary so much (4). Nevertheless, whilst the MCA allows for fluctuations in capacity by being explicitly decision specific, a reservation must remain about how this can deal, on the one hand, with the moments of lucidity, flashes of insight, or awareness that can be very troubling to close observers of people with dementia and a baseline incapacity, or on the other, with the lacunae of absence and apparent incompetence or confusion in otherwise capable people as they process their dying and near the end of life. We will return to this when we talk about multiple selves.

The fourth step in capacity, communication, is equally troublesome. Being *incommunicado* always makes one vulnerable to being considered *incogitato* as emerging research in persistent vegetative, minimally conscious and locked in states is beginning to show (5,6). This reminds us also of how our neat theoretical models or apparently clear and past advance decisions are sometimes only tangentially related to what turns out in the end to be reality.

Autonomy and interests

Understanding autonomy in its various formulations is essential when considering the ethics of ACP. Most basically, autonomy entails having a personal identity, which is able to discover, articulate, and express individual interests. As such a person, we can be free to form and realize what we see as a good life. This is almost cardinal amongst the principles by which western societies such as ours are governed. In other words, the autonomous person is capable not only of such formulation(s), but crucially is given the wherewithal to bring them about through freedoms and entitlements that are legislated. This is the liberal ideal—autonomy as self-determination and self-interest. Interests are merely the expressions of autonomy, and where there are people they will compete and conflict.

This is the classical, individualist or existential view of autonomy, which can emphasize the here and now (I am who I am) and asserts itself through evidentiary interests in which my current desires trump everything. The alternative is the a broader narrative view that looks across the scope of ones whole life and sees who one is now in the light of who one was or may become. We will return to these later.

There is another, complementary way of seeing autonomy relevant to our discussion: the communitarian view. Here, one identifies oneself through relationships—having a sense of self through membership of family, tribe, community, gang, religion etc. We are social animals and human interaction fulfils that need and part of our identity. Nevertheless, the motivation to relate is predicated on some mutual benefit, whether it is culturally embedded or a matter of current need. Even an apparently altruistic interaction, despite being of great worth and desirability, will still be sensitive to the interests of the parties involved. Preferences over place of care and place of death that seem straightforward choices are a case in point, with their dependence often upon informal care networks or family. Hence, in EoLC at least, they are fluid, suggestible, and change to and fro right up until the closing days of life according to what is going on in the group (7).

Viewed from the inside, as per the *existential* views of autonomy, expressions of interests, my rights, needs, and wants are all that matter; whereas from the outside, *communitarian* view, individual interests are freely subjugated according to the impact upon others' personal rights and projects. The common good is what matters. We all live connected lives, and according to the extent of that co-dependency, we may not even see individuality in its radical sense to be either adequate or even coherent. This is the norm in 'hot cultures' where the emphasis is on collective life and community so that a person's identity is tied to that of the group. This is especially marked where the life of the collective body is necessary for individual life itself.

So much for the patient and family, but many other people and agencies also have interests in an individual's EOL care and ACP, believing that because it is personalized, the care is therefore good. Indisputably the patient's best interests should take precedence, but the vested interests need to be seen, owned, and balanced in decision making. For example, a hospital or hospice team may genuinely believe they are acting in someone's best interest if they delay plans for discharge home to die because the 'care package' is incomplete, yet the opportunity is lost for the patient to die where they wanted to be.

Scratching in this way at the surface of what constitutes genuine autonomy might reveal far more about the real world and our relationships than we thought. Egocentric views of autonomy, whilst held by the majority when convenient, are not coherent bases upon which to describe the people that we know ourselves to be—individuals embedded in, formed by, and forming relationships and communities for whom collective values may well trump what we want for ourselves. This communitarian or collective view owes much to feminist ethics through its acknowledgment of the importance of emotion and psychology in the otherwise rather aridly logical analysis of conventional ethical reasoning.

We will not dwell on autonomy *per se* much more and refer you to other commentators (8–10) except to conclude that the real challenge is to deliver care in the broadest terms for people who lack or have fluctuating capacity and limited autonomy. Nevertheless, those unable to be moral agents on their own behalf still have claims as members of society to the same freedoms and entitlements to be cared for in what is believed to be their best interests and protected from harm. So in closing the section on terms, what is meant by words like best, good, and harm and how do we arrive at their definition?

What are goods and harms?

Values, not facts

We are apt to bandy around words like 'good' and 'harmful' and assume objectivity, a universal agreement about their meanings, even though they are subjective, relative terms. Generally there is agreement on arguments, which are arrived at by observation of concrete phenomena or rational thought and that are considered as facts. But values are much less precise, more slippery to define, dependent as they are upon the collective values of those making the judgement. Yet so called scientific truth is still subject to the pervading values of the day (11). Such differences almost always come down not to ones arguments or evidence, but to ones assumptions or premises.

Premisses

As individuals, we often forget that there are other views of the world. Not everyone starts reasoning from the same set of assumptions. Even decisions about appropriate treatments are influenced by our premisses. For example, analgesia seems to be undoubtedly a 'good' thing, but when do we know it is good enough? The patient's capacity may be affected by the pain; their view of good analgesia may change when the acute severity of pain has eased. A relative may not be able to bear the sight of even a transient pain and consider 'good' to be analgesia that eliminates the pain entirely even at the cost of significant drowsiness/capacity. A lawyer making out the dying person's last will and testament might have a different view. A nurse who fears the patient dying soon after an injection of the analgesic (even though such injections don't kill) might consider the death her fault and that any analgesia as death approaches as a bad thing. So what is 'good' here, what measure are we to use? Some guidance will come from considering who gains from an action or decision, yet even that is subjective and open to inherent bias from other premisses.

Similarly judgements of what is harmful have the same vulnerabilities. There can be times when what seems harmful, or is deemed harmful, is in reality inconvenient for a particular interest. A patient refusing a fourth line palliative chemotherapy with significant toxicity and small expectation of disease remission may be judged to have been spared a real harm by those who fear the false hope, the side effects, and the distraction from coming to terms with their death. But those with a duty to protect NHS budgets may feel such treatment is harmful in a different way as they act as advocate for the unseen patients who compete for the same limited resources. And a researcher thinking of the patients in the future who may gain from the knowledge perhaps gained from trying the treatment will have another view.

Futility

The concept of futility, attractive at first sight for its apparent objectivity to those struggling with finding the correct way through decision making, only throws one back on the same issues. Labelling an intervention as futile (and therefore to be decided against or not to be pursued) is value laden. The precepts that inform these values are wholly subjective, emanating entirely from collective values or worse still one person's interpretation of those values. What rule says that a one in one hundred chance of success is futile when a one in ten, or a one two chance, is not? What rule allows us to suggest the quality of life is likely to be so poor that trying to prolonging it is futile?

Quality of Life

On the face of it one may claim that we can be pretty clear about poor quality of life. Anyone who peruses medical notes on dying patients and those with severe multi-system illness will soon come across such judgements. But when we are trying to decide what decision might maximize quality of life or even if there is any real quality of life there at all, it is a perilous area and arguably ACP might hinder as much as help. Asked if life with Locked in Syndrome (LIS) was consistent with any worthwhile quality of life most people would be clear it was not and an Advance Care Plan might quite justifiably incorporate such views. Yet, there are well known examples of people living a life they consider worthwhile with such profound physical limitations. This inner life, entirely within the mind, can be precious even when the connection to or ability to manipulate the outside world is extremely limited. People adjust amazingly well and two thirds of people with LIS consider their quality of life to be good (12). So whose judgements must we rely upon, and when were these judgements made?

How much harm is a person allowed to wish upon themselves? We accept a person's freedom to accept great risk, hardship, and suffering without society needing to intervene. For example, despite seeming to be unwise by some, a person with capacity can insist on going home to squalid and dangerous conditions, the MCA explicitly protects the freedom to make unwise or eccentric decisions. Yet it is important to recognize that neither law nor ethics allows anyone to insist on someone else doing something to them that is knowingly of net harm (i.e. you can't make me do something to you that I think is harmful). Freedom comes at a price. When someone with capacity makes a valid ADRT that price is clear, but there are more subtle ones too, especially upon those around that person.

Some hazardous activities such as SCUBA diving have a safety concept of the 'Incident pit' where a series of individually inconsequential errors or events, which could easily have been managed but escape notice, gradually tip a person deeper and deeper into a situation which is desperate by the time stock is taken. The same process often applies in gradually deteriorating health and capacity. There is rarely any one catastrophic event and even the diagnosis may take considerable time. Trying to decide when decisions should be made, who should make them and the applicability of ACP in these slow deteriorations is not easy. Which may be worse, to default to the tidiness of ACP which seems to offer clarity in the face of a likely different current perspective or person, or to trust those on the spot to judge and balance the evolved situation? Either route includes the possibility of facing unwanted treatment.

There is no watertight answer to these dilemmas other than to recognize the inherent contradictions and flux in the process of considering what is good or bad, beneficial or harmful.

Dignity

Dignity is recognized to be fundamental to care and efforts are made actively to enhance dignity in healthcare (13,14). Dignity involves a recognition of true human worth, of valuing a human being for all that is worthwhile about them. Unbridled freedom is not the same as dignity. If a person who is suffering from a temporary delirium tries to walk naked in a public place it is not undignifying to stop him, quite the reverse. His inherent worth makes action to prevent such uncharacteristic behaviour necessary even at the expense of freedom. Allowing a poor choice for the wrong reasons diminishes dignity. As discussed earlier, the judgement here about what is 'for the wrong reasons' may be difficult but must include a normative view of that person's worth. We accept that society is entitled to a view about a person's intrinsic value—as Kant said, people are 'ends in themselves' and Schweitzer said that the way in which the vulnerable are treated reflects on a society's civilization. This means that a broader view of a human's value is valid that reflects things other than the persons' individual perceptions of themselves, or our views of their capacity or capability.

To summarize so far, in a culture of relativism, finding absolutes is a fool's errand, except to say that in terms of entitlements, these must necessarily be societal and normative goods e.g. the right to health care, life, and education. Second, autonomy finds its expression in a person's interests— what counts as important to them; alongside one's leaning to evidential autonomy would be experiential interests, and alongside the integrity view will be critical interests that will prioritize the sweep of one's life rather than immediate gratification etc. Third, the tensions, choices and balance necessary to be an individual and citizen in turn will both restrain and preserve, not what is good or harmful in my eyes, but the extent to which I can realize goals through freedom from interference or through the assistance that comes with society recognizing that 'x' is sufficiently good and necessary in the circumstances to be an entitlement.

Let's move on now to the central moral challenge to ACP, the matter of what we mean by self.

Building the theory

Are we the same person as time passes or minds change?

Past events and the person we once were, over whom we have no control now, shaped the present person we are and influence our future. This relationship lies at the heart of the moral debate about ACP for a future and arguably unknowable self.

Shakespeare noticed this long ago through Jaques who dolefully notes that our final self may be in 'second childishness and mere oblivion…' and it seems that he assumes this to be a bad thing. The prospect of needing to be fed, of being unable to remember even whether one has been fed, of being wholly dependant but oblivious as to why, may fill us all with some disquiet if not terror. But how shall the person I might be, in the actual event, view things? Will I care then or just now? If I have a catastrophic brain injury and plunge suddenly into such a state, how long is it right to allow adjustment before withdrawing treatment if an ADRT is in place? What if an ADRT forbids ventilation or does not account for the possibilities of improvement? Say my incapacity might be temporary, but my 'current self's' ADRT dictates that I cannot be sustained until that capacity returns? What if adjustment and improvement takes years, as the literature is clear that it does? Or in the face of no improvement, what if my demented self seems now to have the *joie de vivre* that my current, capable self doesn't have and never anticipated? Is it merely a question of my diminished capacity in the future making the earlier decision more powerful? Can and should I proscribe now for then? If I do, does it imply that my interests are only based in the present and not the overall sweep of my life or the future, possible contemporaneous state and interests of that self? If you like I may even be saying my current state, and the anxiety it is engendering as a contemporaneous emotion, trumps the emotions or feelings of that future self. Am I entitled to amputate, reject, or even kill that future self and that part of my identity, which after all is just as much part of the sweep of my life as any other? If that is so then there is an implication that I am less of a human being, my value becoming less with diminishing insight or intellect and cognition. This then implies a categorization of humanity where some, and their views, are worth less than others. Furthermore we often assume a global deterioration in these matters but even here it is not that simple. People have good days and bad days, have islands of awareness and of insight. Many of the drives and mental or spiritual burdens people carry can change and diminish. So when we are troubled by contact with someone who we once knew and is now utterly changed by dementia yet is tranquil and content: whose trouble is it, the patient's or ours the witnesses? Whose distress might we be treating if we elect to withdraw or not offer treatment—ours or theirs? These are all dizzying and disturbing thoughts when fired as a salvo of possible problems.

Thankfully, for some people there is little conflict of interest between the present and future self, because decisions regarding ACP are more clearly cut because of values or beliefs that guide them and offer equilibrium in the face of uncertainty. For others some decisions cannot be made or are never made, even when circumstances such as sudden deterioration and death prevail. In the absence of ACP some may be content simply to abdicate decision making to others.

So, how strong is the grip of autonomy upon advance planning? Let us continue to build theory. Keep in mind that we are on an ethical quest to find what, if any, moral authority we or others have in determining what happens to us when capacity is lost.

Ropes of continuity, strands of connectedness

Much has been written in the theoretical literature on identity in its various forms. It is one of the cardinal questions of metaphysics. For brevity, we draw on some of the substantial relevant commentaries of the subject as fitting portals into the source texts (9). We have drawn heavily from MacLean's review in particular as it addresses our theoretical dilemma, whilst falling short on the clinical insight and application that we are able to apply (15).

Reductionist views

The theorists begin by distinguishing our physical identity, i.e. our biology/body, from the cognating, self-conscious person that one would call me-the-person, the components and distinguishing parts of which are memories, experiences, decisions etc. that form the narrative of our life. Both change constantly in response to our environment and the 'slings and arrows of outrageous fortune' such that we find that over time we change generally by shades of degree—a series of overlapping selves—but also by type as we forget more distant selves or reject proximate selves through shifts and changes in values, beliefs etc. These shifts in one's paradigm are particularly important in real life.

Munday reported that preferences for place of death frequently changed over time and were often ill defined or poorly formed in patients' minds. Preferences were often described as being co-created in discussion with the patient or, conversely, inferred by the health professional without direct questioning or receiving a definitive answer from the patient. This inherent uncertainty he believes challenges the practicability, usefulness, and value of recording a definitive preference. For our purposes the inference is that the self is too fragile or mercurial to project reliably into the future.

Derek Parfit gives a key account of this position of multiple selves in an analysis using thought experiments and logic (16). Parfit suggested that it was possible, indeed likely, that a recognizable, apparently singular individual, was in fact a succession of different selves. Whilst these selves shared a common ancestry, they could be entirely different and unknown to each other, because whilst continuous, they were not necessarily connected—much as a hemp rope is a single entity whilst consisting of many short overlapping but discrete fibres, many of which have no contact or connection together—for these selves to be connected required a psychological link through memories and experiences (17). What matters at a particular point in an individual's identity then, is the psychological connectedness and strength of relationship between these strands of self rather than any chronological continuity. Consequently we are strangers to some of our ancestral selves despite occupying the same biological and biographical space. We see this of course in that we cannot connect with or remember many things in our past, whilst others are 'as though they happened yesterday'; and in other ways, we say 'to forgive is to forget', or that we had a conversion experience or moment of revelation that changed the course of our life and we say 'I was never the same again'. With that event or purpose we may have terminated the connections and therefore the moral authority or even the existence of that self for subsequent selves.

This compelling account questions ACP as an expression of autonomy. It places the weight clearly with experiential autonomy—the here and now over integrated autonomy across a lifespan. Ancestral selves are strangers and cannot, therefore, have any moral authority over the present self through any advance decisions. There are of course problems with Parfit's account, but the analysis survives in its claim that there is no moral basis from the perspective of autonomy to justify ACP or AD (15). Furthermore, Parfit's conclusion invites us to consider something very uncomfortable: that there can also be a living human who is no longer a person, a 'dead man walking'.

This brings us to what may be called "a non-person argument" where one may claim that the person inhabiting a body is dead. We will suspend judgement on this claim for now to stay with the relevant moral point, which is the proposition that there may be survivorship interests between selves—what Kuhse would call a death with a body that merely remains biologically active (e.g. if one believes in truly vegetative states). The argument is that the previously competent past self has an interest in the vestigial body as much as one has in the disposal of one's own corpse. Of course it begs the question of when that death has occurred and the equally troubling alterative that the state may decide that it is society's interest for the body to die or be killed (if such terms continue to have meaning).

Tragically there are views that see nobility in a patient ending their life because they are demented on the grounds that they are a burden to themselves, their families, and the NHS (18).

Those of us who encounter dementia every day, will of course find this pretty unpalatable since the problem so often, in even the most advanced case, is not that there is no-one at home, but that they can't open the door. Our defensible position is that we are not to harm whoever is there whether we can contact them or not.

But back to our main moral question: ultimately, the incompetent person ends up the property of someone—either of the previous and possibly stranger-self or of the state. The unanswerable question for this moral justification is 'when does an autonomy no longer matter, and therefore when could it have mattered at all'? Seeing as it does matter, this argument fails to overthrow Parfit, since it merely substitutes autonomy with the tyranny of one or other self over its chronological sibling selves.

Reductionist analyses such as these assume that people can be unbundled into mind and body, but as MacLean points out, other conceptions see the person as greater than the sum of her component parts, that there is some unifier that makes a whole person more than her mind and body—as some would say, 'man is more than a computer made of meat' (19). These are the ideas that the mind and consciousness are something more than the brain, but because this line of reasoning, as a source of moral authority, relies on beliefs about transcendence and theology, we may find ourselves derailed. So let's step back and look to see instead if a conception of life, as greater than its component parts, through narrative and biographical views, and ideas of autonomy as the integral of a series of selves, offers a way forward independent of beliefs about the soul.

Non-reductionist views of a life

'When I was a child, I used to speak as a child, think as a child, reason as a child; when I became a man, I did away with childish things.'

1 Cor. 13:11, New American Standard Bible

Quante calls perspectives that look across the sweep of a life 'a thick concept of autonomy' and Dworkin, the integrity view—by this they mean the values, character, and convictions are what matter along with the goals and plans that sculpt ones whole life, not the day-to-day things of the here and now. This is offered as a justification for the competent self to extend these aspirations to times when that competent self is no longer there. Whilst it is entirely worthwhile to build a life that has an overall meaning and coherence and this is not to be denied anyone, it doesn't give any more help on the autonomy question, for the issue remains: not that there is a whole life, but which bits of that whole have moral authority over other bits? Well, the problem remains: that high or thick views of autonomy as the project of a whole life, still relegates the failing autonomy of a dementing self to a second class subject (or even object) powerless to resist the project of criteria interests that it may no longer hold or value outside its 'there and then'. Of course, one may modify what one may determine in advance with tests, exceptions and societal values, but they don't alter the type of bottom line, merely where it is placed, i.e. one that cannot be justified morally on the grounds of autonomy, or equality for that matter.

To summarize, common sense and philosophy tell us that we are not the same person as time, experiences, and choices pass, and that no matter how hard one tries, decisions about a future self made by a former one, irrespective of intellectual gymnastics and ingenuity, cannot be justified morally on the grounds of autonomy, because one self or other trumps and either way, autonomy is the loser. We still remain stuck with whom to benefit or harm, the present or previous self. This does not mean that our moral intuitions are entirely wrong. ACP/ADRT may still be good and is probably the 'least worst' option. Fortunately, some rescuers are at hand and Korsgaard's idea of our authorial agency as 'Unifier of Successive Selves' moves us towards positions that begin to feel like the real world and engage more coherent, pragmatic and traditional analyses with a chance of success.

A compromise?

Since autonomy *per se* cannot justify ACP, what are the other sources of moral authority that the competent self can claim? One is very practical—a call to humanity, pragmatism, and the rich context of the incapable person within a whole life and its relationships, gives the competent self weight for no other reason than that's the way things are in the situation; and the competent self is as good a place to look for guidance as anywhere, not least because the competent self is the most informed of the past, and probably the best to guess how a future self may see things (20). The justification here, then, may be that it is right because it works as an intuitive idea of good in the web of a society and its current values. Nevertheless, there is now space for other legitimate interests to enter the ring. For example, beyond immediate social connections, beneficent interests and duties exist. We see them in the patient doctor relationship and other social contracts stimulated by various social or professional duties of care.

Is there a parent in the house?

MacLean makes a persuasive offer to take a different view and see the person from the incompetent, rather than the competent end. This is appealing because it seems just and looks to some symmetry across a life from one childhood to the next. It views the problem, not from the obsessional egocentricity that liberal autonomy fosters, but from the obligations that one, as a competent self, has for the welfare of a future unknown and possibly incompetent and vulnerable self. This is similar to the role of a parent and considers the ACP/ADRT through that lens. One is connected by being part of the same life, sharing the same body and history, and obligations exist intuitively between the past, present, and future phases of a person's life towards themselves. There is also an established justification and normative structure in the parent child relationship for decisional authority, which in principle at least, could apply to a parental relationship between competent and incompetent selves. This type of relationship and its governance and viability as an approach already exists in Law where parents have decisional authority, but they do not have absolute power (21). And on MacLean's account, neither should the former self.

So far so good, but there are limitations. In this type of parenthood, it is not the dynamic, observing carer relationship modifying a view as autonomy emerges; it is the other way around and one can only anticipate and guess scenarios and responses. We do not know what lies ahead. Whilst the decisional authority is there it may then need to be trumped on the grounds of unintended consequences due to unforeseen contexts. At this point, as with the law in relation to minors, others with guardian interests may come into play, particularly if they are part of the collective autonomous identity of the subject through Parfit's psychological connectedness (biological/biographical family) and within their family, or group, or finally through duties of care established by the state. Of course whatever of the new self is able to contribute, and can be accessed, also has a say. So, where is the moral justification for all this?

Taking the obligation position rather than the autonomy/rights position, one has cogent responsibilities towards an incompetent self, because one is recognizably connected either psychologically and at least physically and this connection is necessarily worthy of respect in its own right: the sounds and senses of a soul that may on occasion recall and share common connections that are a life's shared narrative are both observable in the lives of countless patients and of moral import. Hence, ACP/ADRTs that are conceived and orientated explicitly to the interests of a future self and that do not simply rehearse the autonomy of the ACPs author's current interests projected onto that future person are justified on these beneficent grounds.

Next, because the 'parental authority' is now one of interest in a beneficent sense, not ownership, such authority is accountable to other interests or parties that bring additional moral weight. Since decisional authority is not absolute, but *prima facie,* others with legitimate interests, and ultimately the MCA's Court of Protection, can police it and those with nefarious vested interests of their own are also likely to be flushed out.

This approach also accounts for one of the more troubling real world examples familiar to specialists, that autonomy had no chance of addressing and was a recent challenge for one author. This is the person whose life journey has taken them full circle in terms of beliefs or values. We will call him John.

This story begins in the spiritual devotions and faith of childhood and adolescence with a view to a life in the ministry. It is not to be; faith is destroyed by a brutal, personal tragedy in early adulthood; bitterness and the self-hatred of survivor guilt take hold, and finally find form in an ADRT made as soon as John has a diagnosis of which incapacity will probably form a part. This is reviewed regularly but never changed. He is clear that no complications, no matter how reversible, are to be treated actively even if this leads to an avoidable death. John also states that if he loses capacity, there are to be no religious symbols around during his remaining life and if a funeral or committal has to be held it must be secular. However, as his incapacity deepens, this gentleman's memories connect so vividly to a distant past beyond his tragedy that he is able to leapfrog the pain and bitterness of his derailed life to see again through his youthful, faithful eyes. He returns to his hymn singing and his language, such as it is now, is almost entirely spiritual. He appears entirely happy and settled most of the time. When distressed, he calls out for 'the old wooden cross'. Staff have found one around the care home and it gives him relief. Sadly, John was estranged from his family when well, but they have recently been in touch. They remember the violent angry man and the current one is a very welcome though puzzling one. His brother remains amazed to see the 'old John' again.

The family are happy and those that care for him now know only the man before them. The author of the ADRT, which is a couple of years old now, is a stranger; the current self is comforted and reassured by the very things that the adult antecedent rejected, and on suffering a painful and distressing urinary tract infection, he is treated with the agreement of family and staff and remains well.

We are managing the patient before us, informed by his past, but not ruled by it. The consensus of those with guardianship has trumped. The parental modelling allows this and can respond to such complexities. Autonomy cannot do it alone.

Practical implications

'The forceps of our minds are clumsy forceps, and crush the truth a little in taking hold of it.'

First and last things; a confession of faith and rule of life, 1908. HG Wells

Assessments

Good, safe and robust ACP demands assessments and reviews including quality of life, timescale, chances of recovery, rate of change, disease trajectory, capacity (where relevant), and practicality. There are real difficulties here, especially with the gradual and variable 'incident pit' situations that test the quality of decision-making. Relying on apparently objective tests and assessments can produce false reassurance: people may be more impaired cognitively than we suppose. When decisions do have to be made it is mandatory to have a clear appreciation of their limits and not to give a simplistic notion of individual autonomy too much emphasis. The person actually before us, as opposed to the person who made the ACP, also has some say.

Fluidity

A key practical consideration is a sense of the fluidity and contingency of the situations that ACP tries to deal with. Like evolution, ACP must recognize that where someone is, may neither be where she would want to be, nor where she may end up when that ACP is enacted. Those assisting with ACP must pay substantial attention to this fluidity and contingency. A plan may seem wholly reasonable and accurately reflective of the wishes of that person when it is made, but may become a burdensome impediment in the unknowable and contingent future.

Time matters

How settled is a person's wish, how transient is the plan or desire expressed? Evidence about interpreting expressed desire for death shows how an apparently settled wish may be a reaction to a particular moment or symptom that can change once the moment has passed (22). Decisions need to be taken within a realistic timescale but with an awareness of potential transience. End of life decisions rarely need to be taken quickly. Even with cardiopulmonary resuscitation (CPR) it is important to avoid a false notion of choice. It can be presented and dealt with in ACP as a real choice—switch the person back on or not? In reality the chances of 'success' in CPR with deranged metabolism approach zero (12). What seems like a real choice may in reality be no choice at all, and the process of choosing whether to opt for CPR in ACP might prove a distressing and point-less charade. For people with capacity they always have the ability to review, amend, or withdraw any preference or decision. The appetite for ACP in people near the end of life may sometimes be less than is sometimes supposed. Some elderly people become resistant to the idea of discussing planning for serious illness wishing to take things 'one day at a time' (23). Whose agenda is being met if such discussions are insisted upon, at particular times and are used as the sole quality markers of EOL care?

Capacity: broader understanding about decision making

Capacity can vary over time. People change too and the decisions they encounter and the influ-ences that affect judgement also vary. The person's beliefs and behaviours may be greatly influ-enced by many factors and at different points of their life or illness including by their symptoms or the needs of people close to them such as their family. We need to think more broadly, 'Whose capacity are we considering?' Is it the person before the illness, the one early on in her illness, later on, or at the very end?

Legislation

The MCA is clear about its own scope, tests of capacity, assessments for best interest and the valid-ity of an ADRT. The MCA and the broader aspects of law must underpin any discussion around the care of a person to ensure that the correct interpretation of ACP is made, especially which components are legally binding. A mismatch of statements and actions can be central to under-standing whether the ACP is still valid in more than just legal terms. A person may have wished to have all steps taken to prolong their life under all circumstances and said so in an ACP. In the uncharted waters of their deterioration a constant plucking at or attempts to remove a feeding tube might be more than physical irritation with the device itself. Such actions may represent a real clue to the unknowable working of the mind now inaccessible. Looking for internal consist-ency of statements and actions is important. Finally in any difficulty or dispute over a best interest decision, there are ample mechanisms for arbitration and ultimately the wisdom of the Court.

Conclusion

The process of drawing up and discussing Advance Care Plans is valuable beyond price and for no other reason than to help people reflect on and prepare for the end of their life. However, it is not out of autonomy, but our parental duties to that future self. Thought, care, love, and honesty can be given a framework and some future-proofing provided that continuing conversations can occur and there are regular reviews such that the ACP is as proximate and connected to the future person as possible. But no piece of paper can hold that subtlety and emotion without a risk, a considerable risk, of disempowering and diminishing a person's true evolving and contingent wishes. However, the shadow of economics is growing long and feeling cold. It is the risk that documents can be used wrongly as a utility or proxy for good care at the end of life, or their existence even made a criterion for receiving services, that has the capacity to transform ACP in the wrong hands into a howling wilderness.

References

1 Higginson I and Sen-Gupta G (2004). Place of care in advanced cancer. *Journal of Palliative Medicine*, **3**:287–300.

2 Grond S, et al. (1994) *Prevalence and pattern of symptoms in patients with cancer pain: a prospective evaluation of 1635 cancer patients referred to a pain clinic.* Journal of Pain & Symptom Management, **9**:372–82.

3 Irwin S, et al.(2008) *Unrecognised cognitive impairment in hospice patients: a pilot study. Palliative Medicine*, **22**:842–47.

4 Glaser B and Strauss A (1968). *Time for Dying* 270. Chicago: Aldine Publishing.

5 Laureys S and Boly M (2008). The changing spectrum of coma. *Nature Reviews Neurology*, **4**:544–546

6 Boly M, Coleman MR, Davis MH et al. (2007). When thoughts become action: An fMRI paradigm to study volitional brain activity in non-communicative brain injured patients *NeuroImage*, **36**(3):979–92

7 Munday D, Petrova M, and Dale J (2009). Exploring preferences for place of death with terminally ill patients: qualitative study of experiences of general practitioners, community nurses in England. *BMJ*, **338**:b2391.

8 Downie R and Calman K (1994). *Healthy Respect*. 2nd ed. Oxford: OUP.

9 Dworkin R (1993). *Life's Dominion*. London: Harper Collins.

10 Ikonomidis S and Singer P (1999). Autonomy, liberalism and advance care planning. *Journal of Medical Ethics*, **25**:522–7.

11 Fleck L (1981). *Genesis and Development of a Scientific Fact*. Chicago: The University of Chicago Press.

12 Bernheim (2008). COMA science group. Available from: www.comascience.org.

13 Chochinov HM, et al. (2002) Dignity in the terminally ill: a cross-sectional, cohort study.[comment]. *Lancet*, **360**(9350):2026–30.

14 Lethborg C Aranda S, and Kissane DW (2008). Meaning in Adjustment to Cancer: A Model of Care. *Palliative & Supportive Care*, **6**:61–70.

15 Maclean A (2006). Advance Decisions, Future selves and Decision-Making. *Medical Law Review*, **14**(3):291.

16 Parfit D (1986). *Reasons and Persons*. Oxford: OUP.

17 Sperry R (1984). Consciousness, Personal Identity and the Divided Brain. *Neuropsychologia*, **22**:661–73.

18 Bannerman L (2008). Baroness Warnock: Euthanasia abroad would mean a 'two-tier death service' *Times* 4 October.

19 Polkinghorne J (2003). Science and Theology in the Twenty-First Century. *Journal of Religion and Science*, **35**(4):941–53.

20 Hughes JC (2001). Views of the person with dementia. *Journal of Medical Ethics*, **27**(2):86.

21 Legal case: Lord Fraser in Gillick v. W. Norfolk and Wisbech AHA (1986) A.C. 112 at 170.

22 Chochinov HM et al. (1999). Will to live in the terminally ill.[comment]. *Lancet*, **354**(9181):816–819.

23 Carres J, et al. (2002). Planning for death but not serious future illness: qualitative study of housebound elderly patients. *BMJ*, **325**:125–27.

Section 2

Context in the UK

Chapter 7

Advance Care Planning for the end of life

Claire Henry and Sheila Joseph

All people approaching the end of life need to have their needs assessed and their wishes and preferences discussed and a agreed set of actions reflecting the choices they make about their care recorded in a case plan
Department of Health End of Life Care Strategy 2008

This chapter includes:

- Introduction and national context to the importance of Advance Care Planning (ACP) in the Department of Health End of Life Care Strategy in England
- Background publications which have highlighted the need for ACP
- Issues surrounding ACP
- Resources to support the process of ACP
- Practicalities of implementation
- Further developments
- Conclusion.

Key points

- Advance Care Planning is delivered as a process of discussion between an individual and their care provider, irrespective of discipline, with or without their carer/family involvement
- Outputs may include a statement of wishes and preferences, decisions to refuse treatment, and/or Lasting Power of Attorney
- Guidance from Health and Social Care Staff has been published
- Further work is underway in areas of education, communication, and information transfer.

Introduction

In England, as in other parts of the world, Advance Care Planning is becoming increasingly important as a means to improve care for all people nearing the end of life. The Department of Health End of Life Care Strategy (EoLC) was published in July 2008 and provides a comprehensive framework aimed at promoting high quality care for all adults approaching the end of life in all care settings within England (1).

Approximately half a million people die in England each year with most of those deaths (58%) occurring in NHS hospitals. Thirty five per cent of deaths are at home (including care homes), 4% in hospices, and 3% elsewhere. This contrasts greatly with the situation a century ago when most deaths occurred at home. As a result of these changes, society as a whole is less familiar with the events surrounding death and less open to discussions about death and dying.

One of the key aims of the EoLC Strategy is to ensure, as far as possible, that services meet the needs of people approaching the end of life. Of course, different individuals have different ideas about the parameters of a 'good death'; this may be based upon religious or spiritual beliefs, personal circumstances, family dynamics, or other factors. But for many the common factors in attaining a 'good death' have been found to be:

♦ Being treated as an individual, with dignity and respect

♦ Being without pain and other symptoms

♦ Being in familiar surroundings

♦ Being in the company of close friends and family.

Advance Care Planning is a key part of this process if needs and preferences are to be met. 'All people approaching the end of life need to have their needs assessed and their wishes and preferences discussed' (1). These will then be recorded so that every service involved in supporting the individual will be aware of their priorities; preferences and choices 'will be taken into account and accommodated wherever possible' (1).

The Strategy recommends Advance Care Planning as a helpful way to achieve this. For some the outcome may be a general statement of wishes and preferences about what is important to them about how they are cared for or where they wish to die. Others may wish to be more specific about future plans by taking the decision to make an advance decision to refuse treatment or refusal of resuscitation.

Background publications

In recent years a number of publications have identified the need for implementing an Advance Care Planning process for staff, patients and carers and the means by which it can be attained. Box 7.1 includes some of the most significant Department of Health policy publications in England in this area.

Box 7.1 Policy publications on ACP in England

2001   National Service Framework for Older People (7)
2003   *Building on the Best: Choice, responsiveness and equity in the NHS* (8)
2004   National Institute for Health and Clinical Excellence (NICE) Guidance: *Improving supportive and palliative care for adults with cancer* (9)
2005   *National Service Framework for Long Term Conditions* (10)
2005 and 2007   *Mental Capacity Act 2005 Code of Practice* (11)
2008   The NHS Next Stage Review: *High quality care for all* (12)

Led by Lord Darzi this emphasized giving people more control and influence over their health and healthcare that was personal to them. The Review also states that by 2010 everyone with a long-term condition will have a personalized care plan, agreed by the patient and a named professional, providing a basis for the NHS and its partners to organize services around the needs of individuals. Services should be organized around patients 'and not people around services'.

> ## Box 7.1 Policy publications on ACP in England *(continued)*
>
> 2009   National Audit Office *Report on End of Life Care* (13)
> This report on value for money within NHS expenditure on end of life care suggests that the wishes of people approaching the end of their life are not always made clear to those who need to know. Such data should be captured in the electronic summary care record, or other means, to document and share accurate patient information on preferences. This information should be regularly updated and shared with all providers across the health, social care, independent, and voluntary sectors who influence decisions about where and how patients receive care.

Issues surrounding Advance Care Planning

Definition

There was a requirement to clarify commonly used terms and agree definitions. This was achieved whilst undertaking a review of the ACP process which then led to the production of a guidance document by the NHS End of Life Care Programme *Advance Care Planning: A Guide for Health and Social Care Staff* (2007) (9). The final definition of ACP—together with other key issues such as an advance decision and statement of wishes and preferences—was agreed by a working party of clinicians and academics (Fig. 7.1).

It was emphasized that ACP is a process of discussion between an individual and their care provider and the process is more important than the specific tool used. Outputs include: a statement of wishes and preferences, an advance decision to refuse treatment (ADRT), and a named advocate or LPOA.

Barriers to implementation

There are, and will continue to be, a number of barriers facing clinicians and policy-makers wishing to implement ACP.

In particular it has to be borne in mind that although the aim of the ACP process is to support and implement people's wishes at the end of life, there may be circumstances that prevent this goal being achieved. For instance:

- People may not be given an appropriate opportunity to consider their best options, based on the best available information
- It may not be possible to have clear and open discussions between professionals and those receiving care
- There may be cultural barriers to free communication
- Professionals may not have the skills needed to initiate and complete the ACP process
- People's preferences and priorities may change as they approach death
- Although people may prefer to be cared for at home, they would want the assurance of high quality care and not to be a burden on their families and carers
- People who live on their own may actually prefer to die where they can be certain of not being alone.

Staff competences

Staff who assist with ACP will need to have core competences to ensure individuals and their families can be supported through the process in a timely and sensitive way. It is important that

Advance Care Planning

ACP is a process of discussion between an individual and their care providers. Irrespective of discipline. If the individual wishes, their family and friends may be included. With the individual's agreement, discussions should be:

• Documented
• Regularly reviewed
• Communcated to key persons involved in their care.

Examples of what an ACP discussion might include are:

• The individual's concerns
• Their important vaues or personal goals for care
• Their understanding about their illness and prognosis, as well as particular preferences for types of care or treatment that may be beneficial in the future and the availability of these.

The difference between ACP and care planning more generally is that the process of ACP will usually take place in the context of an anticipated deterioration in the individual's condition in the future, with attendant loss of capacity to make decisions and/or ability to communicate wishes to others.

Statement of wishes and references

This is a summary term embracing a range of written and/or recorded oral expressions, by which people can, if they wish, write down or tell people about their wishes or preferences in relation to future treatment and care, or explain their feelings, beliefs and values that govern how they make decisions. They may cover medical and non-medical matters. They are not legally binding.

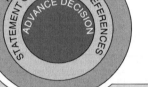

Advance decision

An advance decision must relate to a specific refusal of medical treatment and can specify circumstances. It will only come into effect when the individual has lost capacity to give or refuse consent.

Careful assessment of the validity and applicability of an advance decision is essential before it is used in clinical practice. Valid advance decisions, which are refusals of treatment, are legally binding.

Lasting Power of Attorney

A Lasting Power of Attorney (LPA) is a new statutory form of power of attorney created by the MCA (2005). Anyone who has the capacity to do so may choose a person (an 'attorney') to take decisions on their behalf if they subsequently lose capacity.

Fig. 7.1 Advance Care Planning: a guide to health and social care staff, 2007.

health and social care professionals recognize their own levels of skill in this area as well as their limitations.

The following competences have been identified by the ACP guide development group:

◆ Awareness of the context in which ACP may be appropriate

◆ Awareness of ACP

◆ Awareness of advance decisions to refuse treatment and relevant guidance

◆ Good communication skills

- Informed consent and the ability to provide sufficient relevant information
- Awareness of legal and ethical issues—Mental Capacity Act 2005, Code of Practice
- Technical skills and knowledge
- Good relationship building
- Knowledge of local resources

Resources to support Advance Care Planning

The National End of Life Care Programme in England has been instrumental in developing a number of resources in response to some of the challenges discussed. They include material for staff, individuals and their carers.

Resources for health and social care staff

Advance Care Planning: A Guide for Health and Social Care Staff 2007 (revised 2008) (9,10)

The Advance Care Planning Guide was initially developed as part of the three year (2004-2007) End of Life Care Programme. The aim of the original 2007 document was to clarify the definition of ACP and related terms and to provide guidance on core competences, education, and training. A revised version in 2008 also took into account the implementation of the Mental Capacity Act 2005, and the Mental Capacity Act 2005 Code of Practice, published in October 2007 (6). See also *www.opsi.gov.uk/acts/acts2005/20050009.htm*

Some of the key learning within the guidance relates to documentation, the timing and context for ACP, and the principles of the process (see Chapter 8).

National End of Life Care Programme website: Advance Care Planning section

The National End of Life Care Programme has expanded the ACP section of its website to help provide the additional support and information that professionals require.

The aim of the site is to provide an overview of guidance related to ACP with special reference to the Mental Capacity Act 2005, identify different aspects of ACP and sources to support professional practice and education, and provide a guide for discussion of ACP in clinical practice and supporting user education/information. See *http://www.endoflifecareforadults.nhs.uk/publications/pubacpguide*

Advance Decisions to Refuse Treatment: A Guide for Health and Social Care Staff 2008 (11)

Following the publication of the Mental Capacity Act 2005 Code of Practice, the Department of Health and Social Care Institute of Excellence commissioned additional guidance on section 9 of the code which relates to advance decisions to refuse treatment.

The legislative framework for advance decisions to refuse treatment is complex. This guide, produced by the National End of Life Care Programme in conjunction with the National Council for Palliative Care, is intended to clarify the law for professionals and offer additional practical information to enable them to support anyone who chooses to consider making an advance decision to refuse treatment—regardless of their age (over 18 years old), race, faith, gender, sexual orientation, gender identity, disability, or preferences.

The guide contains the full text of section 9 of the Code of Practice, dealing with advance decisions to refuse treatment, together with additional commentary and relevant information. It also refers to other sections of the Code of Practice as well as identifying additional links and resources (see Chapter 9).

Resources for individuals and their carers

Planning for Your Future Care - A Guide (12)

This patient information booklet has been developed by the National End of Life Care Programme in conjunction with other stakeholders to provide a simple explanation of the process of ACP and the options open to individuals should they choose to discuss their wishes and preferences. It may also help as a tool for professionals to use when taking the first steps in initiating a discussion.

The booklet defines ACP as 'a process of discussion between you and those who provide care for you, for example your nurses, doctors, care home manager or family members. During this discussion you may choose to express some views, preferences and wishes about your future care.'

From the individual's point of view some of the key elements of this process are:

+ Opening the conversation
+ Exploring your options
+ Identifying your wishes and preferences
+ Refusing specific treatment, if you wish to
+ Asking someone to speak for you
+ Appointing someone to make decisions for you using a Lasting Power of Attorney
+ Letting people know your wishes.

The National End of Life Care Programme and the NCPC has also produced a downloadable patient information leaflet based upon earlier work from Mid Trent (*Advance Decisions to Refuse Treatment: A Guide for Patients* (13) written in question and answer format in an attempt to address some of the queries patients may have if they want to take the ACP process to the stage of making an advance decision.

Practicalities of implementation

How can staff use this guidance to ensure they are enabling patients to make the best possible decisions at the end of their life?

There is no set format for recording an ACP discussion, although having an individual's wishes documented will prove helpful to those involved in their care. Professionals involved in supporting someone who wishes to discuss ACP should avoid using a prescriptive method of interview and recording.

ACP may be instigated at any time by either an individual or a care provider but may be most appropriate at certain key points in the individual's life. A care provider may initiate the discussion following a 'cue' given by the individual, such as an expression of worry about the future. Whatever the trigger, the professional leading the discussion will need to follow some basic principles and have the appropriate skills to take the discussion forward.

Timing/context

There can be many events that might trigger the beginning of this process. These could include:

+ A life-changing event such as the death of spouse or close friend or relative
+ Following a new diagnosis of a life-limiting condition
+ During assessment of the individual's need
+ Multiple hospital admissions
+ Following admission to a care home

Principles/process

It is important to remember that this is a voluntary process. No pressure should be brought to bear. In addition the content of any discussion should be determined by the individual concerned.

All health and social care professionals should be open to any discussion which may be instigated by an individual and know how to respond to their questions. They should only instigate the discussion if they have made a professional judgment that the ACP process is likely to benefit the individual's care.

Discussion should focus on the views of the individual although they may wish to invite their carer or another close family member or friend to participate. Some families are likely to have discussed preferences and would welcome an approach to share this discussion. Confidentiality should always be respected.

It should also be borne in mind that ACP requires that the individual has the capacity to understand, discuss options available, and agree to what is then planned. Health and social care professionals should also be aware of, and give a realistic account of, the support, services, and choices available in the particular circumstances.

Should an individual wish to make a decision to refuse treatment (advance decision) this should be documented according to the requirements of the MCA 2005.

Finally, professionals need to be aware when they have reached the limits of their knowledge and competence and know when to seek advice.

Case study: trigger point for an ACP discussion

Mr James is seriously ill in hospital and approaching the end of his life. His illness means that he drifts in and out of consciousness but when conscious he is still able to be quite coherent.

On one occasion when Mr James was unconscious his daughter asked those caring for him to arrange for her to become his representative as his Personal Welfare Power of Attorney and manage his financial affairs. Those caring for Mr James are concerned and unsure what to do, so they seek the advice of a colleague who has received training in the Mental Capacity Act Code of Practice. The advice is that Mr James' opinion should be sought at a time when he is conscious and has the capacity to make decisions for himself. A Personal Welfare Lasting Power of Attorney can only be created by someone who has the mental capacity to do so and cannot be made on their behalf should they lose mental capacity.

When asked, Mr James, for personal reasons, did not want his daughter to act as his representative so he was encouraged to have this recorded in his notes.

Case study: exploring options

Mrs Smith lives with her daughter, son-in-law, and two young grandchildren. She knows she is approaching the end of her life and would like very much to remain in her home. Despite this she feels that she must go into a nursing home before she reaches the final stages of her life in order to save her family any extra work or upset. She is particularly concerned about the effect that dying at home would have on her grandchildren. The idea of making arrangements to go into a nursing home is causing her a great deal of worry.

Mrs Smith has not told her family her wishes so she does not know how they feel about the possibility of looking after her. She has not asked her doctor what support is locally available to help her stay in her own home, what support there is for the children, or if there are any alternatives to a nursing home available to her.

This is an appropriate time for her to have an Advance Care Planning discussion with the health or social care professionals. Finding out all the options available to her and then discussing them openly with her family may help Mrs Smith make her plans and put her mind at rest.

Future developments

NHS end of life care quality markers

In response to a request for the development of unified quality standards in end of life care, including some of reference to this discussion (see Box 7.2) the Department of Health, with input from the Strategic Health Authority pathway chairs, developed quality markers for end of life care in all settings.

The common assessment framework for adults

This is a generic approach to assessing the health and social care needs of individual adults. This will aim to support improved coordination and information sharing around multidisciplinary assessment and care planning.

Core competences

A large number of health and social care staff working across all settings have at least some role in the delivery of care to people at the end of their life. But all will require the necessary knowledge, skills, and attitudes if they are to play their parts effectively.

Skills for Care and Skills for Health have been working collaboratively to define the core principles and competences required by each staff group. The four areas of development are: training in communication skills, assessment of a person's needs and preferences, ACP, and symptom management.

E-learning

The e-Learning for Healthcare (eLFH) project was launched in January 2009. The aim is to develop 60 hours of learning materials based on the four common requirements identified for

---

Box 7.2 Advance Care Planning and the DH quality markers in end of life care

QM 1.37 All providers have processes in place to identify the development needs of all other workers (registered and unregistered, including volunteers) across health and social care who require end of life care related training. They should take into account the four core common requirements for workforce development (communication skills, assessment and care planning, ACP, and symptom management) as they apply to end of life care.

QM 2.2 All GP practices to demonstrate:

They have mechanisms in place to assess and document the needs of those approaching the end of life (e.g. use of the Gold Standards Framework or equivalent) and to discuss, record, and (where appropriate) communicate the wishes and preferences of those approaching the end of life (ACP).

QM 3.5 All acute hospital providers to demonstrate:

That they have mechanisms in place to discuss, record, and (where appropriate) communicate the wishes and preferences of those approaching the end of life (ACP).

QM 5.2 All care homes to demonstrate:

That they have mechanisms in place to discuss, record, and (where appropriate) communicate the wishes and preferences of those approaching the end of life (ACP).

workforce development and will support the Core Competences Project with a specific module developed in ACP. All NHS staff as well as social care staff and those working in care homes and hospices will have access to this learning where appropriate. Given the large number of staff involved, this will be a key element in the delivery of training.

Conclusion

There are now real opportunities and resources to address the fundamental issues in the planning for future care by, with, and for patients, and to involve and integrate with agencies working on similar issues. This will involve learning from the experience of others and taking positive steps to monitor and evaluate outcomes.

This is a complex challenge for communities and societies requiring the active involvement of the real people at the heart of the care services: the public, patients, carers, and health and social care professionals. In particular there must be an active promotion of choice, access, and real benefit from services to those who have been, or are at risk of discrimination, including vulnerable people with mental health and learning disabilities.

Further research on ACP is also needed, both to evaluate the effect of ACP discussions with individuals and the outcomes these discussions/planned interventions may have on future care or treatment. We also need to know how well integrated ACP has become in health and social care professionals' education, training, and core competences.

Further resources

Department of Health (October 2007). *Single Assessment Process*, DH, London.

Department of Health (October 2007). *Treating Older People as Individuals*, DH, London.

Department of Health (2009). Care Service Improvement Partnership. *Common Assessment Framework for Adults*, DH, London.

For further information on the National End of Life Care Programme see also www.endoflifecareforadults.nhs.uk/eolc/eolcpub.htm

For further information on the Mental Capacity Act 2005 Code of Practice see also www.opsi.gov.uk/acts/acts2005/20050009.htm

References

1 Department of Health (July 2008). *End of Life Care Strategy: promoting high quality care for all adults at the end of life*, DH, London.

2 Department of Health (May 2001). *National Service Framework for Older People*, DH, London.

3 Department of Health (December 2003). *Building on the Best: choice, responsiveness and equity in the NHS*, DH, London.

4 National Institute for Health Clinical Excellence (March 2004). *Supportive and Palliative Care Guidance*, NICE, London.

5 Department of Health (2005). *National Service Framework for long term conditions*, DH, London.

6 Ministry of Justice (April 2007). *Mental Capacity Act 2005 Code of Practice*, London.

7 Department of Health (June 2008). *High Quality Care for All - Next Stage Review*, DH, London.

8 National Audit Office (November 2008). *End of Life Care*, **National Audit Office**, London.

9 NHS National End of Life Care Programme (February 2007). *Advance Care Planning: A Guide for Health and Social Care Staff*, London.

10 NHS National End of Life Care Programme (revised 2008). *Advance Care Planning: A Guide for Health and Social Care Staff*, London.

11 NHS National End of Life Care Programme & National Council for Palliative Care (September 2008). *Advance Decisions to Refuse Treatment: A Guide for Health and Social Care Staff*, London.

12 NHS National End of Life Care Programme (March 2009). *Planning for Your Future Care – A Guide*, London.

13 NHS National End of Life Care Programme (February 2009). *Advance Decisions to Refuse Treatment: A Guide for Patients*, London.

Chapter 8

The implications of the Mental Capacity Act (MCA) 2005 for Advance Care Planning and decision making

Simon Chapman and Andrew Makin

This chapter includes:

- ◆ An overview of the MCA's impact on end of life care
- ◆ Setting the MCA in the current context of policy and practice
- ◆ How the MCA can
  - be used to improve care
  - enable people to express and protect choices
  - empower and enable the professional and/or the proxy decision maker
- ◆ An introduction and explanation of the role of the IMCA and how it might apply to Advance Care Planning (ACP) and End of Life decision making
- ◆ An explanation of the legal and ethical process involved in reaching best interest decisions, especially for potentially vulnerable people in care homes and other settings.

Key Points

- ◆ Planning ahead: using Advance Care Planning to identify and protect their preferences and choices should they lose capacity in the future
- ◆ Assessing a person's capacity to make decisions (including making Advance Care Plans)
- ◆ Implementing Advance Care Planning: making decisions on behalf of someone who lacks capacity
- ◆ The IMCA is a new provision in English law with a specific role and statutory rights
- ◆ IMCAs are not decisions makers but ensure the correct process has been followed for a decision to be reached in the best interests of the person who lacks capacity
- ◆ There are areas to be tested in case law especially in the interpretation of Serious Medical Treatment that will clarify the role and requirement to involve an IMCA
- ◆ Advance Care Plans which include expressions of preferences and wishes (including treatment decisions) will greatly help both the decision maker and IMCA arrive at reasonable conclusions about what is in the person's best interest.

Summary

The Mental Capacity Act (MCA) 2005, which applies in England and Wales, but not Scotland or Northern Ireland, provides the statutory framework within which Advance Care Planning must be used.

This legislative context is important. It means that ACP is not simply a practice option, that organizations or professionals can provide if they choose to do so. Instead, people can make Advance Care Plans as of right and professionals must respond to them appropriately. The MCA provides a supportive framework within which adults can express and protect their choices and preferences about their future care, should they lose capacity to make their own decisions.

On 16 July 2008, the morning of the launch of the End of Life Care Strategy in England, the then Secretary of State for Health, Alan Johnson, was interviewed on BBC Radio 4's *Today* programme and said:

> 'The most important objective is to ensure that people's individual needs, their priorities, their preferences for end of life care are identified, they are documented, they are reviewed, they are respected and acted upon wherever possible. Now that message has to go out everywhere within the NHS and I think that's the important starting point for everything else . . .'

Subject to the additional proviso that this message should not be confined to the NHS but to health and social care services in all sectors, this was a very clear affirmation of the importance of both care planning and ACP in improving end of life care.

The End of Life Care Strategy lays great emphasis on introducing ACP. The Mental Capacity Act is therefore a vital legislative support for that policy goal.

Background

The impact of the Mental Capacity Act

The impact of the Mental Capacity Act on ACP and end of life care can be seen from this list of some of the issues that it covers:

+ Statutory check-lists:
    * to assess people's capacity
    * to determine their best interests
+ An underlying duty to take all practicable steps to support people so that they can make their own decisions
+ There is an emphasis throughout on person-centred care
+ Duty to consult relatives and carers about a person's best interests
+ People's preferences and choices about their future care must be taken into account when they lose capacity
+ Advance decisions to refuse treatment
+ There are new types of proxy decision-making and advocacy: lasting powers of attorney and independent mental capacity advocates
+ It is accompanied by a new Code of Practice to which paid carers must have regard
+ There are two new criminal offences: wilful neglect and ill-treatment
+ There is new administrative and judicial architecture: a new Office of the Public Guardian and Court of Protection.

The MCA is increasingly understood and implemented and is now beginning to have a significant impact on health and social care. It has a very broad range: it covers every decision made by or on behalf of people with impaired mental capacity, including financial decisions about property or investments, decisions about place of care, day-to-day living, and decisions about medical treatment.

Anecdotal evidence suggests that the MCA is better understood in some settings and areas of practice than others. Concern is sometimes expressed about the extent to which it has been incorporated into some acute hospital settings.

Planning ahead: using ACP to identify and protect their preferences and choices should they lose capacity in the future

There are a number of ways that a person with capacity can use MCA provisions to identify and in some cases protect their choices about their future care and treatment, should they lose capacity to decide for themselves:

- They can nominate people whom they would like to be consulted when decisions are being made

- They can identify people whom they would not wish to be consulted

- They can make statements about their preferences and choices to inform and assist people who may later have to make decisions about their care or treatment. These statements must be taken into account when best interest decisions are made in relation to them

- They can appoint another person (or more than one person) to consent to or refuse treatment on their behalf, by giving a Personal Welfare Lasting Power of Attorney

- They can identify specific treatment(s) that they wish to refuse, and any circumstances in which they want that to apply—an advance decision to refuse treatment (ADRT).

A person may do one of these, or any, or all of them in combination. Together they create what is in effect a statutory toolkit for ACP, which an adult with capacity can use at any time of their life (2). Those who subsequently provide care and treatment to them will need to respond appropriately and in accordance with the MCA.

Some people will do some of these things before they ever become ill. For others, the experience of living with a life-threatening condition may lead them to ask what they can do to control or influence their future care. In all cases it is important for them and everybody concerned to remember that people's wishes and preferences change over time and that any Advance Care Plans they have made should be kept under review. Both they and anybody providing care to them should revisit any Advance Care Plans that have been made on a regular basis.

This section of the chapter considers what people need to do to use ACP in anticipation that they might lose capacity, and the factors they should keep in mind. It is written with their perspective foremost. The later section, on implementing people's Advance Care Plans, considers how others should respond to those Advance Care Plans, once the person who made them has lost capacity to make a particular decision.

Nominating people to be consulted

Under the MCA it is possible for people to nominate others who should be consulted about their best interests, should they lose capacity at a later stage. Those nominees must be consulted if practicable to do so. They will not be decision-makers, and this is not the same as creating a proxy decision-maker under a Lasting Power of Attorney (see below). Equally, it is possible to identify people who should not be consulted. One example of this might be a close family member, who in ordinary circumstances might expect to be consulted, but whom the person believes that, for whatever reason, they would not be able to give reliable insights into the person's best interests.

Making statements about preferences and choices

This is the area in which the relationship between legislation (the MCA) and practice (ACP) is most apparent.

The MCA states that a person's wishes, feelings, beliefs and values, including any written statement that they made whilst they had capacity, must be taken into account when assessing their best interests if they have lost capacity to make a particular decision (3). Compare that with what is included in the following definition of ACP(author's emphasis added):

An ACP discussion might include:

+ the individual's **concerns**
+ their important **values** or **personal goals** for care
+ their understanding about their illness and prognosis
+ their **preferences** for types of care or treatment that may be beneficial in the future and the availability of these (4).

So a person can make an Advance Care Plan which includes statements about their choices and preferences, in the knowledge that such statements must be taken into account by anyone who makes a decision about their care or treatment should they lose capacity. Unless they amount to an advance decision to refuse treatment, these statements will not be legally binding. However the person who makes a decision must take them into account and, if they do not follow them, be prepared to explain why not if challenged. This is powerful legislative support for ACP.

The MCA refers in particular to written statements about people's preferences. That is not to say that verbal statements are not valid; they may be very powerful. However it is always wise for people to record their wishes in writing. If they make verbal statements to professional care providers they should be recorded in people's notes.

The Preferred Priorities for Care Plan has been developed to help professional carers work with people to make Advance Care Plans (5).

Lasting Power of Attorney

The change from Enduring Powers of Attorney (EPAs) to Lasting Powers of Attorney (LPAs) is one of the most significant aspects of the MCA. It had always been possible to appoint a proxy to make decisions about your property and affairs using an EPA. The LPA extends that so that it is now possible to appoint people to make decisions about personal welfare, which includes your health and social care. At present more property and affairs LPAs are being registered than personal welfare LPAs (6). As a result many health and social care professionals have not encountered a personal welfare LPA. However it is likely that their usage will increase.

A Lasting Power of Attorney is a type of agency arrangement. It is formal. Attorneys can only be appointed by using a prescribed form, which can be downloaded via the Office of the Public Guardian website (7). The LPA form must be registered before it takes effect, and a fee is payable (8).

There is some flexibility. An individual can appoint more than one person as an attorney, and can appoint different attorneys to make different kinds of decision. People should only give LPAs to people that they trust. They should not be placed under any pressure to give anybody a Lasting Power of Attorney.

Anyone deciding to create an LPA, would be well-advised to discuss their wishes with the person to whom they have given the LPA (the 'donee'), to tell them what they would want to happen. This might include making a written statement about their preferences. Like any other decision-maker, the donee will be required to make decisions in the best interests of the person who gave them the LPA ('the donor'), and this will include taking into account any statements the donor made whilst they had capacity. Lasting Powers of Attorney are governed by sections 9–14 of the MCA. Further information about LPAs can also be found in Chapter 7 of the Code of Practice.

Advance decisions to refuse treatment (9)

More information about advance decisions to refuse treatment can be found in Chapter 9. The information in this chapter is intended to describe how advance decisions to refuse treatment fit into the overall range of options available to a person who wishes to do ACP. Of the many important things to understand about advance decisions, the first is that this area of law applies only to decisions to refuse treatment. It does not apply to requests, and it does not apply to non-treatment decisions. People can of course make Advance Care Plans which include requests and which cover issues other than their treatment, for example about their place of care. However, whilst such preferences must always be taken into account, they will not legally binding in the same way that an advance decision to refuse treatment can be.

Relationship between Lasting Powers of Attorney and advance decisions

It is possible both to give an LPA to somebody and to make an advance decision to refuse a specific treatment. If a person does both, the rule is that the one done later is the one that counts. So, if a person gives an LPA to a relative and subsequently makes an advance decision, the advance decision should be followed.

Offering and recording Advance Care Planning: professionals

Advance Care Planning is a right that people can exercise if they want to. However it is voluntary. For some it will be a valuable reassurance to know that their preferences and choices have been recorded and will be used in decision-making about their care should they lose capacity. Others may find it difficult or distressing to consider their future. People should be offered the opportunity to make Advance Care Plans if they wish to, but they should not be compelled to make them.

Health and care professionals will need training in ACP and communication appropriate to their level. Those whose role it is to offer ACP and open discussion about it will need training in how to do that and in the way that any tools, such as the Preferred Priorities for Care documentation, should be used. It should be remembered that some members of staff, such as care assistants, may spend considerable time with a person. The insights and information they gain from conversations with people for whom they are caring may provide very valuable assistance and evidence when it comes to assessing those people's best interests. Their line managers and employers should recognize the potential for this, and support all their staff so that they can contribute to care and decision-making and be ready to record and report significant conversations.

Implementing Advance Care Planning: making decisions on behalf of someone who lacks capacity

Capacity

The starting point is assessing the person's capacity. If a person has capacity to make a decision, they should be enabled to make that decision. Advance Care Plans should only be considered when the person is assessed as not having capacity to make a particular decision, even with support. The MCA contains a statutory framework for the assessment of a person's capacity (10).

Mental Capacity, the key points:

◆ A person's capacity should be assessed on a decision by decision basis

◆ A person's capacity must not be assessed merely by reference to the person's age, appearance, condition, or aspect of their behaviour

◆ There is then a two-stage test:

  • Diagnostic: there must be an impairment or disturbance of the mind or brain

  • Functional: there must be impaired understanding, judgement, memory, or ability to communicate which amounts to incapacity

◆ A person must be supported so that they can make their own decisions so far as possible.

Decision by decision basis

A person's capacity should not be assessed on a blanket basis so that they are regarded as either having capacity or not (unless they are unconscious, or close to it, or locked-in). Instead, capacity must be assessed on a decision-by-decision basis.

Decisions range enormously in terms of importance and complexity. A person might have the capacity, with support, to make a range of simple decisions which together would have a significant impact on their daily experience of care. For example a care home resident may be able to decide the following: what to wear; what to eat; where to sit; who to talk with; whether to read, watch television, or go outside. They might not be able to make complicated financial decisions about investments.

Maximizing capacity

This is covered in detail in other chapters. If the decision does not need to be made immediately or in an emergency all reasonable attempts must be made to maximize capacity, for example treat any reversible medical problem or find and provide specialist communication assistance. This might mean new ways of working, organizing ward routine, staffing differently, or learning new methods of communication. There is a duty to support people to make their own decisions, which will mean that anybody who has assessed that a person is unable to make a decision will need to be able to show that they took all practicable steps to support that person, if challenged about it.

Person-centred assessment: capacity and best interests

The MCA's provisions about assessing both capacity and best interests contain the same prohibition against assessing a person simply by reference to their age, appearance, condition, or any aspect of their behaviour which may lead to the making of unjustified assumptions about them. These are often summed up as 'do not discriminate', and are in the same line as other rights-based legislation; in the care context they emphasize the importance of being person-centred and carefully assessing the individual.

Legal obligation to act in best interests

If, even with support, the person is assessed as lacking capacity to make a particular decision, then any Advance Care Plans must be considered. In summary this will mean:

◆ If it is a decision about treatment, assessing whether there is a legally-binding advance decision to refuse treatment

◆ In the absence of that, making a decision in the person's best interests.

The MCA sets out a statutory check-list about what must be taken into account when assessing a person's best interests. This will include any Advance Care Plans they made which contain evidence about what they wanted to happen, or not. There is also a duty, where practicable, to consult anybody who is a carer for that person or interested in their welfare, about what their views are about the person's best interests. This will almost always include family members.

Who is the decision-maker?

This is a vital question, and there is potential for considerable misunderstanding, distress, and conflict where this is not clearly addressed. In particular, there is a risk that relatives will carry the burden of making best interests decisions which are not theirs to make, albeit that they should be consulted about them.

Where there is no proxy decision-maker

Although it is expressed in convoluted language, the result of section 5 of the MCA is that the person who is responsible for the decision is the person who implements it. Section 5 states that a person (D) can do an act in relation to the care or treatment of another person (P) if D reasonably believes both that P did not have capacity to make the decision and that the act was in P's best interests. So for example, where a decision has to be made about the withdrawal of medical treatment at the end of life, the decision-maker is the doctor who withdraws the treatment. However, family members must also be consulted if that is practicable.

Where there is a proxy decision-maker

Where there is a proxy decision-maker either under a Lasting Power of Attorney or because the court has appointed a deputy, that person is responsible for making the decision. They must still follow best interests and consult family members and those close to the person where practicable.

Decisions can be challenged if it is felt they cannot be justified by reference to the person's best interests, using the factors identified in the MCA (section 4).

Decisions by health and social care professionals

In cases where clinical decisions need taken urgently for a person who lacks capacity it is the senior clinicians responsibility to ensure correct treatment and care is delivered. This might include reversing any cause of incapacity and stabilizing the patient's condition so that the patient can recover, regain capacity, and then make their own decision. The law makes provision for clinicians to take decisions especially where there is reasonable doubt e.g. the existence, validity, and applicability of an advance decision to refuse treatment. It is important to also understand that there might be decisions that relate to urgent and important social care issues e.g. the safeguarding of a vulnerable adult (who lacks capacity). There are formal mechanisms in England and Wales to achieve this by a partnership agreement with Health, Social Care, and the Local Authority. This is important especially if the vulnerable person requires admission to a care home. The same principles and statutory requirements of the MCA must apply to any decision to protect and offer care to such a person.

Independent Mental Capacity Advocates (IMCAs)

IMCAs are not decision makers. They are required to be involved in specific decisions for people without capacity and who are unbefriended. See later in this chapter.

Criminal offences

The MCA introduces the two new criminal offences of wilful neglect and ill-treatment of people lacking capacity. 'Neglect' and 'ill-treatment' are not defined. The Courts will have to decide what level of neglect or ill-treatment is so serious that there should be a criminal sanction. For example, how long can a person be left unchanged in soiled clothes and bed-clothes before that mounts to wilful neglect? At what point does shouting by an exhausted carer trying to feed a person with dementia become ill-treatment?

The reverse litigation risk

One significant, but as yet untested, potential of the Mental Capacity Act to support ACP is that it creates what can be called a 'reverse litigation risk'. The best way to illustrate this is by an example.

A frequently-reported scenario is that in which a care home resident has expressed the wish to die peacefully in the care home, but that an out of hours GP without direct experience of caring for that person calls an ambulance and insists on them being taken to hospital, relying on concepts of defensive medicine and avoiding a perceived risk of litigation. However, where the resident had left a well-documented wish to die in the care home it should be possible for the care home staff to challenge that decision on the basis that the resident's best interests should be informed by their previously expressed wish that they wanted to die in the care home not in hospital. The GP would have to justify the decision to transfer the resident to hospital on a best interests basis, and could face subsequent complaint or challenge if unable to do so.

In other words, there is a reverse side to the traditional 'defensive' decision to admit to hospital—a new litigation risk of failing to take account of an Advance Care Plan. This point is made not to raise the spectre of countless litigation risks, but to emphasize that the better course is not to practise defensively and admit to hospital, but to focus on assessing the individual and deciding where their best interests lie.

Introduction to Independent Mental Capacity Advocacy (IMCA)

The Mental Capacity Act (MCA) 2005 supported by the Code of Practice in 2007 included new roles for those supporting people who lack capacity to make decisions for themselves: the Court Appointed Deputy (CAD), the Lasting Power of Attorney (LPA) which replaced the Enduring Power of Attorney, and the Independent Mental Capacity Advocate (IMCA). The Act also defines the role of the decision maker who will make these decisions. In practice of course it is often a multi-disciplinary team, but one individual is designated as having the responsibility to decide what is in that person's best interest. This decision can be, and often is, part of some form of an Advance Care Plan.

Five Statutory (MCA) principles which must be exhibited in every decision:

1 A person is assumed to have capacity unless it is demonstrated that they lack capacity

2 A person is not to be counted as unable to make a decision until all reasonable steps have been taken to help him make a decision

3 A person is not to be treated as unable to make a decision merely because he makes an unwise decision

4 All decisions made on a person's behalf must be made in their best interest

5 When considering the decision or act to be done, the decision maker must look for the least restrictive way of carrying out that decision or act.

Whilst the LPA and the CAD can have a wide range of powers, depending on what the donee (the individual who has since lost capacity) or the Court has granted, there are specific conditions under which an IMCA may be involved, and others in which involvement is optional:

◆ demonstrably lack capacity to make a particular decision at the time it needs to be made.

◆ be in the words of the Act 'unbefriended', i.e. have no-one to consult on their behalf such as a spouse or close family member. The exceptions to the 'unbefriended' rule are explained later in this chapter.

There are two kinds of decision where the involvement of an IMCA is mandatory. Either there is a proposal to place the individual in a place of long term care—for 28 days or more in an NHS establishment; for 56 days or more in a private care setting—or there must be a proposal to carry out Serious Medical Treatment (SMT). Serious medical treatment also includes withholding and withdrawing treatment, which we look at more closely later.

In April 2009 a further requirement was added: that an IMCA be instructed where Deprivation of Liberty issues are being considered. This is unlikely to be a factor in ACP decisions, but even where deprivation of liberty is part of the scenario it is legally a separate issue. The authorization to deprive a person of their liberty for the purposes of treatment does not authorize that treatment, and treatment plans will be made separately.

In two further areas of decision making there is the option, as opposed to the requirement, for the decision maker to instruct an IMCA. These are for safeguarding procedures, and for care reviews. For safeguarding only, the absence or presence of a friend, a spouse, or anyone else, is immaterial if the decision maker wishes to instruct an IMCA. In addition, for any decision the decision maker can disregard family or close friends if they are thought to be 'inappropriate to consult'. This cannot be because the decision maker disagrees with that person or persons: there has to be a good reason such as that person having an ulterior motive, perhaps a financial interest in the client. The family member might have mental health needs themselves, live in another country, or have fallen out with the client. In such circumstances the decision maker can and should instruct an IMCA.

When considering ACP one can see how safeguarding issues might collide with decisions to withdraw treatment, especially if there are conflicting family views over the matter. The Act also introduced the specific criminal offence of abuse by neglect, and if there is a perceived difficulty the decision maker could reasonably ask an IMCA to provide an independent point of view.

ACP decisions made by proxy—a decision maker—are likely to be in an institutional setting. There are many people who have advanced conditions like dementia who will have an extensive loss of capacity and are also unbefriended, who will be receiving ongoing support either in an NHS institution or more likely a care home. It is these people who are likely to become vulnerable and to have complex health and social care needs, including those related to the end of life. It is for these reasons this chapter will emphasize this particular aspect.

Specific decisions require specific decision makers

In the absence of capacity or a nominated proxy with appropriate delegated authority, medical treatment decisions will be taken by the clinical team, for example a surgeon with the multidisciplinary team will decide if an operation should be undertaken. This decision will be informed by a best interest assessment that might include discussion with an IMCA where appropriate. For other decisions, e.g. the change of accommodation from hospital to a care home, the decision maker would probably be a social care manager. Rarely, there might be a move to a higher level facility for symptom management, which would be a clinical decision. The requirements for referral to an IMCA were described earlier.

The role of the IMCA and making the Mental Capacity Act work

Most people understand advocacy as a support to the individual, to encourage and help them in making their own decisions. The generic advocate is usually (though not invariably) instructed by the client. In some circumstances an advocate might help a person with a specific need/vulnerability to have some say in how their lives are run. This role is not obligatory, and not statutory. The IMCA role is statutory and obligatory in the circumstances described above, and the IMCA is instructed by the statutory sector (although anyone can make an initial referral to the service). The role is primarily to ascertain and put forward the individual's point of view, and secondarily to ensure that the Act is complied with. It is not an ongoing support; the IMCA will reach a conclusion about what the person wants and submit a report to the decision maker as evidence of that person's best interest.

> IMCA: statutory rights
> - the right of private consultation with the client
> - the right to access all relevant clinical and social care records
> - the right to request a second medical opinion
> - the right to challenge a decision if that is felt to be appropriate, up to the Court of Protection of necessary.

The first thing that the IMCA must check is that the individual's lack of capacity to make this decision has been satisfactorily demonstrated, on the balance of probabilities, by the decision maker. In fact, the IMCA should not have been instructed until this has been done. The IMCA does not carry out the capacity test, or make the best interest assessment, but has to be satisfied that these have been done in accordance with the Act and its Code of Practice. The capacity assessment is central to the protection which the Act affords both the individual and the decision maker. If there is any doubt, the person is presumed to have capacity (you are innocent until proven guilty), and the IMCA has no further part to play.

It is essential therefore that the assessment follows the correct form. The Act makes it clear that the test of capacity relates to a specific decision. The capacity to decide what to eat does not imply the capacity to decide what to wear; the incapacity to make a will does not mean the incapacity to consent to surgery, or indeed vice versa. Where there is a requirement for a complex and demanding decision the test of capacity for that decision might need to be performed by a person with appropriate competence. Capacity is not about mental illness or diagnosis. For example: any one of us, however mentally acute, could lose capacity to make decisions after too much alcohol. Capacity is, as the Act specifically defines, the ability to make a relevant decision, for whatever reason, *at the appropriate time* (my emphasis). This means in turn that it does not have to be a mental health professional who does the assessment, although the more serious the decision, the more senior and experienced the decision maker will be, and in some cases the decision maker might welcome the opinion of an expert. In some circumstances an expert might be required to help maximize the capacity of the individual by facilitating communication, using specialist skills or equipment.

Historic assessments and diagnoses are of limited value but can act as an indicator that an assessment might be necessary; degenerative conditions do not signify that a person who lacked capacity a year ago automatically lacks capacity today. Those of us who have worked with dementia are aware that people apparently lost in deep impairment for years can still be remarkably apposite at times. The person has to be assessed at or around the time that the decision needs to be made. Where capacity fluctuates the decision should be delayed if possible until capacity is improved. It may be necessary for the afore-mentioned intoxicated person to sober up before asking them to make a decision. This concept applies to patients who have a temporary loss of capacity from delirium.

There is a presumption in the Act that the decision maker will carry out the capacity assessment. The Code of Practice states (4.38) that: 'The person who assesses an individual's capacity to make a decision will usually be the person who is directly concerned with the individual at the time the decision needs to be made'.

To be exact, the decision maker has the responsibility to see that the assessment is carried out. We can see however that communication is a critical part of the assessment, and it is usually preferable for a professional carer who knows the individual well to practice that communication. Those who work with people with learning difficulties will be particularly aware of the idiosyncrasies which people can develop in their speech and body language.

The IMCA then must ascertain what they believe to be the client's point of view. This can be difficult if the client cannot express themselves, and if there is no-one to speak on their behalf other than professional carers. The IMCA must gather evidence from wherever seems appropriate: from written records, from the client's body language and 'stream of consciousness' verbalizations, from professional carers who have known the individual a long time, from social groups to whom the client has belonged, from family or any one close to the person to help the IMCA to build up a picture of his client. Perhaps the most difficult issue is that of a client's past expressed wishes.

Identifying the person's wants and needs

Medical treatment

The IMCA, like anyone else, runs the risk of being swayed by apparent circumstance. The Act cautions against using subjective criteria such as diagnosis, personal history, or physical appearance to determine best interest. When it comes to the suggestion of withholding or withdrawing treatment the judgement may be made: 'it must be awful to be like that', and indeed for some people life with dementia is a perceived torment, as they struggle to make sense of what is around them. This does not necessarily mean that they would be better off (whatever better off means) without treatment.

Advance decisions and refusals of treatment

This is covered in detail in Chapter 9, but it is important to discuss aspects of this in this chapter and how it might affect the role of the IMCA. Many people make a range of decisions about the future which range from simple issues to complex medical treatments about life sustaining treatment. The terms 'advance directive' and 'living will' are still in common usage but they have been superseded in English law by advance decisions to refuse treatment (ADRT). They will be useful evidence for the IMCA, and may be very useful expressions of preference describing what the individual would like, but the individual cannot direct what should be done for them. The decision in the Leslie Burke case (R (Burke) vs GMC and others (ECtHR) 2006) has made it clear that a patient's demand for a treatment, especially one which a doctor believes would not be in the patient's best interest, does not have to be met. The right granted by the MCA is the right to refuse treatment.

Charles Foster, a barrister specializing in medical ethics, has pointed out the use of the present tense in section 4:1 of the Mental Capacity Act 'in determining for the purposes of this Act what *is* in a person's best interests' and believes the interpretation and intention are quite clear.

The Act does not ask what this person's best interest was when they made the ADRT, on the presumption that a person with capacity to make such a (valid) decision knows their own best interests. It seems clear that the intention is to look at this person at the present moment, just as the test of capacity applies to the present, the time at which the action needs to be taken ensuring that the ADRT is still valid.

Section 4:6 of the Act states that the person's 'past and present wishes and feelings' (including written statements) must be taken into account by the decision maker. Not necessarily followed; merely taken into account. Foster cites the Court of Appeal decision in R (on the application of Burke) vs General Medical Council (July 2005) (a decision handed down before the Mental Capacity Act came into force, but after it had received the Royal Assent), which seems to follow the same reasoning:

> While section 26 of that Act requires compliance with a valid advance directive to refuse treatment, section 4 does no more than require this to be taken into consideration when considering what is in the best interests of a patient (1).

Kitwood argues (1997) that personhood remains in dementia, and that in caring for people with dementia we need to connect as individuals with that person to understand them (2). But who is that person? Is it the same person who wrote the ADRT believing that they would never want to live with dementia or be put in a home? Can it be argued that as he or she did not foresee that they would be happy in their new personhood the terms of the ADRT are no longer valid or applicable? The law recognizes only that the person who made the statement has now left the body, and that it therefore falls to a decision maker to implement what seems to have been their decision. It does not recognize that another person might have taken their place, with perhaps other needs and priorities. An experienced advocate, Roger Milthorp of Cloverleaf Advocacy in West Yorkshire expressed it thus: 'we are oppressed by the person we used to be'.

Many advance decisions will be both valid and applicable and the decision maker will have no difficulty in justifying implementing them. It would be foolish to claim that an ADRT could be set aside because the person with dementia or acquired brain injury was contented, but it would be equally dangerous to assume that the ADRT must automatically be followed without question. The tension between section 4 and section 26 may be an anomaly which case law will eventually resolve, but until that time these are debates that the decision maker will have to go through to decide true best interest of the person in front of him.

The IMCA, meanwhile, has to make a decision on the personhood of the individual, the person who truly needs to have their interest safeguarded. As with the decision maker, what they discover is only evidence, and must be weighed accordingly against all other evidence. This may lead to conflict with a decision maker who sticks rigidly to another interpretation of the Mental Capacity Act.

Serious medical treatment: at what point is an IMCA required?

The difficulty here is that the IMCA is to provide evidence for a specific decision which needs to be made now, and not for ongoing support, whereas what we are trying to do is plan for contingencies which have not yet arisen. The IMCA service is not a blue light service and in any case, in an emergency the doctrine of necessity applies as always. The danger with that doctrine for our purposes is that it can lead to a form of Ulysses syndrome: action for action's sake; investigation done for investigation's sake. Leaving decisions until they become imperative means that neither the IMCA nor the ACP has much to offer to a person in a coma in the last days of life. A doctor who does not know the patient's background may feel it necessary to act. It is said that the two hardest things in medicine are to say nothing and to do nothing.

Serious medical treatment (SMT) is broadly described but not defined in the Act. Examples such as the amputation of a limb, chemotherapy, and heart surgery are given in the Code of Practice. More importantly, for our purposes, the definition of SMT includes withholding and withdrawing treatment, including Do Not Attempt Resuscitation (DNAR) orders. The Regulations to the Act, section 4:2 define SMT as 'treatment which involves providing, withdrawing, or withholding treatment in circumstances where—(c) what is proposed would be likely to involve serious consequences for the patient'. It is likely to be these decisions with which the IMCA will be involved when considering an ACP, and again in the care home, where there is less opportunity to consult with a wider multidisciplinary team. The General Medical Council (UK) guidance on withholding and withdrawing treatment has been revised (2010) to include the provisions of the Mental Capacity Act 2005.

It is worth emphasizing the nature of the specific decisions relating to cardiopulmonary resuscitation, as many perceive this to be a SMT. The expression 'do not attempt resuscitation' should relate to a medical decision not to offer a treatment to attempt resuscitation where there is little chance of success (grounds of medical futility) and/or it is considered ethically unjust; for example to resuscitate a person whose death is expected, in known circumstances, e.g. a diagnosed terminal illness in the last days of life. Once we are clear that it is only an attempt, the ethical position shifts towards the rightness of the clinician making a reasoned judgement, rather than taking it on themselves to decide life versus death, which is how the layman—and the patient—might see it.

It seems at first clear, because it is specified, that a decision to withhold or withdraw treatment with resultant serious consequences would require the instruction of an IMCA (if the IMCA conditions were satisfied) to safeguard the patient's interest. It becomes less clear when examined more closely because it also specifies providing treatment with serious consequences. And what is a consequence? Does one assume that consequences are by definition negative, because of that word 'serious' in the Regulations, or can serious consequences be good ones?

The MCA Code of Practice uses an example of heart surgery to try and clarify this definition of SMT. Carrying out heart surgery usually results in a satisfied patient who might live longer; not carrying it out usually will result in increased symptoms and an earlier death. It could be argued by the strict application of Regulation 4:2(c) therefore that heart surgery is not after all serious medical treatment, because the proposal has no consequence other than a scar and the resumption of normal life. For both lay people and professionals this argument is not logical: the consequence of treating is almost invariably less serious than the consequence of not treating: the correct balance is of benefit to risk. It is on these grounds that the current provision in English law with regard to the definition of SMT and application of the law is subject to further clarification.

IMCA: supporting the vulnerable and frail person in a care home

The same rules and indications for instructing an IMCA apply in care homes as any other setting. The increased prevalence of cognitive impairment, affecting decision making in the very old and frail, means that this group is particularly vulnerable. Government awareness raising programmes, via statutory social care services, have raised the awareness of the MCA and Deprivation of Liberty, and although there is a range of competencies of staff working in or supporting people in care homes, it is more likely that IMCAs will become involved. For day-to-day decisions the decision maker is a member of the care home staff; for more serious decisions such as ACP or withholding or withdrawing treatment, although care home staff can contact the IMCA service, someone from the statutory sector, such as a GP or social worker, must arrange for an IMCA to be instructed.

Experience confirms that many people are happy to be approached about care planning, including their wishes or preferences and decisions relating to treatment at the end of life. It is considered better practice to begin such discussions when they are clinically stable and death may not be imminently anticipated. Some people entering into long term care will remain there for the rest of their lives, which of course includes the end of their lives. It is perhaps in this context of the long term relationship that a more supportive approach to ACP can take place. Difficult conversations may become easier, including introducing the concept that there may one day come a point at which it is reasonable to withhold, or not to offer treatment. Best practice would usually involve professionals with medical competencies to inform such a discussion relating to treatment, but this is not a requirement in law. People are allowed to make such decisions even if they seem unwise. Specific tools to support ACP in care homes are covered in Chapter 12. For most residents of a care home death is a process and rarely a sudden event; usually a dwindling over many months or even years. If ACP should begin with the pre-admission assessment, then the awareness that at some time treatment may be withheld or withdrawn must be built into that plan. For all except DNAR orders, which will have immediate force, this can be done without the input of an IMCA, but for DNAR the situation is more clear cut and such a decision could be made early, based on the likelihood of success and resultant quality of life (although the latter has to be approached with caution).

Case study 1: The apparent utility of initiating futile treatment

A 92 year old woman living in a care home has been becoming increasingly frail over many months. She has been seen by a number of doctors who have treated minor intercurrent illnesses; most noting in their records this overall decline. No decisions about medical treatment or care planning have been made, although her carers are aware and expect that the woman may only have weeks or months to live. She is found one morning by a carer, she is not breathing and there is no pulse. Resuscitation is started, an ambulance is called, she is rushed into hospital to die on a trolley in the emergency department, among complete strangers, in a corridor somewhere. Relatives arrive just too late, and have to find a nurse who knows where the body is. The doctors and nurses then tell the relatives that she died despite trying their best to resuscitate her.

In case study 1 is there an apparent utility in initiating a futile treatment? The professionals might have thought, so as it might have been easier not to make an ACP anticipating the death, which included provisions not to offer resuscitation. Is the application of treatment for the patient or for the protection against litigation of the professional? Whose best interests were being given preference? New guidance from the General Medical Council about End of Life Care helps to set out the expectations of doctors' duty of care and clarifies professional standards of practice.

With its emphasis on a good death, in a place of choice, with acceptance of the inevitable, and treatment appropriate to that acceptance, the End of Life Care Strategy is the antithesis of the sudden rush to the hospital, with its serious consequence for the quality of your last hours and minutes. The consequences in this case study are potentially very unsatisfactory to many concerned where potential pain, distress, disorientation, and loss of dignity have impacted in the last few minutes of life. In identifying serious medical treatment therefore I would hold that it is the consequence both of treating and of not treating that we have to examine.

There will always be decisions as to the efficacy of treatment, the burden versus benefit, and indeed concordance of the person without capacity, and this will have been a regular feature of treatment up until now. The difference is that we acknowledge we are no longer attempting to maintain some kind of stability, but actively managing a foreseeable end. In this we come to the best interest decision.

The best interest decision

This chapter has identified the role of an IMCA. Central to that role is understanding the best interest process, which both protects the vulnerable person and guides the decision maker.

At the heart of the Act is the principle that all decisions taken for someone who lacks capacity must be taken in their best interests. Best interest is not defined because it will vary between individuals. Guidance on reaching the decision is given, but the best we can conclude from the Code of Practice is that we will know best interest when we see it. Once again we come to subjective judgement, the very thing that the Act attempts to do away with.

Although the best interests process in the Act (section 4) states that decisions must not be motivated by a desire to bring about a person's death, section 5.33 of the Code of Practice to the Act says that:

> Section 4:5 cannot be interpreted to mean that doctors are under an obligation to provide, or to continue to provide, life-sustaining treatment where that treatment is not in the best interests of the person, even where the person's death is foreseen. Doctors must apply the best interests checklist and use their professional skills to decide whether life-sustaining treatment is in the person's best interests.

Physicians down the years will be familiar with Clough's Last Decalogue: 'Thou shalt not kill; but need'st not strive officiously to keep alive'. Nothing in the Act removes this judgement from the armoury of the clinician. Section 4:1(b) of the Act cautions against unjustified assumptions about best interest, but does not example what might justify an assumption. Might there be justified assumptions?

Best interests checklist:

- Encourage the person to participate
- Consider the chance of the person regaining capacity at some point
- Do not make assumptions about the person's quality of life
- Consider the person's previous expressed wishes, beliefs, and values
- Gather evidence on wishes, beliefs, and values from relatives, close friends, or persons with power of attorney
- If there is no such person appropriate to consult, an IMCA must be instructed
- If the decision concerns life-sustaining treatment, you must not be motivated in any way by a desire to bring about the person's death.

Having accepted the risk we should still examine what subjective evidence there is. The Code of Practice does not permit us to make assumptions about a person's quality of life. Nor are we permitted to make judgements such as 'if he could tell us he would say . . .' Nonetheless it has to be acknowledged that this is frequently a guide to conclusions around best interest, especially when informed by the opinion of experienced professional health and social care staff.

Case study 2: Best interests—withholding and withdrawing treatment.

How do we make assumptions about quality of life when the Act does not allow us to do so?

Alan is 61 years old, but has a long history of alcohol abuse which has left him both physically and cognitively impaired, with severe liver failure. He was admitted to hospital for treatment of recurrent chest infections which required several courses of treatment. For a time he was ventilated via a tracheostomy and was only weaned off ventilation with difficulty. He cannot swallow safely, only being allowed six teaspoons of pureed food three times a day, receiving his main nourishment via a nasogastric tube.

His consultant physician felt that it may be time to stop active treatment. As Alan had demonstrated a lack of capacity to consent to treatment a referral was made to the IMCA service. The referral included the statement by the consultant:

'With a background of alcohol abuse and cognitive impairment and his current situation of marked frailty and slow stuttering improvement, the prospect of a return to a reasonable quality of life seems poor and therefore continued active treatment could be considered intrusive and unwarranted'.

Is this a justified assumption about a person's quality of life, or how that quality seems to him?

The IMCA made a number of subjective judgements in turn:

- Alan reported to the IMCA that he felt 'lousy'. This is hardly an indication that he found life not worth living, more of an indication of his physical health and mental state. Yet it was one of several pointers.

- All staff (nursing and medical) concurred independently that his quality of life was poor and that he has, in the words of one nurse 'been done no favours' by repeated attempts to postpone an expected death.

- It would be wrong to infer from his history of alcohol abuse the stereotypical view that he has not been happy in his life, but it may be a further pointer to the fact, and that this may also contribute to his present expression of 'lousy'.

- Although potentially a circular argument, the consensus of those attending him was that his prognosis was poor, and that withdrawing active treatment would not so much cause his death as cease postponing it.

- Continued life preserving measures such as antibiotic treatment and ventilation for repeated chest infections have not reversed the declining health but have only slowed the progression, Alan becoming frailer and at more risk of sudden decompensation and death. In terms of his overall wellbeing, nothing has been gained.

- He has repeatedly pulled out his nasogastric tube. Whilst this might only be carphology it is an indication that he is distressed by at least one aspect of his (life sustaining) treatment.

Prognosis is one part of the assessment of the IMCA, but it is very significant in the decision maker's conclusion.

The IMCA concluded:

There is nothing separately in his wishes, feelings, beliefs, and values that would indicate that we are justified in making assumptions about his quality of life. Taken together however, it is a large body of evidence to suggest that life is burdensome to him and, importantly, will not improve. The balance of probabilities would seem to be:

1 that the decision maker is right, when considering his overall best interest, not only in deciding not to escalate treatment, but to suggest withholding further antibiotic treatment even though it should seem to be clinically indicated.

2 that assumptions about his quality of life are justified in terms of section 4:1(b) of the Act.

In case study 2 there was little but assumption to guide the decision maker, although from a purely clinical perspective treatment was possibly futile, at best only marginally successful. But clinical perspective is only part of best interest—guidance to physicians antedating the Act has stressed this for years, and the Act includes it, bringing largely pre-existing perceived good practice writ into statute.

There have been a number of judgements in the courts about quality of life and intolerability, but they acknowledge that the court cannot compare the 'worst' of lives with actual death. Although Alan's health was damaged, and his prognosis poor, how would one argue that we should not attempt to save his life? Because he was confused or because we did not think it would work? Either way, what has that to do with his best interest? The most desperately ill person might claim that it was in their interest to prolong life as long as possible, and there are few more subjective judgements than the idea: 'we should put him out of his misery' (or allow him to slip away without intervention). How do we know how miserable he was? He said he felt 'lousy', but we all feel lousy when we have the flu or a hangover. Would he feel better if the next treatment was successful?

It has to be a reasonable belief based on the balance of probabilities. The aggregation of evidence pointed to an overall poor quality of life; although any one factor could have been dismissed on its own, together they tilted the balance of reasonable belief. External influences such as the effect on third parties, or care staff conscientiously being unable to participate in withdrawing treatment, or even a shortage of resources, are only factored in after the best interest decision is reached, and not used to determine the best interest, even though they may then turn the decision around.

The IMCA will report their conclusions to the decision maker, who will use it as evidence in deciding the person's best interest. The decision maker is legally required to take into account the IMCA's report: to all intents and purposes it is the voice of the person who has lost capacity and in some ways carries the same weight as the individual's own opinion. This does not go as far as the right to refuse treatment on someone's behalf, but might include evidence that a person does not want treatment. The decision maker can refute the IMCA's conclusions if that is what they believe they must do, but they must show very good reason to do so. The IMCA primarily assesses wants, not needs, and they might run counter to best interest. It is one of the central roles of the IMCA to point out that best interest is not merely clinical best interest. The IMCA might even have to propose a point of view which they privately acknowledge to be absurd or unrealistic, but which is nonetheless what they believe this individual wants.

IMCA: helping to understand process versus outcome

Much decision making in health and social care is outcome driven, for better or worse, by measurable targets, but as Einstein said: 'Not everything that can be counted counts, and not everything that counts can be counted.' We have to live with immeasurable uncertainty, and that can seem counter intuitive when becoming involved or making such serious decisions by proxy.

We, including IMCAs, want to believe and sometimes assume we do get it right. We may fall into the trap of assuming that the outcome of a good death is what our decision making is about, but this sometimes hard to define goal of an ACP may appear differently for every member of the decision making group, and the Code of Practice forbids the kind of presumption: 'if I were in that position I would want . . .' The explanatory notes to the Act add, Paragraph 28: 'Best interests is not a test of "substituted judgement" (what the person would have wanted), but rather it requires a determination to be made by applying an objective test as to what would be in the person's best interests.'

We cannot guarantee an outcome in making decisions for other people. The IMCA cannot guarantee that the best decision is made, not least because the best is undefined and indefinable. By following the processes in the Mental Capacity Act we are more likely to arrive at, not necessarily the best decision, but the optimum decision. Process, not outcome, is the safeguard for the vulnerable person.

Knowing and practising skills involved in the process is essential for individuals and teams. To undermine the process is to deprive the vulnerable person of their voice. Enshrining the principles in everyday practices to the extent where they may be non-deliberate or subconscious, even for those instances where there is easy consensus, will prepare us for the occasional case which is exceptionally challenging. Clinicians might believe it is part of their usual practice to use this approach but when appropriately challenged it is not easily demonstrated as exampled by 'best interests' and end of life care. Implicit team consensus in familiar scenarios can lead to false assumptions linked to automatic actions (we always know what 'good' end of life care means; we always do it this way because it is 'right'). The skill of an IMCA when this is occasionally seen is to encourage the team to step back and re-evaluate the situation with more objectivity. The role of the IMCA by virtue of being an outsider allows powerful scrutiny which then can facilitate joint learning.

Conclusion

Advance Care Planning and End of Life decisions must follow a robust ethical and legal framework. Sometimes ethically there are no right answers, only right questions. There are statutory requirements to follow, due process that will maximize the protection for both the vulnerable person and those making decisions on their behalf. The role of the IMCA is specific and when applied appropriately can enhance the decision making process. The IMCA has the authority to challenge a decision taken by a professional for a person lacking capacity, including referral of the case to the Court of Protection. Many hope this is the action of last recourse and would represent the failure to reach a local resolution. This chapter has introduced new concepts presented by the Mental Capacity Act which have yet to be properly defined through legal challenge.

Provided we follow the capacity assessment and best interest process as defined in the Code of Practice, we will arrive at reasonable conclusions. For all its faults, the Mental Capacity Act is a good piece of legislation which protects the rights of both client and decision maker in a way not done before. As to section five of the Act, protection for the decision maker, the worth of a doctor or nurse is not measured merely by how well they avoid risk or litigation, rather by how well they serve the needs of the individual for whose wellbeing they are responsible. Fortunately for us this Act, this process, does both.

Further resources

NHS End of life care: *Planning for your Future Care—a guide* (2009). http://www.endoflifecare.nhs.uk/eolc/files/NHS-EoLC_Planning_future_care-guide-Apr2009.pdf

National Council for Palliative Care. *Good Decision-Making.* www.ncpc.org.uk/publications

www.adrtnhs.co.uk. This website contains valuable resources for both patients and professionals on Advance Decisions and many related end of life care issues.

The Mental Capacity Act 2005. *Independent Mental Capacity Advocates (General) Regulations* (2006). http://www.opsi.gov.uk/si/si2006/20061832.htm

The Mental Capacity Act 2005. *Code of Practice* (2007) London. http://www.publicguardian.gov.uk/mca/code-of-practice.htm

References

1 Foster C (2005). Burke: A tale of unhappy endings. *Journal of Personal Injury Law: JPIL* Issue, **4**(5):293.

2 Kitwood T (1997). *Dementia Reconsidered: The Person Comes First.* Maidenhead: Open University Press.

3 Section 4 of the Mental Capacity Act 2005 (MCA)

4 Henry C and Seymour JE (2007).*Advance Care Planning: a guide for heath and social care professionals.* National End of Life Care Programme, Leicester. (Revised 2008)

5 Preferred Priorities for Care document Version 2 (December 2007) which can be accessed via http://www.endoflifecareforadults.nhs.uk/tools/core-tools/preferredprioritiesforcare. Accessed on 28 October 2010.

6 Office of the Public Guardian, Annual Report 2007 -8, which can be accessed via http://www.publicguardian.gov.uk/docs/opg-annuual-report-2007-08.pdf. Accessed on 28 October 2010.

7 www.publicguardian.gov.uk

8 Details of the fees currently payable in respect of Lasting Powers of Attorney can be accessed via www.publicguardian.gov.uk/about/fees.

9 Advance Decisions to Refuse Treatment: a guide for health and social care professionals (2008) authors: The National End of Life Care Programme and the National Council for Palliative Care. Access via: http://www.endoflifecareforadults.nhs.uk/assets/downloads/pubs_Advance_decisions_to_refuse_guide.pdf Last accessed 28 October 2010.

10 Sections 2 & 3 of the Mental Capacity Act 2005. See also the National Council for Palliative Care publication: "Good Decision-making – the Mental Capacity Act and End of Life Care" (2009); purchase via www.ncpc.org.uk/publications

Introduction

People might make a variety of advance decisions that might apply to a range of issues about their health, welfare, finances, or other person matters. This chapter concentrates on the advance refusal of treatment.

Background to advance decisions and care planning for end of life

This chapter starts with a quote from Ernest Hemingway that emphasizes the importance of listening to people. Most people, especially those living with challenging physical or mental health illnesses, value above all being listened to. It is the first and most important part of the caring relationship and the real understanding to offer personalized care comes from this. 'Failure to listen' is one of the most common causes of complaints and errors in healthcare systems.

In the context of ACP it is paramount we respect the autonomy of the 'Decision Maker' by first listening well and then supporting their preferences and decisions. This must be done using the principles of good clinical practice and professionalism. In the UK the NHS and Social Care promote personalized care, the offer of choice, the maintenance of privacy and dignity, and ensuring that services are safe and effective. Our society and the law confirm our right to consent to or refuse treatment and care. Consent for treatment and care cannot be given if the person has lost mental capacity to make that specific decision. Advance decisions to refuse treatment (ADRT) and Advance Care Plans help in such circumstances to ensure the right outcome.

Advance Care Planning (ACP) has already been defined (1). The discussion may help both the person and care providers to have a better and mutual understanding, and lead to:

◆ an advance statement—a record of values and preferences

◆ an advance decision to refuse treatment, ADRT

◆ the appointment of a Lasting Power of Attorney, LPA (can be a nominated representative for health and welfare).

It must be clearly understood that in English law a patient cannot demand a doctor to give a treatment that is unlawful or futile especially those that would be considered as assisted suicide and bring about an unnatural death.

What is an advance decision to refuse treatment?

Some people may decide that they wish to make sure that they do not receive specific treatment(s) at some future time and an ADRT is defined as 'a specific refusal of treatment(s) in a predefined potential future situation'. The MCA enables them to make an advance decision to refuse specific treatment in the future when they have lost capacity to make their own decision.

Such an advance decision will be legally binding on the person's carers, if all the requirements of the MCA have been met 'at the time that the decision needs to be taken'. An advance decision to refuse treatment that complies with all the MCA's requirements will be as valid as a refusal of treatment by a competent patient, and must be respected in the same way.

Please note that terms like 'living wills' and 'advance directives' have been superseded in English law and for the rest of the chapter the term advance decisions to refuse treatment (ADRT) is used.

Whilst ACP has been used for some time in North America, there has been relatively little experience in the use of ACP in the United Kingdom. However, with legislation in the form of the Mental Capacity Act (2), and NHS initiatives aimed at increasing uptake of ACP (1), it is likely that health and social care professionals will be faced more and more frequently with ACP scenarios.

Chapter 9

Advance Decisions to Refuse Treatment (ADRT)

Ben Lobo

'When people talk, listen completely. Most people never listen.'
Ernest Hemingway

Help the person to talk by being a good listener, but most of all, be a good learner. They may only tell you once.

This chapter includes:

♦ Introduction

♦ Background to advance decisions and care planning for end of life

♦ Specific context: English law, society and culture
  • Mental Capacity Act 2005: helping real people make real decisions

♦ Related topics
  • Advance Decisions to Refuse Treatment (ADRT) and children
  • Decisions relating to cardiopulmonary resuscitation
  • Assisted suicide

♦ Moving forwards
  • Raising public and professional awareness
  • Implementation: systems
    ▪ Education and professional development
    ▪ Evaluation: patient carer and professional outcomes.

Key points

♦ The public have increased awareness and expectations of about 'achieving a good death'

♦ National End of Life Strategy promotes Advance Care Planning and related tools including Advance Decisions

♦ People in England and Wales now have a legal right to refuse even life sustaining treatment

♦ Professionals must respect a valid and applicable ADRT which is legally binding

♦ ADRT for most is best taken in context of ACP

♦ ADRT/ACP must be supported by good clinical practice, professional development, and service redesign

Much of the evidence base for ACP comes from North America; in interpreting the evidence we have been mindful of the differences between the two healthcare systems. An important distinction is that the North American system is less paternalistic and decision making more patient centred, whereas in England and Wales, it is clearly established that doctors are not obliged to provide treatments which are clinically inappropriate (3). US legislation also requires that all individuals admitted to a care home are offered ACP. Preferences are less likely to change if they have been discussed with a doctor (4). Even so, up to one-third of individuals will change their Advance Care Plan over time (months-years), influenced by changes in diagnosis, hospitalization, mood, health status, social circumstances, and functional ability (5,6).

There is no good evidence that the completion of an ADRT leads to the denial of appropriate health care (7,8–13) or increases mortality (8,14–16).

Specific context: English law, society, and culture

From statute to real choice

Healthcare staff must understand and implement the new law relating to advance decisions to refuse treatment presented by the Mental Capacity Act 2005. The MCA came into force in 2007. It is supported by a Code of Practice: Chapter 9 of the Code relates to advance decisions. Everyone must comply with the requirements of the Act and Code.

The legislative framework for advance decisions to refuse treatment is complex. In 2008 the National Council for Palliative Care and the national End of Life Care Programme published a guide on Advance Decisions to Refuse Treatment. This guidance helps to clarify the law for health and social care professionals and to offer additional practical information to enable them to support people who may choose to consider making an advance decision to refuse treatment.

Advance decisions to refuse treatment that meet all the requirements of the Mental Capacity Act will be legally binding on health and social care professionals. The person making an advance decision to refuse treatment must take account of the following formalities:

- Specify the treatment. They can use layman's language, but they should identify a specific treatment. For example, 'I refuse all life-sustaining treatment' does not specify a treatment; 'I refuse cardiopulmonary resuscitation' or 'I refuse assisted ventilation' does.

- Specify the circumstances in which they want the refusal to apply, unless they want the refusal to apply in all circumstances. Some people may wish to refuse a particular treatment in all circumstances, for example because of religious or ethical objections, or because of allergy. Many people however will wish to refuse a treatment in some circumstances, but not others. If that is the case, they must specify the circumstances in which they wish to refuse that treatment. If they specify any circumstances, all the circumstances must exist at the time the decision about the treatment needs to be made for the advance decision to be legally binding.

- Special rules apply if they want to refuse life-sustaining treatment:

  - The person must state that the advance decision is to apply to the specified treatment even if their life is at risk.

  - The advance decision must be in writing, signed either by the person making the advance decision or by another on their behalf and at their direction, and signed by a witness.

People should be very careful to be clear about the circumstances in which they want to refuse a particular treatment. For example, a person with MND or MS might decide that they wish to refuse antibiotics in the event of a chest infection, but not if they had a urinary tract infection. If

ιce decision should specify that antibiotics are being refused on one circumstance but
:r. This makes advance decisions to refuse treatment quite distinct from other aspects
ιe latter may include requests or other statements of wishes about future care and treat-
h statements of values, wishes, priorities, or preferences about what is to be done should
n lose capacity at some point in the future must be taken into account as part of an over-
nterests assessment but are not legally binding.

guidance states the legal requirements necessary for any advance decision to be valid and
ιble and provides commentary to help with the sometimes difficult task of assessing whether
an advance decision is binding.

vill often be helpful for the person to discuss their advance decision with a healthcare profes-
al. If necessary this professional may give advice or support during this process about how to
κe the advance decision. This may also be an opportunity to discuss the person's future care
d treatment. It is really important that the person who has made an advance decision commu-
cates this to relevant people and organizations to ensure that its existence is known and for
rofessionals to check the validity and applicability when it becomes active.

A quick summary of the Mental Capacity Act (2005) code of practice: advance decisions to refuse treatment

- An advance decision enables someone aged 18 and over, while still capable, to refuse specified medical treatment for a time in the future when they may lack the capacity to consent to or refuse that treatment.
- An advance decision to refuse treatment must be valid and applicable to current circumstances. If it is, it has the same effect as a decision that is made by a person with capacity: healthcare professionals must follow the decision.
- Healthcare professionals will be protected from liability if they:
  - stop or withhold treatment because they reasonably believe that an advance decision exists, and that it is valid and applicable
  - treat a person because, having taken all practical and appropriate steps to find out if the person has made an advance decision to refuse treatment, they do not know or are not satisfied that a valid and applicable advance decision exists.
- People can only make an advance decision under the Act if they are 18 or over and have the capacity to make the decision. They must say what treatment they want to refuse, and they can cancel their decision—or part of it—at any time.
- If the advance decision refuses life-sustaining treatment, it must:
  - be in writing (it can be written by someone else or recorded in healthcare notes)
  - be signed and witnessed, and
  - state clearly that the decision applies even if life is at risk.
- To establish whether an advance decision is valid and applicable, healthcare professionals must try to find out if the person:
  - has done anything that clearly goes against their advance decision
  - has withdrawn their decision
  - has subsequently conferred the power to make that decision on an attorney, or
  - would have changed their decision if they had known more about the current circumstances.

> ## A quick summary of the Mental Capacity Act (2005) code of practice: advance decisions to refuse treatment *(continued)*
>
> ◆ Sometimes healthcare professionals will conclude that an advance decision does not exist, is not valid and/or applicable, but that it is an expression of the person's wishes. The healthcare professional must then consider what is set out in the advance decision as an expression of previous wishes when working out the person's best interests (see Code of Practice, Chapter 5).
>
> ◆ Some healthcare professionals may disagree in principle with patients' decisions to refuse life-sustaining treatment. They do not have to act against their beliefs. But they must not simply abandon patients or act in a way that that affects their care.
>
> ◆ Advance decisions to refuse treatment for mental disorder may not apply if the person who made the advance decision is or is liable to be detained under the Mental Health Act 1983.

Real choice, real responsibility

The Act and Code of Practice clearly define that the responsibility for making an advance decision lies with the person making it. The person retains the right to make an advance decision even if it appears unwise and if valid and applicable it must be acted upon. For most people the process that leads up to making the decision requires the careful balance of both benefits and risks. These are described in the Guide.

Table 9.1 simplifies the overall process of identifying the need, making, implementing, and evaluating the outcome of an ADRT. This might not be the case for many people involved in making an ADRT. It does, however, demonstrate there are number of important factors that can

Table 9.1 The overall process of identifying the need, making, implementing, and evaluating the outcome of an ADRT

Process	Comment
Patient/Person	Often best supported by a key worker which might include the generalist or a specialist professional either at home/community, in hospital/hospice or another environment e.g. care home
Trigger	This might be a routine review, new diagnosis, bereavement, admission to hospital, or other assessment
Process of preparing ADRT	Help and specific resources might be required to write the ADRT to ensure that it is valid and applicable
Implementation and Dissemination of ADRT	Telling people and organizations might be a challenge. Patients might require support
Reviews	This might be planned or triggered by an event or change in circumstances (e.g. the advent of a new treatment)
Outcomes	This is difficult to measure unless there is shared information across care pathways

influence the decision. Again it must be stressed that ethical dilemmas, cultural sensitivities, and society can play a significant role. Simple stipulations from patients can bring about tremendous personal and or professional stress, 'This is my (valid and applicable) ADRT. Don't tell the wife!' Confidentiality, privacy, and dignity must be maintained even if the decision might be considered as 'unwise'.

Case History

P has progressive and distressing symptoms because of her motor neuron disease. P understands that her prognosis is poor and she will potentially require help with her breathing and artificial nutrition and may loose capacity at any stage to make such a decision. P has discussed the situation with her husband. P does not want her life to be extended by the use of specific treatments including cardiopulmonary resuscitation or artificial ventilation or feeding. She writes her ADRT with the support of her key worker. She checks that her ADRT meets the legal requirements. She asks her key worker for help to tell local health professionals including the ambulance service.

P was reassured that she has made this decision. P's husband and family were involved and supported her. P achieved her wish to die with dignity and on her own terms.

Comment: For P an ADRT was made in the context of ACP and in expectation of a natural death. Her prognosis was easier to predict. P was very clear what she didn't want and when. For other people with different challenges it might be harder to predict prognosis. Some people might wish to make an ADRT some time in advance of a possible event, illness, or deterioration. Some people make decisions based on values or beliefs we don't share, these can sometimes result in blanket refusals, e.g. because of my religious beliefs I never want to have a blood transfusion even if my life is at risk. Any professional must check that no matter what is implied the ADRT exists, is valid, and applicable. If it complies with the requirement of the law and there is no evidence to question it, the ADRT must be respected.

Related topics

ADRT and children

The Mental Capacity Act 2005 and Code of Practice 2007 describe that only adults (18 and over) have the right in law to make an ADRT. In 2008 in England, Hannah Jones, aged 13 decided that she wanted to refuse a heart transplant. This transplant was essential to maintain her life. The decision to refuse this treatment was challenged by her local health trust. The High Court ruled that she had been able to make an informed decision and her right to refuse this treatment must be respected. This challenges the age restriction as laid down by the Act and draws parallels about the wider issues of the ability to consent to treatment. There are many children that are expected to die from a variety of 'natural' reasons. Existing practice requires a consensus with the patient, family, and care team. Resuscitation is not performed and the patient is allowed to have a natural death. In circumstances where there is a wider dissemination of the Advance Care Plan which includes allowing such a death a much greater level of scrutiny is brought to bear. Despite the primacy of good clinical practice and medical professionalism the care team must demonstrate they are compliant with the requirements of the law.

ADRT and decisions relating to cardiopulmonary resuscitation

This subject is addressed in more detail in Chapter 10. It must be emphasized that the MCA and related legislation/policy sets about empowering and enabling many more people to take responsibility and make their own decisions about their lives and welfare. For people who have capacity (or have a nominated proxy decision maker e.g. Lasting Power of Attorney) good clinical practice would require the professional to have a discussion with this person to explore this type of decision. For some people it might be inappropriate and unethical to enter into a discussion this type. If a healthcare team considers that CPR has no realistic prospect of success then they may decide it is not to be attempted or offered. In these circumstances this decision is made by the healthcare team and is not an advance decision to refuse treatment made by the patient. DNAR orders should not be used as a convenient short cut to circumvent open discussion of end of life decisions. The senior clinician in charge of the patients care must take the responsibility to assess the situation, correctly apply an ethical and culturally sensitive approach to formulate an agreed clinical management plan. If the patient has not got the capacity to decide for themselves about decisions then a proper best interests assessment must be done that meets the statutory requirements in the Mental Capacity Act. In emergency situations where a decision has to be made quickly without wider consultation the senior clinician must act and then be able to defend the decision later.

The British Medical Association, the Royal College of Nursing, and the Resuscitation Council have published a joint statement on decisions relating to cardiopulmonary resuscitation which considers these issues in more detail. Professionals should refer to that statement. Further commentary is also contained in the National Council for Palliative Care's publication: *The Mental Capacity Act in Practice: Guidance for End of Life Care.*

Assisted suicide

Although suicide was decriminalized in 1961 assisted suicide (including physician assisted) in this country remains an illegal act. Attempts to change the law have failed despite a significant amount of public support. Experiences in other countries including the Netherlands and Switzerland have demonstrated both the benefits as well as the risks in having such legislation. Recent test cases challenging English law have been made. This includes cases where carers/families have helped another member of their family travel to Switzerland for a physician assisted suicide.

Following the instructions of the Law Lords the Director of Public Prosecutions (DPP) for England and Wales stated on the 23 September 2009,

> I am today clarifying those factors of public interest which I believe weigh for or against prosecuting someone for assisting another to take their own life. Assisting suicide has been a criminal offence for nearly fifty years and my interim policy does nothing to change that . . . There are also no guarantees against prosecution and it is my job to ensure that the most vulnerable people are protected while at the same time giving enough information to those people, like Ms Purdy, who want to be able to make informed decisions about what actions they may choose to take.

The public interest factors in favour of prosecution identified in the interim policy include that:

◆ The victim was under 18 years of age

◆ The victim's capacity to reach an informed decision was adversely affected by a recognized mental illness or learning difficulty

◆ The victim did not have a clear, settled, and informed wish to commit suicide; for example, the victim's history suggests that his or her wish to commit suicide was temporary or subject to change

◆ The victim did not indicate unequivocally to the suspect that he or she wished to commit suicide

◆ The victim did not ask personally on his or her own initiative for the assistance of the suspect

◆ The victim did not have a terminal illness; or a severe and incurable physical disability; or a severe degenerative physical condition from which there was no possibility of recovery

- The suspect was not wholly motivated by compassion; for example, the suspect was motivated by the prospect that they or a person closely connected to them stood to gain in some way from the death of the victim
- The suspect persuaded, pressured, or maliciously encouraged the victim to commit suicide, or exercised improper influence in the victim's decision to do so; and did not take reasonable steps to ensure that any other person did not do so.

The public interest factors against a prosecution include that:

- The victim had a clear, settled and informed wish to commit suicide
- The victim indicated unequivocally to the suspect that he or she wished to commit suicide
- The victim asked personally on his or her own initiative for the assistance of the suspect
- The victim had a terminal illness or a severe and incurable physical disability or a severe degenerative physical condition from which there was no possibility of recovery
- The suspect was wholly motivated by compassion
- The suspect was the spouse, partner, a close relative, or a close personal friend of the victim, within the context of a long-term and supportive relationship
- The actions of the suspect, although sufficient to come within the definition of the offence, were of only minor assistance or influence, or the assistance which the suspect provided was as a consequence of their usual lawful employment.

The DPP also stated that:

> Each case must be considered on its own facts and its own merits. Prosecutors must decide the importance of each public interest factor in the circumstances of each case and go on to make an overall assessment . . . I also want to make it perfectly clear that this policy does not, in any way, permit euthanasia. The taking of life by another person is murder or manslaughter—which are among the most serious criminal offences.

The great public interest and pressure vocalized by people like Debbie Purdy helped lead to these guidelines. These guidelines are supposed to offer some assurances to people that they will not be prosecuted where there are clear cases of need on humane/compassionate grounds e.g. the public interest factors against prosecution. This unfortunately does not remove all doubt as the guidelines do not represent a guarantee preventing prosecution. The person (who wishes to die) may still feel forced into an earlier decision to enact suicide before the need to involve a third party. This would only 'remove life from years' dying on someone else's terms.

Moving forwards

Raising awareness

Public awareness of advance decisions, and related ethical end of life dilemmas is rapidly growing. Stories of real life decisions continue to be presented in the media. These cases, including young adults and children, have established new precedents in law and brought into sharp reality the nature of peoples lives, the decisions they would like to and have taken, and the challenges they have to get through to realize these decisions. Stories that are dramatized in prime time television series are now part of popular culture.

Implementation

Professional awareness and participation in advance decisions has been for many restricted to specialists in palliative medicine. The medical and wider health and social care profession is being challenged to respond to both the clinical need of the patient and their rights in law.

These professions must demonstrate both the competency and confidence to maintain good clinical practice and comply with the law.

Systems, communication, and documentation strategies

The requirements in law relate to the content and verification by a witness of an ADRT. There are no requirements to use an approved form/format or to inform other parties. It is, however, very important to inform key people, professionals and organizations of the existence of an ADRT as this will increase the chances that it will be recognized and respected. The national guide offers information about this process and an example form. Clearly support from a key worker will help to ensure other parties know about the advance decision and or reviews/amendments and cancellations. ADRT is the patient's own document. It can be copied and inserted into their case notes and shared with other agencies including the ambulance service. As the gold standards framework (GSF) is implemented in care homes in this country and ACP is better understood it is expected that decisions including advance decisions will be more openly approached and the outcomes recorded. It is certainly hoped that essential information like an advance decision or DNAR is included in any future electronic records and is shared with multi-agency partners in health and social care.

Service improvement to deliver choice: end of life decisions registry

In the East Midlands region in England there is an End of Life Decisions Registry to help the ambulance service. An advance decision to refuse CPR or the presence of a DNAR can be recorded. If the ambulance service receives a call about a particular patient with a registered end of life decision they will be prepared on dispatch to offer an appropriate response. This requires a verification process at registration and at the point of care checking the validity and applicability of such decisions. This system has been used to support the care of thousands of patients, including children, across the region without serious untoward incident.

Education and professional development

There has been widespread 'training' on the Mental Capacity Act as part of the national implementation strategy. Although most programmes cover advance decisions they do not often go into enough detail to help to resolve sometimes complex clinical, ethical, and legal issues. An example of a specialist resource on this subject can be found at adrtnhs.co.uk website. This website hosts a modular and interactive educational programme that covers in detail ADRT for health and social care professionals. It also contains many other resources and references that support both the generalist as well as the specialist in delivering end of life care. It encapsulates many ideas and methods that support good practice and emphasizes many important features of communication and documentation.

It is of real importance that organizations understand the competencies required of their workforce to deliver safe and effective services. Although there might be an obvious priority for professionals involved in specialist services e.g. palliative care to become competent and confident it is essential that other services have safe base line knowledge and also understand how to access support and knowledge in a timely manner.

Education and professional development must be evaluated with the same rigour as the implementation of the wider strategy. Evaluations are required as part of performance management for organizations and might be required to be demonstrated to commissioning or regulatory bodies. Clinical audit is one established way to demonstrate performance against expected standards. Audit can be used to help drive up the quality and clinical effectiveness of services and learning.

Outcomes

It is now expected in health care systems that real outcomes or health gains are demonstrated rather than outputs. These outcomes include assessments of more subjective matters about the experience of the patient/carer. Chapter 10 describes in detail the perspective of the patient/carer and how they can be at variance sometimes to that of the professional/organization. Outcomes are now written into contracts with health care providers. End of life care including ACP is described in quality schedules which those commissioning services expect to be met.

Outcomes which can be demonstrated when ADRTs are used

Person/patient and carer related outcomes:

◆ Reassurance that decisions will be respected and acted upon
  • the refusal of life sustaining treatment might allow a natural death and maybe influence the preferred place where this is achieved
◆ Peace of mind knowing that family/friends will not be burdened with decisions
  • Enhanced autonomy through legislative empowerment
  • Better communication with health care professionals
  • Could help carer/family adjust to bereavement.

It is recognized that an ADRT can in some situations cause problems e.g. if there is a disparity in the views of the patient and their carer and thoughts and feelings are unresolved including guilt, denial, regret, loss

Professionals

◆ Better understanding of patient choice
◆ Better informed and clearly documented/communicated patient decisions
◆ Staff empowered to protect autonomy and support the patient's choice by law and policy of their employing organization
◆ Support for good clinical practice increasing the chance for job satisfaction.

Organizations

◆ Clearly defined responsibility to ensure adherence to the Mental Capacity Act and Code of Practice
◆ Fulfil Clinical Governance commitment to pursue good clinical practice, ensure patient/carer and professional outcomes whilst correctly managing risk
◆ Prevent unwanted and possible unnecessary admission to hospital and treatments
◆ Reduce costs of unscheduled care, help predict clinical service demand.

Next steps: three self assessment questions

1 Do you (person, carer, professional, and organization) have the right knowledge and skills about advance decisions to refuse treatment/end of life decision making?

2 Do you have a strategy to acquire and maintain them?

3 Have you got policies/procedures to support safe, effective practice and can you demonstrate this?

Conclusion

Health, social care services, and society in general promote and protect personal/patient choice. The law lays down in statute the rights of the person including that to make an ADRT. With this right comes great personal and professional responsibility and accountability to ensure that the right process is followed and the right outcomes are achieved. ADRT taken in context of ACP for the End of Life is a component of a national strategy to improve services for people to help ensure a good death with dignity and privacy. There is a real opportunity to use this legal and societal imperative to drive the commissioning and provision of health and social care services that respect this autonomy and achieve real results for people. This new legal power can bring significant benefits and when used appropriately minimizes (but never removes) risk.

Acknowledgement

This chapter draws upon the national publication, *Advance Decisions to Refuse Treatment—A Guide for Health and Social Care Professionals*. Although this is not fully referenced throughout, as the national clinical lead for this work I would like to acknowledge this publication and the rest of the team that contributed. I would also acknowledge Dr Simon Conroy for his contribution to this chapter.

Further resources

See also Appendix 1

National End of Life Care Programme & National Council for Palliative Care Advance Decisions to Refuse Treatment: A guide for health and social care staff (2008). http://www.endoflifecare.nhs.uk/eolc/files/NHS-EoLC_ADRT_Sep2008.pdf

NHS End of life care, *Planning for your Future Care – a guide* (2009) http://www.endoflifecare.nhs.uk/eolc/files/NHS-EoLC_Planning_future_care-guide-Apr2009.pdf

A website containing valuable resources for both patients and professionals on Advance Decisions and many related end of life care issues: www.adrtnhs.co.uk

   Advance Decisions Check list http://www.adrtnhs.co.uk/pdf/Advance_Decisions_Checklist.pdf

   ADRT Proforma http://www.adrtnhs.co.uk/pdf/EoLC_appendix1.pdf

NCPC: *Good Decision-Making.* www.ncpc.org.uk/publications

Department of Justice (formerly Dept. of Constitutional Affairs). www.justice.gov.uk

   Mental Capacity Act (2005). http://www.opsi.gov.uk/acts/acts2005/ukpga_20050009_en_1

   Mental Capacity Act: Code of Practice (2007). http://www.publicguardian.gov.uk/mca/code-of-practice.htm

Clinical Decisions Algorithm: The process for making clinical decisions in serious medical conditions in patients over 18 years in Regnard C, Hockley J, Dean M. (2008) *A guide to Symptom Relief in Palliative Care.* 6th ed. Radcliffe Publishing, Oxford.

Patrick DL, Pearlman RA, Starks HE et al. Validation of preferences for life-sustaining treatment: Implications for advance care planning. *Ann Intern Med.* 1997;**127**(7):509–17.

Carmel S, Mutran EJ. Stability of elderly persons' expressed preferences regarding the use of life-sustaining treatments. *Soc Sci Med.* 1999;**49**(3):303–11.

Danis M, Garrett J, Harris R, Patrick DL. Stability of choices about life-sustaining treatments. *Ann Intern Med.* 1994;**120**(7):567–73.

Caplan GA, Meller A, Squires B, Chan S, Willett W. Advance care planning and hospital in the nursing home. *Age Ageing.* 2006;**35**(6):581–5.

References

1 NHS End of Life Care Programme (2007). *Advance Care Planning: A Guide for Health and Social Care Staff*. London.

2 Department for Constitutional Affairs (2005). Mental Capacity Act. London. http://www.opsi.gov.uk/acts/acts2005/ukpga_20050009_en_1

3 R (Burke) v General Medical Council: Queen's Bench Division (Administrative court), 2004.

4 Emanuel LL, Emanuel EJ, Stoeckle JD, Hummel LR, and Barry MJ (1994). Advance directives. Stability of patients' treatment choices. *Archives of Internal Medicine*, **154**(2):209–17.

5 Kohut N, Sam M, O'Rourke K et al. (1997). Stability of treatment preferences: although most preferences do not change, most people change some of their preferences. *Journal of Clinical Ethics*, **8**(2):124–35.

6 Silverstein MD, Stocking CB, and Antel JP (1991). Amyotrophic lateral sclerosis and life-sustaining therapy: patients' desires for information, participation in decision making, and life sustaining therapy. *Mayo Clinic Proceedings*, **66**(9):906–13.

7 Froman RD and Owen SV (2005). Randomized study of stability and change in patients' advance directives. *Research in Nursing & Health*, **28**(5):398–407.

8 Engelhardt JB, McClive-Reed KP, Toseland RW et al. (2006). Effects of a program for coordinated care of advanced illness on patients, surrogates, and healthcare costs: a randomized trial. *American Journal of Managed Care*, **12**(2):93–100.

9 Connors Jr AF, Dawson NV, Desbiens NA et al. (1995). A controlled trial to improve care for seriously ill hospitalised patients: The study to understand prognoses and preferences for outcomes and risks of treatments (SUPPORT). *JAMA: The Journal of the American Medical Association*, **274**(20):1591–8.

10 Lee MA, Brummel-Smith K, Meyer J, Drew N, and London MR (2000). Physician orders for life-sustaining treatment (POLST): outcomes in a PACE program. Program of All-Inclusive Care for the Elderly [see Comment]. *Journal of the American Geriatrics Society*, **48**(10):1219–25.

11 Hammes BJ and Rooney BL (1998). Death and end-of-life planning in one midwestern community. *Archives of Internal Medicine*, **158**(4):383–90.

12 Tolle SW, Tilden VP, Nelson CA, and Dunn PM (1998). A prospective study of the efficacy of the physician order form for life 14 Advance care planning © Royal College of Physicians, 2009. All rights reserved. sustaining treatment [see Comment]. *Journal of the American Geriatrics Society*, **46**(9):1097–102.

13 Danis M, Southerland LI, Garrett JM et al. (1991).A prospective study of advance directives for life-sustaining care [see Comment]. *The New England Journal of Medicine*, **324**(13):882–8.

14 Hanson LC, Tulsky JA, and Danis M (1997). Can clinical interventions change care at the end of life? *Annals of Internal Medicine*, **126**(5):381–8.

15 Molloy DW, Guyatt GH, Russo R et al. (2000). Systematic implementation of an advance directive program in nursing homes: a randomized controlled trial. *JAMA: The Journal of the American Medical Association*, **283**(11):1437–44.

16 Goodman MD, Tarnoff M, and Slotman GJ (1998). Effect of advance directives on the management of elderly critically ill patients. *Critical Care Medicine*, **26**(4):701–4.

Chapter 10

The tough questions: do not attempt resuscitation discussions

Madeline Bass

'There is no ethical obligation to discuss CPR with the majority of palliative care patients for whom such treatment, following assessment, is judged futile.'
National Council for Palliative Care (2002)

This chapter includes:

◆ Development of cardiopulmonary resuscitation (CPR)

◆ Success rates of CPR

◆ Who should make the final decision about CPR?

◆ The CPR decision-making process involved in Advance Care Planning

◆ How to handle a conversation about CPR.

Key Points

◆ CPR is not as successful as many professionals think

◆ CPR should not be offered if it is going to be futile

◆ If patients have capacity they should be given the option to make decisions for themselves if there is a choice

---

Following a process in decision-making can help to know what to do.

The word 'patient' has been used throughout this chapter to represent patients, customers, clients or residents.

Introduction

Cardiopulmonary resuscitation (CPR) has been known in its present form, since 1960. The first time mouth to mouth, closed chest compressions and closed chest defibrillation were used together was in 1960 (Kouwenhoven et al.) and it is this groundbreaking research to which we owe so much. Most people can learn CPR. There is however a significant need to understand the more fundamental and anticipatory question, 'Is CPR appropriate?' This is one key component to Advance Care Planning (ACP) for the end of life.

The original CPR research subjects were victims of sudden, unexpected cardiac or respiratory arrest. CPR for these subjects was associated with good survival outcomes. It is not surprising that the current reported outcomes are quite different because this intervention is offered more widely and is used sometimes irrespective of the poor prognostic factors. Any concerns we have about the correct indication for CPR must be based on an objective appraisal of the evidence. Risk must be understood as it applies to an individual and any blanket decisions e.g. based on age would be discriminatory. In fact CPR is now having a lower success rate than ever because healthcare professionals tend to have an overoptimistic view of its success (1–3) and are increasingly using it inappropriately (4,5).

The ethical dilemma of CPR

It is easy to understand why, for safety reasons, there should be a default position to offer resuscitation where no other decision exists. There should be an active process to consider this decision especially for people at higher risk of a cardiopulmonary arrest. For many people and professionals it is initially very difficult to resolve the inherent paradox about CPR decisions. Usually health professionals ask patients to consent to receive a specific procedure, performed by a named person, with the detailed risks and benefits outlined. For this treatment (CPR) the only decision the patient can make is to refuse to consent to be resuscitated (thus making an Advance Decision to Refuse Treatment). Often there is no guarantee of who will perform the resuscitation and how it will be done. There is little factual basis described on the effectiveness, benefits, and risks in any discussion if it takes place.

There needs to be a paradigm shift in the approach. Decisions by professionals relating to CPR need to be based on clinical evidence and a better ethical justification. CPR should not be offered as a choice to patients where there is no choice i.e. when the decision to not offer resuscitation actually lies with the senior clinician. It is a different ethical and professional challenge to tell people of a decision not to offer them resuscitation, especially if they have a preference for this treatment. It is clear that better communication supported by empowered and enabled professionals must underpin any transaction. Advance Care Planning is best supported by an active process of listening to the ideas and concerns of those involved and ensuring that there are agreed (if possible) and realistic expectations. Hopefully the ultimate treatment decision by the clinician will be more secure by going through this approach.

What about when someone demands CPR?

It is really important to listen to a patient who demands any treatment especially a potentially life sustaining treatment. Behind this demand might be a number of ideas and expectations that may or may not be well founded. For example the patient's (public) perception of CPR may be different to health professionals as the media can present biased and factually incorrect portrayals. Very rarely seen are the negative consequences of futile attempts, especially for patients where it is a lengthy and 'violent' process that only delays an inevitable death with profound loss of dignity, increased pain, and distress for all concerned.

English law does not allow a patient, or their proxy, to demand treatments which are likely to be futile (i.e. have no benefit to the patient, only side effects). This includes CPR. This means that if the medical team are as certain as they can be that CPR will not be successful, it should not be offered. It is an expectation that professionals will be more proactive in asking patients about their preference and wishes as part of making an Advance Care Plan. Professionals cannot start this process including discussions about CPR without knowing how to manage very specific hopes and aspirations of patients that cannot be met. Any decision that is made about treatment, especially CPR, must be specific and in the context of the circumstances that apply to that individual.

A decision made against CPR is often called Do Not Attempt Resuscitation (DNAR) and only applies to CPR, not to other interventions, treatments, and care.

Futility and CPR

What is meant by the word 'futile' and how does this apply in CPR? Here are some more detailed definitions of 'futile':

- 'When treatment offers no benefit to the patient because maximal therapy has failed and physiologic improvement is impossible' (6). In terms of CPR this would mean that it would not be successful, because the patient is so unwell, and that the patient will not improve from it.

- '… when important goals of care cannot be achieved although other goals might be.' (7) This means CPR would not be successful but other goals, such as comfort and good palliative care, can be. Perhaps healthcare professionals forget that death is actually normal, that life will end for all of us, so it is important that death is diagnosed and appropriate care received to ensure a good death.

- '… if reasoning and experience indicate that the intervention would be highly unlikely to result in a meaningful survival for that patient' (8). Once it is recognized that the person is dying and that their heart will stop as a result of an expected, irreversible, occurrence then CPR will not be successful. It is worth remembering that following an arrest most patients require a (brief) period of specific observation, either in CCU or ITU. If such a transfer of care would not be appropriate then CPR should not be attempted (9).

A palliative care consultant said something to me some years ago which I have always remembered, 'What you need to ask yourself is this: is this arrest the first thing which has happened to somebody, i.e. it is completely unexpected? If so, then CPR may have some success so it is appropriate to attempt it. However if an arrest is the last thing to happen to somebody, i.e. as part of the dying process, then CPR will not be successful as all other major organs in the body have also stopped working.' Looking at CPR in this way fits with the Gold Standards Framework (GSF) surprise question: 'Would I be surprised if this person were to die in the next few weeks/days?' If the answer is no then a decision needs to be made about CPR, remembering that it won't be successful when the person is dying. Instead the new goals of treatment and care should be explained, such as comfort, and being in their preferred place of care with whom they want present. The NCPC (10) state that there is no ethical obligation to discuss CPR with patients for whom it is thought to be futile.

Patients, family carers, and even some professionals, may request futile CPR because of guilt, unrealistic goals and expectations, misunderstanding of CPR, a mistrust of doctors, the need to have tried everything, denial that the patient is dying, communication difficulties, or conflicting values and beliefs, culture, and religion.

The medical team, however, 'must be as certain as they can be that CPR will not be successful' (11). Another question which may be helpful is this: 'Does this patient present as a person for whom arrest would be unexpected and sudden and for whom the medical team is as certain as they can be that CPR would be successful?' If the answer is yes then CPR should be offered and discussed with them to see if they would want it. If the answer is no, then it should not be discussed with them as a treatment option.

Patient choice in healthcare

The 'choice' reality for some patients has been on the basis of serendipity e.g. where you live; which doctor or hospital you attend; socio-economic and cultural factors including what you look and sound like; linked with the ability to work a system. Patient choice was enhanced by the advent of the Patients Charter (12), and subsequently it has rightly become more prominent. This charter in part counters the culture of inappropriate medical paternalism where patients were often not told all their treatment options, and many did not think to ask because they felt that 'the doctor is always right.' There has to be balance to prevent the undermining of appropriate professional opinion and behaviours. Professionals must maintain and promote the highest standards of care and not be frightened or threatened. There will always be situations where there will be bad news, this includes telling a patient that their health has deteriorated and CPR will not be offered. We must remember that the general public often come with little medical knowledge. Yet we expect them to make sometimes complex decisions about their health and future. If we as a society believe in choice we must resource choice. The first resource must always be appropriate communication to truly inform patients. It is difficult enough for people to make decisions about subjects they know little about, but when it concerns their own future we forget the effects of stress, anxiety, and worry on how people are thinking.

Success rates of CPR

Before the statistics are presented it is essential to consider success in the wider context. Success depends wholly on how it is defined and this may be very different for the patient compared to the professional. Professional publications tend to quote success as either 'initial success' or 'success to discharge'. CPR might be perceived as a success by the professional if they are discharged but might be a complete failure by the patient if they did not want CPR in the first place and are left with a potential complication of that 'success' such as hypoxic brain injury and disability. Professionals must understand the difference between outputs (numbers) and outcomes, especially patient and carer related outcomes.

Initial success is defined as the patient being able to independently maintain their heart rate, blood pressure, and breathing. Success to discharge means that they survive long enough to leave the hospital. The statistics for these outcomes are quite diverse. Quotes vary from 16.5% to 65.7% initial success and 0% to 29% for success to discharge (13–17). The statistics quoted in the latest CPR decision-making guidelines (9) state 15–20% success to discharge for all hospital arrests (18), and only 5–10% success to discharge for all community arrests (19). CPR statistics are very different due to the variables in the research groups, and this is about as specific as it gets in terms of whether CPR should be offered or not. CPR should only be offered if there is felt to be even a small chance of success.

CPR will be most successful in those with reversible medical conditions (20). We should also be mindful of 'post-resuscitation disease' (21) i.e. the effects of resuscitation on those who survive which might include broken ribs, pneumothorax, neurological damage, memory loss, etc. From personal experience my mother in law was resuscitated whilst being treated for bilateral pneumonia. She survived and was discharged to live the following two years of her life bedbound in a nursing home, on continuous oxygen, then developed cancer of the oesophagus, and had severe memory loss to the extent she often could not recognize her children. So, yes there was initial success and yes there was success to discharge but the post-resuscitation disease left a previously capable lady (who never wanted to go in a care home and who had wanted to join her husband since he had died 30 years before) to end her days in a way she would not have wanted. If she had been asked, or her family consulted, the CPR decision would have been no.

A useful tool to help in resuscitation and treatment decisions is the GSF Prognostic Indicator Guidance. It clearly states how the prognosis for malignant and non-malignant disease may progress, as well as in dementia. This can be a useful tool in identifying those patients for whom CPR may not be successful.

When is CPR appropriate?

CPR is appropriate when it may be successful (not futile), and when the patient (or their legal proxy) has not specifically refused it. CPR is most successful when the arrest is witnessed, basic life support is commenced immediately, defibrillation is carried out as soon as possible for ventricular fibrillation (VF) and pulseless ventricular tachycardia (VT), and the patient's prognostic indicators are good (22). Other proven positive predictors are:

+ Non cancer diagnosis
+ Cancer patients without metastases or limited metastases
+ Not housebound
+ Good renal function
+ No known infection, particularly of the chest
+ Normotensive (i.e. normal range of blood pressure)
+ Generally robust health (23).

Experience supports that when evidence/indicators are objectively considered the same answer to the GSF Surprise Question is reached. When there are multiple negative prognostic indicators it is not a surprise that death occurs sooner and that CPR would be both a futile treatment and be unsuccessful.

It used to be that if no decision had been made CPR would always be attempted on a patient who arrested. Unfortunately with the latest CPR guidelines (9) there is still some confusion. These state: 'Where no explicit decision has been made in advance there should be an initial presumption in favour of CPR… *But* if CPR would not restart the heart and breathing it should not be attempted'. They go on to say that if the patient is adamant they want CPR then it should be offered, 'but that at the time of arrest the decision will be reviewed.' I interpret this to mean that to the patient and family, yes, of course we will uphold your decision and give CPR; but as soon as the patient arrests the decision can be reversed. This does nothing to maintain the truth-telling, honesty, and trust which healthcare professionals should be aiming to achieve with the patient-professional relationship. Instead CPR should not be offered as a treatment option in the first place. Even if the patient demands it, it should not be offered and they should be made aware of why not. We are so frightened of litigation, or anger, or of requests for second opinions, yet we should maintain our belief that what we are doing is right for that patient. We would not offer a patient an operation which was not thought to be appropriate, so why do we offer CPR? Unfortunately many healthcare professionals are unaware of any CPR guidelines, and some areas do not yet have a resuscitation policy, so the old practice of carrying out CPR as the default continues, yet with no evidence-base for it.

When is CPR inappropriate?

CPR is inappropriate when it expected to be unsuccessful (futile), and when the patient (or their legal proxy) has specifically refused it. Research on CPR shows outcomes are dependent on:

+ The place the arrest occurs
+ How long before CPR was started, either basic life support (mouth to mouth and chest compressions) or advanced life support

- Any post-arrest complications which may occur in those who are revived
- The condition of the patient before arrest
- The condition of the patient when they were discharged from the hospital
- Any pre-existing co-morbidities, or metastatic disease
- How experienced the professionals involved in the resuscitation are.

We should remember that CPR is resuscitation, not resurrection (24). Inappropriate CPR itself can have several negative consequences (25): distress to the relatives, an undignified death, demoralization for the professionals involved, and an inappropriate use of resources.

So who makes the final CPR decision?

The Joint Statement on Decisions Relating to CPR (9) accepted as national guidelines state that the final decision is down to the senior clinician in charge of the patient's care, according to local policy. What happens when there is no clear resuscitation policy? Consider how this might apply to a care home? If the responsibility still lies with the senior clinician say the general practitioner (family doctor) to which the person is registered, is this doctor going to make this decision and be in a position to review appropriately?

What happens if no CPR decision has been made and the person arrests but that senior clinician is not available to make the decision? Then it is down to the senior person in charge of that patient at that time. 'Senior' is a very relative concept. In a care home situation this could be a recently qualified nurse on night duty, at home it could be the out of hours or locum doctor. In these situations access to the patient's medical notes and information might be limited and that 'senior' clinician may not be able to or want to make a decision. CPR is commenced, an ambulance is called, and the person is sent to hospital. Is there always time and the ability during this process to contact family or discuss with members of a multidisciplinary team? Even if the senior clinician is the one to make the final decision, it does not mean they have to be the one to lead the discussion: any health or social care professionals involved in the patient's care can take the lead, particularly as the patient may raise the subject with someone who they feel they trust, but who cannot make the final decision.

Blanket policies are no longer legal or ethical, because where a person lives or is cared for in a certain setting should not influence whether or not it is appropriate for them to receive CPR.

Senior clinicians must act as strong and supportive leaders and work effectively with their teams. The Joint Statement (BMA et al.) describes that once the senior clinician has made the decision this should be supported by their senior colleagues. Circumstances and subsequent decisions often do change e.g. other treatment might reverse the immediate physical condition and improve the chance of CPR being effective. Senior clinicians must accept responsibility but there must not be a culture of blame. Every decision and every consequence of that decision must be professionally managed. This does not stop actions to investigate and address clinical negligence or unprofessionalism.

CPR and ACP for the end of life

This chapter has already considered aspects of CPR in the context of ACP. Other chapters go into detail about the changes in law in England and Wales with the advent of the Mental Capacity Act (26) which enshrines the patient at the centre of the decision-making process. It formalizes what was already being done by many good health and social care professionals, considering what the patient/person themselves wants. ACP and end of life decision-making translates into opportunities for the patient as well as the professional to say what they would, or would not like to happen.

Again other contributors in this book describe in detail the components of ACP including making advance statements and advance decisions to refuse treatments. The views and decisions of a patient can then be recorded. The formalization and strengthening of a person's right to make a valid advance decision to refuse even life sustaining treatment such as CPR trumps any other decision maker.

This chapter has already described the role of the patient in a CPR decision and where it is ethical and also practical to include them in this process. If the patient has capacity and is voluntarily willing to make a decision to refuse CPR an ADRT should be made, not a DNAR. DNAR should only be used when the clinician for transparent reasons has to impose such a decision on a patient (e.g. for a patient who has no mental capacity to make this specific decision, no valid and applicable ADRT, or no legal proxy). The DNAR should be made with the involvement of the multidisciplinary team if there is time and as part of a best interest's assessment.

The new legal statues and existing laws on confidentiality can generate new challenges. The person with capacity can make an end of life decision and stipulate that this decision has been made in the strictest confidence and at the exclusion of other people close to the patient e.g. family. Again the responsibility associated with these new powers lies squarely on the shoulders of the decision maker, the patient. Professionals cannot break confidence but they can offer ongoing support and advice that might address any underlying interpersonal differences to facilitate a future discussion by the patient when they are ready.

Where there is consent, active or strongly implied ACP only really works effectively when key people are told of the plan including that the patient is dying and that CPR will not be successful. Otherwise family carers, however much they recognize the person is dying, may still ring the emergency services at the point of death because they think CPR is the norm. Health or social care professionals should not make assumptions that others will recognize the person/relative is dying. It is important that professionals use the 'd' (dying/death) word when talking with them.

Facilitating resuscitation decisions

No matter what the stage of the decision-making process, the patient's best interests should be uppermost at all times, not the professionals', or family carers'. Therefore when deciding about CPR decisions, it is not enough to talk to the family carers to see what they want. Patients should always be consulted first, and they could have someone with them if they wish. It is best to establish early on before results of important discussions need to take place. By asking, 'Are you the sort of person who likes to know what is going on? If so, would you like anyone with you when we discuss things with you, and who would you like this to be?' This means professionals can plan ahead to meet these requests.

So, once you know the decision-making process there are certain phrases and questions which may be useful when discussing CPR with patients and/or their representatives. One way to approach any such discussion is to use a model for breaking bad news. My personal favourite is the model used by Buckman et al. (27) available here http://theoncologist.alphamedpress.org/cgi/content/full/5/4/302. It is called the SPIKES model and is easy to understand and follow. Buckman stated that a person who was good at breaking bad news was someone who got it wrong less often: therefore it is important to remember that there will be times when leading such a conversation will never go as you would like: this does not mean that you have done anything wrong, simply that the news given has been difficult for the receiver(s) of that news to comprehend. The SPIKES model represents:

Setting up the interview

Perception: This is where the patient (or their nominated representative's) perception of what is going on is discussed

Invitation: It is important to see if the patient still wants to know the full picture

Knowledge: this is where the patient is told the information

Emotions

Summary: a summary of the next step should be given.

SPIKES and other techniques are discussed in Chapter 23.

Reviewing the decision

The guidelines simply state that the decision should be reviewed regularly. Some professionals choose to do this at a set time, but I feel it should be reviewed according to that patient's condition. Whenever they are seen by a healthcare professional it should be reviewed. If that decision changes it needs to be communicated to those concerned and anyone recipient of the previous decision.

Case History

Janice is a 55 year old lady with metastatic breast cancer. She is now bedbound and being cared for at home by her husband. She is weak and frail, and has a chest infection. When the district nurse next visits, Janice asks whether CPR will make her feel better than she does at present: her sister is travelling to see her from Australia and will arrive in three days and Janice wants to be around to see her. The nurse sits with Janice and goes through the situation with her, using the SPIKES model. It is clear that although Janice knows she is dying she thinks CPR will still be given, will be successful, and will make her feel better than she does now. The nurse gently explains that because Janice is so unwell, CPR would not be appropriate now, and that it is more important she receives good care. The nurse also explains that CPR does not improve someone's condition, and in Janice's situation it would not be successful. Janice is very upset, but the nurse sits with her and her husband and listens to her distress and concerns. Janice wants a second opinion so the nurse contacts the GP, who discusses it with the palliative care consultant who has been involved in her care. The nurse lets Janice talk to the GP on the phone, and he also listens to her concerns (the nurse does not want to leave the house until the decision is discussed fully, as she realizes something may happen before she next visits). The nurse documents the decision on a DNAR form, and communicates it verbally with all those involved once she is back in the car, and then faxes a copy to everyone once she is back in the office.

Although this may seem impossible to achieve because of the time element involved, it is certainly something which professionals, not just nurses, can do. The nurse followed the SPIKES model and in summary made sure everyone else knew the situation and that the form was left in the house where it could be easily seen. She allowed Janice's distress but did not back down from the decision made. She even allowed a second opinion and made sure the senior person in charge of Janice's care made the final decision, i.e. the GP. This means that Janice has every possibility of staying at home and of not receiving inappropriate CPR, which would be undignified and distressing to her husband.

Conclusion

It can be seen that CPR decisions may be complex and highly emotive. But by following the correct decision-making process, by not using false reassurance, and by being honest and direct, CPR decisions can be made appropirately. This can result in the patient having a dignified, and a good death.

Further resources

Gold Standards Framework 'Thinking Ahead' document: available from Gold Standards Framework website: http://www.goldstandardsframework.nhs.uk/AdvanceCarePlanning/ACPandGSF (accessed 24 June 2010).

References

1 Miller DL, Gorbein JG, Simbartl et al. (1993). Factors influencing physicians in recommending in-hospital cardiopulmonary resuscitation. *Archives of Internal Medicine*, **13**:1999–2003.

2 Ghusan HF, Teasdale TA, and Shelley JR (1995). Limiting treatment in nursing homes: knowledge and attitudes among medical directors. *Journal of the American Geriatrics Society*, **41**:SA65.

3 Wagg A, Kinirons M, and Stewart K (1995). Cardiopulmonary resuscitation: doctors and nurses expect too much. *Journal of the Royal College of Physicians*, **239**:20–24.

4 Ewer MS, Kish SK, Martin CG, Price KJ, and Feeley TW (2001). Characteristics of cardiac arrest in cancer patients as a predictor after CPR. *Cancer*, **92**:1905–1912.

5 Bains J (1998). From serving the living to raising the dead: the making of cardiac resuscitation. *Social Science and Medicine*, **47**:1341–1349.

6 Lo B (1991). Unanswered questions about DNR orders (Editorial) *JAMA: Journal of the American Medical Association*, **265**:1874–75.

7 LeVack P(2002). *Making Judgements Based on the Concept of Futility*. NCPC, London.

8 American Thoracic Society (1991). Withholding and withdrawing life-sustaining therapy. *Annals of Internal Medicine*, **115**:478–85.

9 British Medical Association (BMA), Royal College of Nursing (RCN), Resuscitation Council (UK) (RCUK) (2007) *Decisions Relating to Cardiopulmonary Resuscitation. A joint Statement from the British Medical Association, the Resuscitation Council (UK) and the Royal College of Nursing,* BMA, RCUK, RCN, London.

10 National Council for Palliative Care (NPCP) (2002) *Ethical Decision-Making in Palliative Care. Artificial Hydration for People Who are Terminally Ill.* NCPC, London.

11 Regnard C and Randall F (2005). A framework for making advance decisions on resuscitation. *Clinical Medicine*, **5**:354–60.

12 Department of Health (1991). *The Patient's Charter*, DOH, London.

13 McGrath RB (1987). In-house cardiopulmonary resuscitation after a quarter of a century. *Annals of Emergency Medicine*, **16**(12):1365–68.

14 Vitelli C, Cooper C, Rogatko A, and Brennan M (1991). Cardiopulmonary resuscitation and the patient with cancer. *Journal of Clinical Oncology*, **9**:111–115.

15 Karetsky PE, Karetsky M, and Brandsetter RD (1987). Cardiopulmonary resuscitation in intensive care unit and non-intensive care unit patients. *Archives of Internal Medicine*, **155**:1277–80.

16 Varon J, Walsh GL, Marik PE, and Fronum RE (1998). Should a cancer patient be resuscitated following an in-hospital cardiac arrest. *Resuscitation*, **36**:165–68.

17 Wallace K, Ewer MS, Price KJ, and Feeley TW (2002). Outcomes and cost implications of cardiopulmonary resuscitation in the medical intensive care unit of a comprehensive cancer centre. *Supportive Care Cancer*, **10**:425–29.

18 Sandroni C, Nolan J, Cavallaro F, and Antonelli M (2007). In-hospital cardiac arrest: incidence, prognosis and possible measures to improve survival. *Intensive Care Medicine*, **33**:237–45.

19 Nolan JP, Laver SR, Welch CA et al. (2007). Outcome following admission to UK intensive care units after cardiac arrest: a secondary analysis of the ICNARC Case Mix Programme Database. *Anaesthesia*, **62**:1207–1216.

20 National Council for Palliative Care (NCPC) (2003) *CPR: Policies in Action: Proceedings of a Seminar to Inform best Practice with CPR Policies within Palliative Care.* NCPC, London.

21 Negovsky VA, Gurvitch AM (1995). Post-resuscitation disease: a nosological entity. Its reality and significance. *Resuscitation*, **30**(1):23–27.

22 Ballew K (1997) *Advanced Life Support Course Sub-Committee of the Resuscitation Council (UK).* Resuscitation Council (UK), London.

23 Newman R (2002). Developing guidelines for resuscitation in palliative care. *European Journal of Palliative Care*, **9**:60–63.

24 Saunders J (2001). Perspectives on CPT: resuscitation or resurrection? *Clinical Medicine,* **1**:457–60.

25 Jevon P (1999). Do not resuscitate orders: the issues. *Nursing Standard,* **13**:44–46.

26 Department of Constitutional Affairs (2005). *The Mental Capacity Act,* DCA, London.

27 Buckman R, Baile W, Lenzi R et al. (2000). SPIKES- a six-step protocol for delivering bad news: application to the patient with cancer. *The Oncologist,* **5**:(4)302–311.

Section 3

The UK experience of ACP: what's happening now?

Chapter 11

Preferred priorities for care: an Advance Care Planning process

Les Storey and Adrienne Betteley

'By putting the patient and carer at the centre of the plan it is hoped that autonomy and control are fostered—factors that many patients perceive as being taken away from them during the terminal stages of disease.'
Storey et al. 2003

This chapter includes:

+ Background and summary of the preferred priorities for care (PPC) document
+ Evaluation and benefit of using PPC
+ Case histories and scenarios
+ Education, training, and mentoring
+ Having the conversation and communication skills
+ Suggestion for getting started with PPC and conclusion.

Key Points

+ PPC is an example of an Advance Care Planning document used to identify an individual's preferences and wishes at the end of life.
+ It can be regularly updated and is held by the individual and can be taken with them if they receive care in different settings.
+ It consists of three main questions providing information about choices, preferences, others involved in care, and what matters to the person that can inform others involved in their care.
+ It can be used to plan further care; (with consent) to share information with appropriate professionals; to provide evidence of patient's wishes should they lose capacity; and to support decisions which may be made with a person's best interest.
+ It has been used since 2007 in England, in various settings, with ongoing evaluation and training resources.

What is the Preferred Priorities of Care (PPC) tool?

Background

Preferred Priorities for Care, formerly known as Preferred Place of Care was originally developed by the Lancashire and South Cumbria Cancer Network as an attempt to evaluate the Community Nurse Education programme (1). However, it was found that the name placed a focus on the place which was inappropriate and did not reflect the value of the tool, so it was revised and renamed as 'Preferred Priorities for Care' in 2008.

Originally PPCs were primarily used in the community by cancer patients who had capacity to contribute to decisions about their end of life care, and were initiated by either community nurses or palliative care nurse specialists. In 2007 it was supported by the NHS End of Life Care Programme, along with Liverpool Care Pathway and Gold Standards Framework, as an example of an Advance Care Planning tool (2). Now PPC is being used in acute organ failure, learning disability, dementia, frail elderly, chronic obstructive pulmonary disease, motor neurone disease, and other neurological conditions in settings as diverse as residential care homes, acute hospitals, hospices, hospice at home, and social work departments in the NHS, private, and voluntary sectors.

The PPC document consists essentially of three open questions, allowing plenty of scope for clarification as part of the Advance Care Planning Process. These questions are:

1 In relation to your health what has been happening to you

2 What are your preferences and priorities for your future care

3 Where would you like to be cared for in the future.

PPC and Advance Care Planning

The Mental Capacity Act (DCA 2005) and the need to develop robust Advance Care Planning processes prompted the need to revise the layout and make minor amendments to the content of the PPC.

The Mental Capacity Act makes it clear that an individual must be involved as far as possible in decision making processes about their care unless it is proved that they lack the mental capacity to do so (3,4). This prompted a revision of the PPC following wide consultation, and the production of guidance by the NHS End of Life Care Programme (5).

Evaluation of PPC

From our experience of working with PPC for over four years and through the development of an evaluation strategy for PPC it is apparent that the process has benefit to individuals, their families and carers, and to health and social care professionals. Specifically the explicit recording of wishes using PPC has been found to result in more people receiving care in their place of choice (6,7). Feedback from areas across the country where PPC has been positive (see Case Study 1).

Case Study 1

In a pilot in Essex, Newton (8) reported that practitioners thought

When the document was introduced to us our feelings at the time were...

'anxiety, trepidation, a good idea, but worried about the extra work involved'

'mixed initially, thinking it was potentially another paperwork exercise'

When we started to use the document we discovered that...

'it was less time-consuming than we thought and the patients were quite positive about it'

'it was a lot easier than anticipated, and provided a way to discuss difficult subjects'

Our experience with patients and families has been…

'some patients were very happy to discuss details, and felt reassured their feelings were known and sent to the necessary members of the multidisciplinary team'

'families have been grateful that their loved ones were able to end their final days in their place of choice'

Using the document has affected our practice in that…

'it encourages open discussion with patient and families and they feel more in control'

'it has resulted in improved relationships with patients'

'we have an early opportunity to discuss patients' wishes'

We have made the decision to continue using the document because…

'it helps improve the quality of care given to our palliative care patients'

'it helps to improve trust with patients and carers'

'it has enabled our patients to be empowered'

Case Study 2

A is 75 year old gentleman who lives with his wife suffers from motor neurone disease. His wife is his main carer, and he has three children who do not live at home but are supportive. He has two carers every evening, day care at the local hospice once per week, and also accesses respite care at the hospice when necessary. The district nurse visits weekly, and he is supported by his GP.

When asked

'In relation to your illness what has been happening to you?' he replied:

'I was diagnosed with MND in May 1987. My symptoms have been slowly progressive over intervening years, predominantly affecting my limbs, but recently with progressive weakness of respiratory muscles and speech, also affecting swallowing. I have lost weight, particularly over the last 12 months.

Have you had any particular thoughts about your care? What would you like or not like to happen?

'I would like to be looked after at home until 'the end'' (his wife wanted to support him in this). In the event of a critical episode, 'I do not want to go to hospital but would want treatment of symptoms with my breathing space kit drugs. I would not want to be intubated or defibrillated'

Place of care: choices

'Primarily at home with my family. If this proved difficult in terms of my wife being able to cope or my symptoms were not relieved then I would prefer to be at the Hospice'.

Death occurred in the place of his choice (home), supported by his wife and family.

Case Study 3

Mrs Y was an 84 year old lady with carcinomatosis. She had recently had several visits to the local hospital, and was very weary of the time in hospital and anxious not to have further treatment there. She was very pleased to complete a Preferred Place of Care document stating that she did not want to be moved 'I wish to stay here for the remainder of my life!'

The community team had not yet faxed the Notice to the multidisciplinary team to notify them of this, when shortly afterwards she contracted a urinary tract infection, and was generally unwell, and slightly confused. As she lived alone, the team contacted the out of hours medical service, concerned about her comfort at home. The ambulance crew was requested to take her into hospital. When they arrived, the crew noticed the Preferred Place of Care document in the home and were informed by her nephew that she was adamant that she wanted to stay at home. Mrs Y, although confused, was able to reinforce this. The ambulance crew realized that she was near to death, and as they had been informed about the document's existence and purpose, they were able to leave Mrs Y where she was, and she died peacefully in her own home a few hours later (8).

Case Study 4

Using PPC to avoid admission from A and E

Mr F had a PPC which was logged with A and E. When he was admitted to A and E the staff were aware of his wishes without him having to wave it around and protest that he wanted to go home. He was seen by the medical staff, the problems dealt with and he went home the same day. This clearly demonstrates the importance of communication between professionals for the person's wishes to be recognized without dispute. It also shows that having an Advance Care Plan or PPC does not preclude going to hospital and being treated for an acute episode and going home again.

Using PPC to facilitate difficult discussions between partners

A patient who lived alone but had good support from his partner completed his PPC with help from the district nurses. We left it with him to discuss with his partner who visited him daily. He had thought that she would care for him at the end of his life. When she read the PPC she realized this and they discussed it fully and changed his preferred place to the hospice if possible. He didn't really have any contact with any other family members and it would've been a lot for his partner to cope with. She explained that she didn't feel able to manage on her own. He had support from hospice at home and the district nurses, visiting the day hospice weekly. He became unwell and was admitted to the hospital where he passed away peacefully. I like this because although the man does not achieve his preferred place of care, the document does facilitate discussion, dialogue, negotiation and communication. To me this is what the PPC is all about. It helped the two people to understand each other's point of view, and come to a mutually agreeable conclusion. He didn't die resenting her attitude and she did not need to feel guilty. It demonstrates the PPC being realistic!

Education, training, and mentorship

Although Advance Care Planning is increasingly used and PPC is now in the public domain health professionals may still require education and training on its use for best implementation. The process of ACP is still heavily reliant upon a health or social care professional initiating the discussion, and this in turn begs the question of whether those staff have the confidence or the necessary skills to have the sensitive conversations related to Advance Care Planning discussions.

A three day training course in ACP was developed in Lancashire and South Cumbria covering such enhanced communication skills and other such courses are widely used across the country (9).

In other areas, where resources are scarcer, training is delivered in differing ways and very often ad hoc.

In general the training needs for staff initiating ACP or PPC discussions include:

- How to have the conversation that leads to initiating the ACP/PPC discussion
- Understanding the document and it's implications in light of the Mental Capacity Act
- Knowledge of the process i.e. how to access the document, and audit.

How to have the conversation

A common problem in palliative and end of life care for health professionals is that of facing difficult conversations around death and dying. Lawton and Carroll (10) suggest that health professionals are more likely to discuss issues around death and dying when the patient asks a direct question such as 'how long do you think I have got?' The National End of Life Care Programme team found that 'confidence levels and communication skills are variable amongst health and social care professionals, and that the lack of openness and honesty with patients around death and dying often hinders good quality end of life care' (11).

In an ideal world, all staff who may be likely to initiate an ACP/PPC discussion would be able to undertake an enhanced communication skills training course including training on how to use the tool in practice. However, this would be extremely costly and is unfeasible in practice.

Some communication skills aids are included in Appendix 2

Case Study 5: Example of a workshop, 1

Jane is well known to you. She has previously talked very openly about having cancer and that one day she will die from this. You have previously completed a PPC with her and noted that she is open about her diagnosis and what she wants.

The second question was also completed when you both discussed her wishes, what she wanted and didn't want. She wanted to pursue all investigations until she was told that her death was now imminent and that at this point she would accept her fate fully.

She had made very clear that she wished to die at home, whatever the circumstances. You noted that the family supported her wishes.

Sometime later, Jane has spent 2 weeks in the hospice for respite care and further investigations of her deterioration. She has deteriorated considerably and the hospice staff contact you because she has requested a discharge home to die.

You begin to make plans for this when you receive a telephone call from the family saying that they cannot manage and that they think it is inappropriate to discharge a dying patient from a hospice.

When you visit the hospice to see the patient and inform the staff of the family's reaction Jane asks you to help her to fulfil her request to die at home. Only one family member supports Jane at this point.

Discuss how you could deal with this.

◆ What factors may be influencing the family's current feelings?

◆ Is it appropriate for the family to decide place of care?

◆ Should anyone else be involved in the decision making process and if so who?

◆ Would it be appropriate to share the PPC document with the family?

Case Study 6: Example of a workshop, 2

Mary is an 86 year old lady who has been a widow for the past 20 years and has one son who lives locally but only visits on occasion to do some shopping for his mother. Mary has no other family, has no support from friends or neighbours but has twice daily visits from a Care Agency funded by Social Services. She lives in a one bedroom bungalow in a small town.

Mary was discharged from the local District General Hospital where she has been diagnosed with breast cancer and multiple metastases and told that there was nothing more they could do for her. On the previous day the GP had been called out by the home care assistant who was worried that Mary's pain was not adequately controlled. When he visited he was very concerned about the fact that she was living alone. He had suggested a nursing home to Mary but she said that she was going to stay where she was and was not going back to hospital again either. The GP was concerned about Mary and referred her to the Macmillan Nurses /D/N symptom monitoring and discussed care options.

Following discussions in your groups please explore the following questions:

◆ When would have been an appropriate time to initiate a discussion using a PPC?

◆ Who would be the most appropriate person to undertake this discussion?

◆ How would you open the discussion?

◆ Who needs to be informed of the outcome of the PPC discussion?

◆ What processes could be put in place to inform people of the outcome of the PPC discussion?

◆ What review process would you put in place?

Suggestions for getting started with PPC

♦ Set up a group to look at implementation locally e.g. involving district nurses, community matron, Macmillan nurse, out of hours services, GP lead, ambulance service, Social Services, hospice staff, care home staff, hospital representation

♦ How will staff access the PPC document? Will it be from a central point or for staff to download from the internet at *www.endoflifecareforadults.nhs.uk/eolc/files/F2110-Preferred_ Priorities_for_Care_V2_Dec2007.pdf*

♦ Will there be a way of monitoring the numbers of documents distributed? Will place of death be monitored? Are audit systems in place within the organization to use data generated to plan care delivery within the locality

♦ Useful to have a place on the out of hours (OOH) handover form to say 'has the person got a PPC?—yes or no'

♦ Link in with education, get PPC on the agenda e.g. prereg courses, training departments, palliative care courses

♦ Ask for it to be put on the agenda of all the GP practices' GSF meetings

♦ Organize raising awareness sessions i.e. grand round

♦ When flyers and posters are produced, have these put up in key places such as GP waiting rooms

♦ Workshops for staff who will be using the document, could involve Specialist Palliative Care team and do interactive demonstration showing how to initiate the conversation as well as basic overview of PPC and a walk through the document.

Conclusion

The PPC is an example of an ACP tool used by an increasing number of individuals in England that has obvious benefits for patients, their families and their health providers. It is clear that using this form of ACP, patients and carers are being included in the decision making process. Families are involved in the decision making process and inappropriate hospital admissions have been averted, nurses have been empowered to challenge decisions about transferring residents for futile interventions and residents have expressed appreciation for being able to record their wishes in a document that can be shared with others.

> For me there is a realization that this document empowers us all. It enables professionals to talk freely about a choice that an individual makes and enables freedom to develop and move teams forward. It assists with coming to terms with choice by communicating, informing and sharing information and the whole idea of collaborative working comes together to enhance the end of life experience of our patients. Tracy Reed (district nurse).

> By opening up discussions with our patients we are in a unique position to help alleviate some of these overwhelming feelings and to help with the transition through to that final destination. The relationships we build when caring for people with palliative and end of life care needs are vital. The PPC can assist with creating an air of openness, honesty and trust. We only have the one opportunity to get this right; assisting people to achieve their final destination in their preferred place is one of the last things we can do for those within our care (Sherwin, 2008) (12).

Acknowledgements

Ann Howard and Chris Pemberton for their significant guidance, leadership, and professional contribution to the development of the original PPC

Community Nurses in Lancashire and South Cumbria who participated in the pilot and implementation of PPC, especially Andrea Docherty

Celia Rhodes (RIP) for her help in developing the Enhanced Communication Skills Course

Mary Turner and Julie Foster for picking up the PPC torch and carrying it forward

David Clark, Mary Turner, and Iris Fineberg for taking up the challenge of evaluating PPC

Justin Wood for initiating the first audit of PPC in Lancashire

Pauline Callagher for promoting the use of PPC for people living with MND

Cathryn Greaves for using PPC with renal failure patients

Jenny Newton, Eleanor Sherwin, and Tracy Reed on West Essex for their resilience in introducing PPC outside of Lancashire and South Cumbria

For all health and social care practitioners who have provided an opportunity for their patients and their families to have a say in their end of life care

And last, but definitely not least, Claire Henry and the National End of Life Care Programme Team for their support in promoting PPC as an Advance Care Plan.

References

1 Storey L, O'Donnell L, and Howard A (2002). Developing palliative care practice in the community. *Nursing Standard*, **18**(8):40–42.

2 End of Life Care Programme (2006). *Advance Care Planning*. NHS End of Life Care Programme. (www.endoflifecareforadults.nhs.uk)

3 Department for Constitutional Affairs. Mental Capacity Act 2005. DCA, London.

4 National Council for Palliative Care (2005). *Guidance on the Mental Capacity Act 2005*. NCPC, London.

5 Department of Health (2004). National End of Life Care Programme. http://www.dh.gov.uk/en/ Healthcare/Longtermconditions/Long-termNeurologicalConditionsNSF/DH_4132992

6 Wood J, Storey L, and Clark D (2007). Preferred place of care: an analysis of the 'first 100' patient assessments. *Palliative Medicine*, **21**:449–450.

7 Storey L, Wood J, and Clarke D (2006). An Evaluation Strategy for Preferred Place of Care. *Progress in Palliative Care*, **14**(3):20–123.

8 Newton J (2006). Management and Outcome of a Preferred Place of Care pilot. *Nursing Times*, **102**(42):32–33.

9 Turner M (2008). Research and Evaluation of PPC, unpublished paper.

10 Lawton S and Carroll D (2005). Professional Development: Communication skills and district nurses: examples in palliative care. *British Journal of Community Nursing*, **10**(3):134–136.

11 Department of Health (2008). End of Life Care Strategy: *Promoting high quality care for all adults at the end of life*. DH, London.

12 Sherwin E (2008). *Preferred Place of Care:West Essex audit results*. West Essex Primary Care Trust.

Chapter 12

Experience of use of Advance Care Planning in care homes

Deborah Holman, Nikki Sawkins, and Jo Hockley

High quality care that incorporates user choice and involvement is a priority for care delivery in care homes. The current emphasis is to transform health and social care through the development of a personalized approach to the delivery of adult care. How care is planned, among staff, residents and relatives in care homes, creates the foundation upon which care planning at times of serious illness, or at the end of life, is based. (1)

This chapter includes:
- The care home setting
- Aspects that have an impact on use of Advanced Care Planning (ACP) in care homes
- Examples of issues
- Use of ACP in the GSF Care Homes Training Programme
- ACP with dementia patients
- Changing care home culture
- Ways forward and recommendations

Key points
- ACP discussions are especially important for residents in care homes in order to clarify and implement wishes and preferences for end of life care.
- Admission to a care home is a key trigger for initiating an ACP discussion.
- Our view is that ACP should become part of mainstream practice in all care homes and offered to all residents. It is our experience that with support and training, care homes can achieve this goal.
- Care homes lead the way in their extensive use of ACP discussions. ACP is routinely used by care home staff than is often recognized, and can be easier to introduce in care homes than in other settings.
- Key challenges for residents include poor means of communication due to dementia/cognitive impairment or physical deterioration.

◆ Barriers to holding these discussions include staff resistance, good communication skills, confidence of staff, sensitivity of timing, and a sense of being at ease discussing dying. Other factors include high turnover of staff; language and cultural differences; lack of time and training.

◆ ACP is greatly appreciated by residents and families when done well. It can reduce crisis admissions at the end of life and thus help reduce hospital costs and ensure the care provided is in line with the person's wishes.

◆ ACP is sometimes viewed initially with uncertainty, but with clear and supportive explanation becomes a reassuring experience for all involved.

◆ The Gold Standards Framework in Care Homes (GSFCH) Training Programme supports and recommends routine offering of ACP discussions to all residents as one of the standards that must be achieved for accreditation.

Introduction

Advance Care Planning is important for all, but is of particular significance for older people in care homes to ensure that their choice for care at the end of life is respected. For many this means being treated as an individual with personal choices and preferences accommodated, and being treated with dignity and respect in familiar surroundings in the company of those who are well known to them. This is no less important for people in care homes, many of whom realize that on entering a care home they will be there for the remainder of their life. Discussions about funeral arrangements have always been part of the admission procedure to a care home; however, focusing on the communication about other aspects of future wishes, and wishes at the end of life, are not so common.

However, where ACP has become part of standard practice, as in those care homes using the Gold Standards Framework (GSF) (2), the impact has been considerable. It may not be widely recognized that care homes are a particularly suitable setting for such discussions, and ideally ACP should become mainstream as a normal part of care in all care homes. Staff sometimes struggle with difficulties in holding these discussions, but once trained and supported, they can grow in confidence and this can become a very natural part of their care. Care home staff often look after their residents over a long period of time and develop strong relationships in which ACP discussions can be a natural part. They are ideally placed to discuss issues about wishes, preferences, and future care. As they help explore resident's thoughts and priorities, this can also be a means of understanding people better and thereby providing better care for them, tailored to their individual needs.

This chapter highlights the importance of implementing a consistent policy of ACP for all residents; of developing the competence and confidence of staff in care homes in relation to ACP, in order to impact practice and improve the lives of residents in their care. It describes the context of care homes and some of the difficulties faced by those who would want to develop such practice. The experiences of both the staff in care homes, and the authors, are shared while seeking to draw attention to the importance of both appropriate training and role modelling of ACP in care homes. The implementation of the Gold Standards Framework for Care Homes (GSFCH) training programme (2) is outlined as a vehicle for helping to underpin the principles for ACP in such a setting as care homes.

The care home setting

Over the last 20 years the care home culture has changed significantly. The Community Care Act (1990) emphasized the importance of caring for people in the community with the aim that it would reduce the dependency on secondary health care service provision in geriatric long stay wards. With this change more private sector care homes opened. To date, there are 18 563 registered care homes providing a total of 453 062 placements in England; approximately 22% of these homes provide nursing care and 78% personal care in a residential care setting (3).

The above Act has changed the focus to less trained staff providing the majority of the care with varying degrees of support from visiting GPs. Many residents in care homes have multiple co-morbidities and complex health and social care needs, including 62% with dementia (4). Because of the large numbers of untrained staff caring in care homes, this poses many challenges in ensuring that the appropriate care is given by staff that are skilled and confident. In the light of this, ACP, or planning ahead can be challenging. Many establishments have a high turnover of staff, and there are cultural and language difficulties for staff with English as a second language.

Around 1% of the UK population now live in care homes for older people, either temporarily or as their permanent home; these challenges are sure to increase with increasing longevity. Recent figures show that 17% of deaths amongst the over 65s in the UK occur place in a care home (5).

Aspects that have an impact on the use of ACP in care homes

Rethinking the excessive use of hospitals

Most people are admitted to a care home when they are no longer able to care from themselves or live independently in their own home. For these people the care home becomes their home where they may choose to remain until they die. However, there is accumulating evidence that significant numbers of residents are being transferred from care homes to acute hospitals in the last days or weeks of life, when this is not necessarily their wish, or in their best interests (6). With the lack of or inadequate ACP discussion, and no plan for proactive care, often a crisis results in an inappropriate hospital admission (Fig. 12.1). 50% of frail care homes residents could have died at home.

Some staff have disclosed that they feel vulnerable when discussing residents' future care plans, as hospital care may sometimes appear to be the right option when residents become ill. This radical change in thinking towards preventing avoidable admissions comes as a surprise to some care home staff, who have become used to hospitals being the safety net of care. 'Some people are too sick to go to hospital—the benefits of admissions can be outweighed by the negative impact of admission, especially for people with dementia.'(8) It also requires a greater emphasis towards more proactive planning of care focussed on the individuals expressed preferences and wishes. This is in line with the trend towards more personalized care.

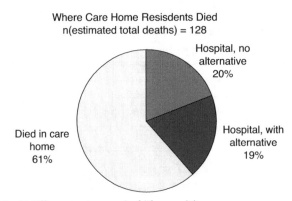

Fig. 12.1 National Audit Office report on end of life care (7).

Cultural differences

Some care homes, particularly in city areas of the UK, have a large multicultural component not only among the staff but also among the residents. Many staff have their own pre-conceptions about the benefit of hospital care, and their own fears and phobias about death and dying. Some have admitted that when they came to work in a care home they were not aware that they would be caring for the dying. This then puts them in a challenging situation when faced with a dying person and even more so when faced with the idea of having to talk about it with residents in the form of Advance Care Planning.

Personal experiences of staff

Many staff who care for the dying in care homes have experienced bereavement themselves and some aspects of their role can become powerful triggers to their own unresolved or newly experienced grief. Staff may feel that they are managing well, but grief by its very nature can 'highjack' a person leaving them overwhelmed and unable to cope. One staff member from Southern India spoke about her own father who had died in the family home and was buried before she was even told that he had died. Many continue at work out of necessity but acknowledge when asked that their own grief does impact their work.

Communication issues

Communication is at the heart of end life care. Talking about death and dying can be difficult for professionals as well as for patients and their carers, but asking patients and noting where they would like to be cared for, and developing an ACP at the earliest available opportunity, is recommended good practice for every resident.

An ACP discussion might include the individual's concerns; their important values or personal goals for care; their understanding about their illness and prognosis; and their preferences for types of care or treatment that may be beneficial in the future. It should be documented and regularly reviewed and communicated to key persons involved in their care. Expressing these wishes at an early stage following admission to the care home increases the chances that they will be fulfilled.

In some instances, with residents who have been living in the care home for many years, approaching a conversation about their advance care wishes towards the end of life can prove more difficult than doing this for each new resident on admission. Staff do need to approach ACP discussions for current residents slightly differently. Informing them and their relatives that this is a new generic policy introduced to improve care for everyone in the home, and that it does not imply impending deterioration or death, can help allay their possible concerns.

The most common reason given by care home staff for not wanting to initiate discussion is that 'they do not know what to say'. Many qualified staff fear answering difficult questions, so when a family member asks 'Is my mother/father dying?' many do not feel they can answer truthfully even though their professional assessment suggests that the person may be within a few days of dying. In our work with staff in care homes, we have found that they regularly express three main fears:

- the fear of making it happen: a self fulfilling prophesy fear
- the fear of upsetting residents and families: some did not have the courage of their convictions using the excuse that it was not their responsibility to give this type of information
- the fear of being misunderstood or misquoted.

With the considerable turnover of staff both at management level and in the general workforce, there is a constant need to ensure that new staff (both nurses and care assistants) are fully aware of ACP discussions. Specific palliative care induction is important for all new staff alongside developing advanced communication skills.

ACP: whose role is it?

In our experience running the GSF Care Homes training programme for over 1000 care homes, we affirm the importance of every staff member being able to handle such opportunistic discussions, but we suggest the home nominates the best people to begin these ACP discussions initially. Many suggest that one of the senior nurses should undertake this conversation, when they have received some training and feel confident in doing so, but others prefer the named nurse or carer for that resident to take the lead, as they are building on a good relationship with the resident.

However, we were delighted to discover that many prefer to support families to have these discussions themselves before admission to the care home and before the ACP discussion with care home staff. Families who are visiting the care home before admission, or later following admission of the resident are informed that holding such discussions is part of the usual procedure within the home and are given an information leaflet to describe what this might mean for them. Many homes write their own introduction to ACP or use the 'Planning for your future care' leaflet from the NHS End of life care programme in England (9). This then helps families feel more at ease in discussing the issues relating to the future care of their relative and can in many ways lead to very special and deeper discussions that otherwise they would have found hard to initiate. This helps to de-medicalize the whole area, bringing it back to essentially being a discussion about living well now, best care, and preferences for the future. Of course some find this difficult and would prefer either not to discuss it at all or for the discussion to be initiated by the senior staff—and of course that is completely acceptable. Some homes have in fact developed a few key questions before this discussion to assess whether the resident might wish to discuss these things or might refuse, and they also record the fact that ACP discussions have been offered and declined or later reviewed on an ACP review sheet.

ACP discussions between an individual resident, a staff member, and usually a relative; are intended to make clear a resident's personal wishes, preferences, beliefs, and values and offers an opportunity for them to say where they would wish to be cared for. It gives them the chance to express their preferences about the kind of care they would like to receive and, even more importantly, how they would like to live their life until the end.

Even if this choice is limited, as when people's previous homes have been sold, it is still important to have the conversation. Some professionals have found it difficult to know when to broach the subject. For obvious reasons, it is best to do so when the resident's health is relatively stable, and not when they are in crisis. It is usually not best to have the discussion at the first meeting but once the person is more settled in the home. Discussions should be recorded in such a way that the resident's wishes and priorities can be reviewed and, with their permission, shared with key people involved in their care, e.g. using one of the ACP tools available (see appendix 2).

DNAR discussions

There can be some confusion about the Do Not Attempt Resuscitation (DNAR) discussions, which are not strictly part of the ACP discussion, as they are related to a refusal of treatment, but can obviously form part of the conversation. This subject does need to be discussed and to be recorded to prevent inappropriate resuscitations attempts. There is now strong evidence of the futility of attempted cardiopulmonary resuscitation in care homes and the extremely minimal chances of success (10). Some may feel there should be a blanket DNAR policy in care homes where there is negligible chance of successful resuscitation. This would help to prevent the inappropriate emergency ambulance call outs, futile attempts at resuscitation, and undignified scenes that distress family, residents, and staff alike. However, an 'Allow Natural Death' policy) (11) is a positive approach where the emphasis is on treating reversible conditions rather than emphasizing the negative DNAR status. This is usually well received and can prevent inappropriate crises when all staff are aware of the policy.

Case Study

An emergency '999' call followed the sudden collapse of an 86 year old lady who was a resident of a care home in rural Norfolk. The home was many miles from the nearest hospital so resulted in the air ambulance being called to aid in the attempt of resuscitation. The helicopter landed on the front lawn of the care home, the emergency team attempted resuscitation, but this failed and the patient was taken to the nearest hospital classified as 'Brought in Dead'. This lady had stated previously if anything happened she 'didn't want any heroics'—a comment which was not explored further with her, recorded, or communicated to others. In the circumstances this lack of communication of her DNAR status had resulted in an undignified death, traumatized family and staff and an inappropriate use of a scarce expensive resources. The staff and the primary care team later reflected on the management and death of this resident, using the Significant Event Analysis template (what went well, what didn't go so well, what could be done better) and agreed as an action point that in future ACP and DNAR discussions in the care home would be offered to every resident, recorded, and communicated appropriately to emergency and out of hours services, to prevent a similar catastrophic event occurring again. This later became mainstreamed and adopted through local policy.

If the resuscitation discussion does proceed, or when having any discussion about medical decisions, it is vital that the resident and, if involved, the relatives have the information they need as to the risks and benefits of resuscitation, so they are able to make an informed decision. Care home staff often lack confidence about discussing medical decisions directly with residents or relatives, in case their words are misconstrued and lead to litigation. Staff tend therefore to have discussions with the GP, or to invite families to complete a questionnaire on behalf of residents.

When asked to indicate how important they felt it was for residents to be consulted about their wishes if their condition deteriorated 80% of care home managers reported that they thought it was very important. However the presence of documented wishes or decisions in care homes did not appeared to support this (1).

ACP in the GSFCH programme

During the GSFCH training programme the theme of ACP runs through all aspects of the training and is mentioned in all four workshops of the programme, and is one of the key 'must do' factors for the accreditation process. It is pivotal in ensuring that the more personalized aspects of care are delivered, not just in discussing care in the final stage of life, but also in clarifying more about how the person wants to live.

A summary of the GSFCH training programme is in Box 12.1, the work is supported with materials, DVDs, the Good Practice Guide, and a before and after 'After Death Analysis' (ADA) Audit (12).

> Introducing Advance Care Planning into our home as normal practice has been one of the most important things we have done—it's crucial to helping us focus on the needs of residents, it helps discussions with families and it changes the way we do everything. Even though it may be hard at first, we would very strongly recommend it for every care home.
>
> Care home matron GSF Phase 3

Box 12.1 The Gold Standards Framework in Care Homes (GSFCH) programme

The Gold Standards Framework in Care Homes Programme grew out of the work of GSF in primary care, but is quite independent of it, with a separately evolved training programme tailored specifically to meet the needs of care homes' staff that has been running since 2004. It is now the most widely used training programme in end of life care. Used by care homes across the UK over 1000 care homes from all parts of the country are now included, with about 100 being accredited each year. The programme is run by the GSF central team but integrated into local areas with facilitator support, and now incorporates the grass roots experience and examples of excellence from this large number of care homes as they care for people nearing the end of their lives.

The programme has three aims:

1 To improve the quality of care provided for all residents from admission

2 To improve the collaboration with GPs, primary care teams, and specialists

3 To reduce the hospitalization of residents, especially in the final stage of life, enabling more to die at home if that is their wish.

Key elements include:

♦ A three stage quality improvement process with preparation and training stage in the first year plus consolidation leading to accreditation

♦ The GSFCH accreditation process 'Going for Gold', managed by Omega, the National association for End of Life Care and supported by Help the Aged/Age Concern, ensures quality assurance using an independent validated process, and leads to many benefits for accredited care homes

♦ A key feature of the training programme is the offering of ACP discussions to all residents with recording of refusal and regular reviewing

♦ It integrates well and leads on to use of other tools used by the NHS End of Life Care Programme e.g. the Liverpool Care Pathway/Care Pathway for the final days and the Preferred Priorities of Care (see Chapter 11) or other Advance Care Planning tools

♦ The work is strongly peer lead and supported, using detailed showcased examples of ways that homes have integrated the work to improve care and practical examples of best practice

♦ It is now evolved into a standardized curriculum and programme, using many resources and DVDs, with a train the trainers cascade process, tailored to meet the needs of local areas

♦ It was initially geared towards nursing homes but also includes residential care homes, learning and physical disability homes, and others.

The GSFCH Programme can be separately commissioned from the National GSF Centre—see Briefing Paper on *www.goldstandardsframework.nhs.uk* or email info@goldstandardsframe-work.co.uk

ACP guidance has been developed both for general usage (13) and for people with dementia (14). The implementation of the Gold Standards Framework (GSF) training programme, adapted and designed for care home staff, has contributed greatly to the ACP process through teaching, and sharing experience and examples in practice. It has helped develop skills in communication with useful prompts and guidance through such documents as the GSFCH 'Thinking Ahead' document or Preferred Priorities for Care tool (PPC) (15). Focusing on the implementation of ACP into practice is one of the key elements of GSFCH and a key standard that has to be achieved for accreditation and receipt of the GSFCH Quality Hallmark Award.

There have been many homes who have completed the Gold Standards Framework training programme where these challenges have been overcome and progress has been made with Advance Care Planning.

Training on Advance Care Planning within the GSF care homes training programme

Workshop 1

+ An introduction and definition of ACP and Advance Decision to Refuse Treatment (ADRT) and the Do Not Attempt Resuscitation (DNAR) or Allow Natural Death (AND) discussions. Affirmation of the importance of seeking the views of residents and communicating to others.

+ A DVD clip of a resident describing her experience of her Advance Care Plan and what it means to her and her family, gives a strong message of how important it is to residents that their wishes are respected.

+ The 'needs based coding' of all residents related to their trajectory of illness linked to the GSF needs support matrices, ensures that the right thing happens at the right time and the right place. Advance Care Planning discussions are commenced when a resident enters the home and are reviewed throughout their care.

Workshop 2

+ Advance Care Planning forms a key topic of this workshop along with means to reduce hospitalization. Further description of communication skills required and the use of the GSF *Thinking ahead* document or other ACP tool is described.

+ 'Gold fish bowl teaching' or role play is utilized, highlighting the importance of good communication skills. The importance of the effective use of role play, although feared by many, enables care staff to actively participate in example scenarios. It also enables them to recognize how useful such an exercise can be in identifying the main issues that people discuss when undertaking ACP conversations.

+ Scenarios can be used in small group discussions as a useful resource.

+ The importance of preparation of themselves as staff for this conversation, the environment, and the resident/family is also covered during this workshop.

+ Sometimes staff build on this to hold other training days on ACP in their home or at a nearby education centre or hospice.

Workshop 3

+ Speed dating sessions with staff from other care homes enables them to feedback on how they have got on since the previous workshop, sharing their experiences with others and ways that they might have overcome challenges and found solutions in practice.

♦ We concentrate here on the difficult discussions as people approach the last days of life, the importance of language used, e.g. using the word 'dying' to avoid confusion over the use of 'poorly' with relatives, enabling care staff to explore ways of improving the communication with residents and relatives at this difficult time.

♦ At this point, the ACP helps to facilitate discussion with relatives and increases the likelihood that the resident's wishes are fulfilled. The workshop encourages again, a linking of the situation with the needs based coding and the needs support matrix.

♦ ACP discussions can also lead into deeper discussions of a more spiritual nature related to the values and priorities of the person and what makes them the person they are. This can include religious manifestations, but is related to the person's inner life and core spirituality.

Workshop 4

♦ This brings all aspects of care together, linking the benefits of ACP discussions with improving the quality of care and reducing avoidable admissions.

♦ The key topic is a focus on Dementia Care, including 'Best Interest Decisions' with those with cognitive impairment who lack capacity to make decisions about their future care. Use of ACP for dementia patients is included.

Consolidation leading to the Accreditation stage

♦ The ACP standard for accreditation states 'An Advance Care Planning (ACP) discussion is offered and recorded for all residents, and may include discussion with their families'.

♦ Accreditation involves self assessment against twenty standards, evidence of attainment in a portfolio, a further After Death Audit (ADA) and an independent visit to the care home by a GSF trained Visitor.

♦ A review sheet helps assessors confirm that ACP is offered to all residents (though some refuse), and keeps a note of review dates.

♦ All findings are reviewed and judged by an independent panel. Then if the standard is achieved the Quality Hallmark Award is given to accredited care homes.

Gold Standards Framework and Advance Care Plan discussion information is part of the admission process and is routinely completed at the six week review, when they have settled in and once trust has been developed. The qualified key worker is responsible for completing the ACP, which is in the resident's file ready to be completed. We have found this to be a successful strategy and greatly assists in the provision of good end of life care

(Matron from GSFCH accredited home 2009)

Box 12.2 Guidance Notes on completing the GSF Advance Care Plan: thinking ahead (16)

1 **At this time in your life what is it that makes you happy?**
   ♦ What do you hope for? What do you enjoy doing?
   ♦ What or who is really important to you?
   ♦ Is there anyone you're especially worried about?
   ♦ Has your illness changed the ways you can get close to people you care about?

Box 12.2 Guidance Notes on completing the GSF Advance Care Plan: thinking ahead (16) *(continued)*

2 **What elements of care are important to you and what would you like to happen in the future?**

- Statements of wishes and preferences can include personal preferences, such as where one would wish to live, having a shower rather than a bath, or wanting to sleep with the light on. Such statements may also include requests and/or types of medical treatment they would or would not want to receive.

- Sometimes people may have views about treatments they do not wish to receive but do not want to formalize these views as an advance decision.

- Discussion should focus on the views of the individual, although they may wish to invite their carer or another close family member or friend to participate.

- Some families are likely to have discussed preferences and would welcome an approach to share this discussion.

3 **Is there anything that you worry about or fear happening? What would you not want to happen?**

- What worries you most about your illness?

- Can you help me understand a bit better?

- What else would help you cope?

- What is helping most at the moment?

- Has being ill made any difference to what you believe in?

- Do you find yourself thinking about what is going to happen to you?

- Are there things that bother you that you find yourself dwelling on?

- Know when you have reached the limits of your knowledge.

- Normalizing can help e.g. 'Many people feel like you'.

4 **Ending difficult conversations but enabling ongoing discussion later**

- Acknowledge emotional intensity of conversation e.g. 'We've talked about a lot of important things today'.

- Help the person to rehearse what they need to do, who to talk to?

- Try and close the conversation on a positive note.

- End conversation in a safe place for them—refer to everyday, practical topics.

- 'What you have said is very important, can we continue this tomorrow?'

- 'Unfortunately I have to leave in five minutes and this is a very important conversation; is there anything else you want to say?'

Examples of questions to ask in Advance Care Planning discussions (17)

- Can you tell me about your current illness and how you are feeling?
- Could you tell me what the most important things are to you at the moment?
- Who is the most significant person in your life?
- What fears or worries, if any do you have about the future?
- In thinking about the future, have you thought about where you would prefer to be cared for as your illness gets worse?
- What would give you the most comfort when your life draws to a close?

Changing care home culture

In a survey of current practice of ACP in care homes for older people a number of areas were considered. These included looking at the process of ACP for residents, the attitudes of managers, how staff were prepared and trained, what factors influenced the process and models of good practice currently in use. Findings from this survey recommended that there was a need for staff development and a wider multiprofessional approach to ACP.

Consideration, other than just training, needs to be taken into account when looking at the most effective way to change practice in care homes. Varying working patterns, particularly where there is no internal rotation of staff, can make capturing all staff for training difficult. High staff turnover can make selection for particular training difficult, especially if the cascade model is used, as those who may access it then leave. The requirement for staff to fulfil statutory training i.e. moving and handling, infection control, can also make it difficult to include extra training around subjects like ACP.

Training the workforce

ACP discussions in a nursing home are led by nurses. Some nurses may have been able to access training, but in a care home providing personal care to residents, this is carried out by the care staff who have had no formalized training. The level of confidence and skills of the workforce reflects the ability of the staff to fulfil this aspect of the GSFCH programme when it is first introduced.

Many staff cited their lack of understanding of the Mental Capacity Act (18) or fear of 'communicating a difficult subject' as a reason to hold back. Therefore breaking ACP down into a process of learning may help dispel their fears. Whilst teaching communication skills is very important, it cannot be done effectively in isolation of end of life care needs. Due to the multicultural context of the care home environment it is very easy for both staff and residents to misunderstand what is being communicated, either through the words used or the tone of voice in which it is said. Often staff do not fully understand the concept of the use of 'open' and 'closed' questions. Sometimes they do not recognize the need to pause after an open question which seeks to elicit thoughts, feelings, and opinions.

It is also important to remember the value of opportunistic conversations. Health care assistants (HCAs) that deliver most of the 'hands on' care are best placed to know the resident's preferences and choices. However, they often perceive themselves to be the least qualified to facilitate end of life care conversations, and as such their contribution to ACP is undervalued. With training HCAs begin to recognize their part in the ACP process and realize that for them it is not about

Box 12.3 A note about Advance Care Planning in dementia

Many of the best practice points generally applicable to Advance Care Planning (ACP) discussions will apply to people with dementia but in addition there are others that need to be taken into account:

Skilled interviewer

Those undertaking ACP with people with dementia will need to have appropriate knowledge and skills to understand the issues in communication in dementia.

The right time

As with all ACP discussions they need to be held at the right time but in dementia these discussions need to be held early on in the illness when the person still has the capacity, cognition, and language to hold meaningful discussions and make informed decisions. Ideally the ACP discussions in dementia should be part of supportive post diagnostic counselling processes within e.g. a memory clinic.

The right place

People with dementia often have visuospatial problems that are associated with their dementia so it is important to hold the discussions in a quiet and unthreatening place with no distractions of noise and interruptions that can hinder their concentration.

Involvement of family

Once a person no longer is deemed and assessed to have capacity, decisions will need to be made in their 'best interest' and the Mental Capacity Act framework for determining best interest applied (see Chapter 8). A Lasting Power of Attorney (LPA) with appropriate authority (Personal Welfare) may be empowered to make decisions on the behalf of a person with dementia based on their knowledge of the person and on what they believe the person would or would not have wanted for themselves.

Take time

People with dementia will require more time for any ACP discussions; these may need to be done over some period of time with some repetition and clarification.

Scenarios

People with dementia may need examples of situations which they need to consider in making an ACP; e.g. Clinical vignettes illustrating cardiac resuscitation or PEG feeding for example for them to conceptualize and apply to their own situation. This has been done using pictures, video clips, and narratives.

Life Story

Much information that is of relevance to developing an ACP can be gained from undertaking Life Story work with people with dementia. Family members can be involved in this work also.

Recording

When a person with dementia does not have the capacity to undertake ACP a note should be made in the ACP document of who was involved in the discussion (e.g. as in the Gold Standard 'Thinking ahead' document). It should be noted that due to cognitive impairment most information was obtained from a named relative/other rather than the person with dementia.

(Karen Harrison Denning, Consultant Admiral Nurse)

their knowledge base as much as about their communication skills in everyday work and the ability to pick up on cues and listen.

The simple learning tool, using the mnemonic SATNAV (19) was developed initially as a teaching tool for GPs and district nurses to help facilitate ACP conversations (see appendix 2). It has proven to be a useful way of helping care home staff to build on their communication approach.

Staff have highlighted that there are two different approaches needed toward ACP in care homes. Whilst introducing the conversation to a new resident has its own difficulties, introducing the subject to those residents who have been in the home for a long period brings its own set of issues. The kind of response staff have been met with is typified by 'Am I dying then?' which initially caught them off guard not knowing how to answer.

Staff who feel that they have communicated well and attempted ACP successfully with residents become more confident at further attempts. They report how residents have commented following an ACP discussion, 'they know what I want when the time comes... I want to be here; with my family with me... they know this is what I want'. Staff measure their 'success' by comments from families who in the bereavement phase comment on how helpful and supportive it was to be 'more prepared' about what might happen. Feedback from residents and families appears to have a great affect on staff confidence and staff moral. Where the death is deemed to be peaceful and comfortable, in the place of choice, and families feel well supported and informed, staff respond with renewed enthusiasm to continue to develop the practice of ACP in their home.

Caring for people with dementia (see Box 12.3)

Staff who care for residents with dementia have difficulty in ascertaining wishes and preferences, especially for those residents who have no family. They also spoke of difficulties that arose when GPs are reluctant to make advanced decisions. Staff are well aware of unnecessary distress that can be caused by sending a person with dementia out of their environment to the hospital and are in many cases keen to have advanced discussions documented. Staff speak of their own distress and powerlessness at seeing residents with dementia being sent to hospital in the last 48 hours of life because of lack of documentation relating to resuscitation status.

ACP discussions can be very helpful for people with dementia (14). Such decisions can take place even though the individual may have quite advanced dementia, as long as they have capacity—the ability to understand and speculate about the decision to be made. Evidence suggests that people with early dementia are interested in participating in ACP discussions, and that they make similar decisions to people without dementia. Therefore we should not hold back from asking people with dementia their views.

Case illustration of ACP and dementia

Marie

Marie received a diagnosis of Alzheimer's disease in the memory clinic. She and her husband Greg, her main support and carer, were referred to the Admiral Nurse Service for post diagnostic support and counselling. Part of this intervention involved discussions about Marie's wishes and priorities, preparing for a time when she may no longer able to express these.

These discussions took place over several weeks; after the initial meeting within the memory clinic all other meetings took place in their home. Marie and Greg felt more comfortable and less pressured when talking about ACP in their own home. The Admiral Nurse introduced both Marie and Greg to the concept of ACP by showing them and talking through various examples of ACP documentation.

Initial discussions involved life story work; through this they were able to articulate what was important to them both, those things that it may be important to know when they are no longer able to communicate such themselves. Both Marie and Greg stated things they 'didn't want to happen' so later on in the sessions the Admiral Nurse expanded the discussions to consider advance decisions to refuse treatment by the introduction of various clinical situations where an ACP would be useful in expressing wishes and priorities e.g. artificial nutrition and hydration.

Whilst the initial intention was to offer Marie the opportunity to consider an ACP for a time when she no longer had the cognition, capacity, or language to do so, both she and Greg went on to develop ACPs and registered them with their GP and solicitor and provided copies to their children.

Developing a learning culture in care homes

Learning in care homes requires a multifaceted approach. Staff may have a wide variety of learning needs based on age, culture, language, and understanding. Knowing that class room training alone will not change practice (20) it is important that this is not the only method employed.

Experience has shown that when trained staff can role model good practice, as a method of learning, staff confidence increases. Role modelling ACP has been shown to allow staff at all levels to sit in on conversations and allow them to contribute at a level they feel comfortable with. It also helps them to feel more comfortable with pauses for silence and expressions of emotions knowing that they are not the only other person in the room.

Care home staff are often undervalued as a group of workers, and yet we have high expectations of them to provide well coordinated person-centred care with often minimal access to training and supervision. The standards of care we expect when caring for all people, particularly those that are vulnerable are high and yet the investment in the carer workforce is disappointing.

The GSFCH programme creates an opportunity to introduce the concept of reflection in practice into care homes using the Significant Event Analysis tool (SEA). This tool is a simple, yet very effective tool to help address issues that arise out of significant events. By asking the three questions 'what worked well?' 'what didn't go well?' and 'what could we have done better or differently?' staff are given a guide to begin talking and hopefully resolving some concerns around their own thoughts, feelings, and practice. This is encouraged to be done both individually and as a team. Some homes produce a small leaflet to enable any member of staff to give their personal reflections on the death of a resident, as a joint process. This is particularly appreciated by night staff and non-trained staff.

A systematic approach to learning that acknowledges and reflects on events should be encouraged in care homes so that after each death in the home staff are given the opportunity to voice their own disquiet.

Conclusion

Advance Care Planning can work well in care homes and can lead to great benefits for residents, relatives and staff. Staff can be supported and trained to learn new skills and grow in confidence to hold such discussions, and additional experiential training days in communication skills required for ACP discussions can be very helpful for all staff.

The GSFCH training programme is a tool that can enable care to be of a 'gold standard' all of the time. It is part of the process in developing a culture where 'this is what we do' becomes the norm. It is an important part of 'raising the level of care to the level of the best'. Coming together at the GSFCH workshops enables the sharing of problems, ideas, good practice, and solutions to many of the challenges this sector of care provision faces on a day to day basis.

The implementation of ACP is one of the key elements to good end of life care, enabling people to 'live well until they die'. This therefore needs to become part of every day practice with staff that are confident with the difficult discussions they have with residents, relatives, and others around end of life care and approaching death. We have explored some of the issues that present challenges in the care home setting such as, access to training etc, building the skills and confidence that are needed to have an effective and meaningful conversation with people approaching the end of their lives.

Recording and communication of ACP discussion should become routine practice in care homes to enable residents to live out the final stages as well as possible, reduce inappropriate hospitalization or intervention, and enable the possibility of greater openness and deeper communication between them and those close to them. Further training is required to support staff to integrate this as normal practice into their homes and to have the skills to undertake these discussions.

The offer of an Advance Care Plan discussion with all residents in any setting is paramount if we are to provide choice of where and how people are cared for and wish to die. If we can get this embedded into every day practice then it is more likely to be achieved. All these aspects can be considered when implementing GSF into everyday practice. To change this in a wider context, there needs to be a greater willingness of all involved to address the needs of improving communication skills, improve collaborative working, and reconsider their documentation process.

> When having the ACP discussion he expressed the fear of going to an unfamiliar place like hospital and his wish to remain with us for the final days of his life. His wishes were established, communicated to others, and were achieved. We all felt satisfied that we had accomplished his wishes for care at the end.
>
> (GSFCH accredited care home 2008, Round 3)

Case study: Transcript of clip from an interview with Iris an elderly resident from a care home, as part of the GSF Care Homes Training Programme

Interviewer	And one of the things that your care home is very good at is the Advance Care Planning.
Iris	That's right.
Interviewer	… which some people find a little bit difficult to talk about. But could you talk to me about the Advance Care Planning?
Iris	I have an Advance Care Plan—with matron we've made one out. She spoke to me about it and said did I mind telling her what I wanted and for my funeral. I said 'I don't mind at all'. So we've made out a complete plan. She knows exactly what I want, and when it does happen I would like to be here when it happens, with my family with me.
Interviewer	And making the Advance Care Plan I guess gives you the power to put those things in place?
Iris	Oh yes, that's right.
	So that she'll be able to do exactly what I hoped for.
Interviewer	And have you discussed that with your family as well?
Iris	Yes. Oh yes, my family know all about it also. They're quite happy with it.

References

1   Froggatt K, Vaughan S, Bernard C, and Wild D (2009). ACP in care homes for older people: an English perspective. *Palliative Medicine*, **23**:332–338.

2   Thomas K and Sawkins N (2009). Gold Standards Framework in Care Homes Good Practice Guide. www.goldstandardsframework.nhs.uk

3   NAO (2008). National Audit Office–End of life care: care home survey results. http://www.nao.org.uk/publications/0708/end_of_life_care.aspx (accessed May 2009).

4   Matthews F and Dening T (2002). Prevalence of dementia in institutional care. *Lancet*, **360**(9328): 25–226.

5   Tebbit P (2008). *Capacity to Care: a data analysis and discussion of the capacity and function of care homes as providers of end of life care.* National Council for Palliative Care. Available from NCPC, London.

6   DH (2008). *End of Life Care Strategy: promoting high quality of care for all adults at the end of life.* Department of Health. Available from: www.dh.gov.uk/publications

7   National audit Office report on End of Life Care Nov 2008. www.nao.org.uk/publications/0708/end_of_life_care.aspx

8   Keri Thomas. *Introduction to the GSF Care Homes training programme.* www.goldstandardsframework.nhs.uk

9   Planning for your future care: a guide. NHS End of Life Care Programme March 2009 www.endoflifecareforadults.nhs.uk

10   *BMJ* DNAR paper to add

11   Goldstandards framework. *Allow Natural Death policy* p47 In the GSF CH Good Practice Guide Sept 09 GSF, UK.

12   The After Death Analysis- www.omega.net.uk

13   Henry C and Seymore J (2007). *Advance Care Planning: A Guide for Health and Social Care staff.* Department of Health, London

14   National Council for Palliative Care (2009). *Out of the Shadows. End of Life Care for people with dementia* NCPC, London.

15   Storey L (2007). Preferred Priorities of Care Documentation. Available from: http://www.endoflifecareforadults.nhs.uk/eolc/ppc.htm

16   Thomas K, Sawkins N, and Holman D. The GSF Care Homes Training programme Good Practice Guide Phases 6/7

17   Horne, G., Seymour J.E. and Shepherd, K (2006). *International Journal of Palliative Nursing*, **12**(4): 172–178.

18   Mental Capacity Act 2005. The Stationary Office, London.

19   Holman D (2009). Personal communication. St Christopher's Hospice. London. SE26

20   Froggatt K (2006). Evaluating a palliative care education project in nursing homes. *International Journal of Palliative Nursing*, **6**(3):140–146.

Chapter 13

Advance Care Planning in the community

Bruce Mason, Dierdra Sives, and Scott A Murray

'It's very fulfilling because it's general practice as I probably
thought it would be when I was a raw recruit as a doctor you
know sort of being a family friend as well as a medical
professional.'
A general practitioner

This chapter includes:

◆ An overview of issues surrounding Advance Care Planning (ACP) in the community

◆ When should you to start ACP in the community? Which patients, when, and who should
be involved?

◆ The barriers to ACP in the community and how to overcome them

◆ Outcomes and benefits for patients, carers, and practitioners; what are they, how can we
measure them, and how can we be sure we have achieved them?

Key points

◆ ACP should be used in the community for patients with all progressive illnesses

◆ ACP should be commenced as early as the patient wishes, but certain trigger are
suggested

◆ Various people may initiate ACP discussions in the community

◆ There are significant barriers to the widespread use of ACP in the community such as staff
resistance, difficulty identifying the appropriate time, time pressures etc

◆ The greatest enabling factor in ACP is a pre-existing relationship between patient and
health care professional

◆ Patients, family carers, and professionals all stand to benefit from better use of ACP
discussions.

An overview of issues surrounding ACP in the community

Until recently, GPs have generally been unaware of ACP and understood end of life care as a series
of progressions from palliative care to terminal care. Research, anecdotal evidence, and what scant
UK studies there are on the subject, indicates that ACP as it is usually defined, has only recently
begun to be practised by GPs in the UK. This does not mean that GPs are not engaged in helping
patients cope; rather what it appears they are doing is having ad-hoc, usually rather reactive

discussions often based on a 'planning for dying' approach rather than living well until dying well. GPs have always had such 'difficult discussions' with patients near the end of life, but this has not previously been formalized into an Advance Care Planning discussion when options, reflections, and preferences may be clarified and openly discussed. With increasing awareness of the requirement to meet patient's needs and preferences, and the recognition that the first step in meeting these needs is to ask the patient, the impetus to clarify such thoughts through more formalized ACP discussions is a key part of the growing momentum of end of life care in this country.

Conversely, Palliative Care Clinical Nurse Specialists (CNSs) working in the community setting perceive ACP as an intrinsic part of their role. They perceive ACP to be an interactive process: maintaining hope is very important while at the same time undertaking discussions about future decline. They generally adopt a patient-centred approach which is individualized and patient led. The timing of these conversations is unique to each individual with nurses accepting that for a small number of patients and families these discussions may not be possible despite their attempts to facilitate them. The current documentation and subsequent communication between professionals of these sensitive conversations tends to be poor, and probably does not reflect all the interactions and nuances involved.

In general, it appears to be the case that ACP is mainly known and practised in the community by specialists, or GPs, or community nurses with a special interest in palliative care. Furthermore what the professionals regard as ACP may often be quite different from what advocates for ACP think it should be. There is little evidence that ACP has been practised in primary care in the UK (1). An extensive literature review by the Royal College of Physicians led them to conclude that although 60–90% of the UK public appears to be broadly in favour of ACP when it is explained to them only around 8% of the public in England and Wales had completed an 'ACP document of any kind.'(1)

Most of the research evidence for the efficacy of ACP in the community comes from North America where an ACP process of some kind has often been required by health insurance providers (see Chapter 17 USA). Whilst some studies do affirm that patients value the opportunity to discuss their future care at a time when they feel well, others were less clear, suggesting that as patients (2) become more ill they may go through lengthy periods of being reluctant to discuss such issues or, simply, not know what to ask about (3–6). There is little understanding of the impact of cross-cultural considerations in ACP in multicultural societies (7).

Some in the USA working in primary care have described scepticism about the merits of ACP and have shown particular concerns about starting 'too early' and overly formalizing the process (8). At the same time, studies have shown that professionals of all types including nurses are often uncertain about their abilities in conducting ACP (9). Finally a matched study of patients and their physicians showed that communication at end of life was only effective around fairly straightforward factual issues (10).

The research evidence, nascent though it is, indicates that there are several challenges to conducting community-based ACP. Difficulties in coordinating care can lead to professionals having incomplete knowledge of a patient's needs and practical difficulties in sharing their knowledge of the patient with other services. The usual pressures of time and resources make conducting a time-intensive activity like ACP particularly difficult, and changing social demographics as well as changing employment practices can make building the necessary relationships between professionals, patients, and carers extremely difficult (11). In addition, the ways in which different types of progressive illness and trajectories of decline need to be addressed in ACP are still poorly understood. Yet the research also indicates that the opportunity to plan future care is valued by patients and carers, and their primary care team would appear to be exactly the professionals best placed to deliver it. Therefore, the value of undertaking such discussions for patients may appear to outweigh its detractors, so in the rest of this chapter, we will spell out some of the issues involved in trying to develop ACP in the community.

Which patients?

All people with a progressive life-threatening illness are likely to benefit from planning ahead at the end of life (12). Thus care planning should be considered not just for people with cancer, but with any life threatening condition and many patients and their carers would really like the opportunity to plan ahead.

But how can such people be identified in the community so that ACP can be considered and discussed? Work done in the USA describing patterns of physical decline at the end of life suggest that the clinical course of patients with eventually fatal chronic illnesses appears to follow three main patterns (13,14). These trajectories provide a way to identify in primary care large and discernable groups of people with similar service needs and barriers to reliably high quality end of life care which ACP can address (Fig. 13.1).

The first trajectory or pattern of decline is the maintenance of good function until a short period of relatively predictable acute decline in the last weeks or months of life: progressive cancer typifies this. The second trajectory, with slow decline punctuated by dramatic exacerbations any of which might end in sudden death is seen more typically in organ failure such as in end-stage chronic obstructive pulmonary disease and in heart failure. The third trajectory is poor long term functional status with slow decline, and elderly patients with dementia, frailty, or multiple co-morbidities fit into this category (15). The GSF Primary Care Programme, suggested in 2005 a breakdown of these into the following: a GP with 2000 patients on average each year will have

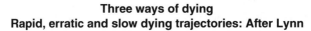

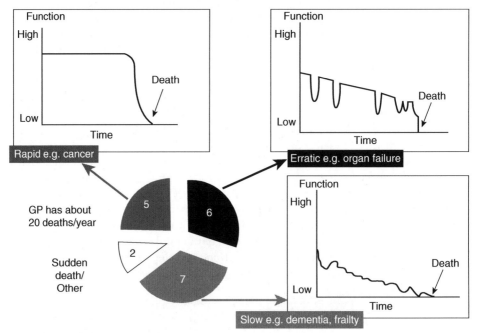

Fig. 13.1 Pie-chart showing typical numbers of deaths for typical GP.

around 20 deaths; five of these are from cancer, about six may be from organ failure and seven or more from the dementia or frailty trajectory. This proportion is increasing, so frailty, multimorbidity is today's biggest killer. Only one or two per year die following an acute event, so sudden unexpected deaths are rare. Thus ACP is relevant in possibly 90% of deaths, but predicting and identifying which patients are in the final years of life is the greatest challenge, particularly for those with multimorbidity and frailty.

In the community we are well placed with electronic records of patients and routine multidisciplinary meetings to identify patients who will benefit with ACP by considering these three groups, and try to recruit patients from each of these trajectories to practice supportive/palliative care registers. People with frailty have a longer period of time when they would benefit from supportive care than the other groups and yet this group of elderly patients are most commonly not involved in ACP discussions, unless of course they enter a care home where this has become normal practice (see Chapter 12). In conclusion, being included on the supportive/palliative care register is a good trigger for considering ACP discussions, and this could therefore become part of standardized good care for all patients nearing the end of life.

When should you to start ACP in the community?

Research increasingly shows that most patients facing death from cancer and conditions such as renal failure and heart failure value the opportunity to discuss the future, although doctors and nurses often hesitate to raise the subject for fear that the patient might lose hope (16). How can we help patients discuss this issue if they want to, and when should we consider trying? Relying on waiting for an exact prognosis to share with the patient is futile, as estimating prognosis is difficult in most illnesses. Ideally, care planning may start even before supportive and palliative care is needed, and is encouraged in long-term illnesses and more recently in 'survivorship planning' for cancer patients.

However, understanding and considering possible likely illness trajectories may help professionals take on board earlier, that progressive deterioration and death are inevitable, and to consider when it is useful to try to begin ACP discussions. Patients and carers also may find understanding their illness trajectory helpful, as they attempt to gain control over their illness by acquiring knowledge about how it is likely to progress (17–19).

General predictive triggers described in the GSF Prognostic Indicator Guidance can also be considered, and the 'surprise question' is proving useful. Looking for specific events such as emergency admission to hospital for organ failure, or admission to a care home to identify for frail elderly people can be used to trigger a care plan. More detailed clinical criteria are given to help identify people with specific conditions who are likely to benefit from extra supportive and palliative care. It is suggested that this guidance and use of the surprise question might trigger patients to be included on the practice palliative care register, and also ensure that every patient on the register is offered such a discussion. Without the clarity of such a systematic approach, many patients might not be able to benefit from better organized care as they near the end of life and might not be given the chance to express their wishes, choices, and preferences in such a discussion. Such discussions may be refused, but opening the space for them is important.

Who should be involved in ACP discussions?

The initiation of an ACP conversation may be most appropriate with the health professional who knows the patient well and this is likely to be someone in Primary Care. There is a need to individualize the process and listen to the patient's story. However to be able to make decisions much of the information being sought by patients requires knowledge of the illness trajectory and in patients with a complex disease a good understanding of likely future scenarios, and this may require more specialist knowledge. In community palliative care, patients and carers initiated conversations with those professionals with whom they felt they had established rapport and trust. Most of these conversations took place in their home away from busy hospital/clinic environments. Patients and health professionals perceived this helped these discussions but was not essential. More important was whether the patient perceived the health professional to be comfortable with end of life discussions. In our study of community palliative care nurses we found that the nurses undertook these discussions with patients while at the same time working closely with GP and other specialists to access information. In addition, such discussions must be recorded and appropriate information given to others involved in their care, perhaps through a patient held record, Thinking Ahead documents, etc or through the use of electronic summary care records, which are increasingly used e.g. Patient Care Summary (PCS).

Barriers to ACP in the community

There are various barriers to implementing ACP in the community: from the most broad sociocultural issues to the idiosyncrasies of each practice. These include:

Hope and Fear

One of the most frequently mentioned concerns among health professionals when it comes to discussing end of life care in general and ACP in particular is the fear of 'destroying hope' among patients. Research with patients, however, indicates that patients value the chance to discuss and plan for the future and that ACP can increase not decrease hope, by 'normalizing' life again so that the fear of the unknown can reduce, and pragmatic plans can be initiated (12). Resilience is described by some as maintaining a sense of 'realistic hope' (20) to be able to both 'hope for the best but still prepare for the worst', which therefore can help reduce the crisis activity that might result from the understandable position of denial (16). Additionally, patients suffering from progressive diseases tend to maintain several 'narratives' about the disease and are able to both 'fight' the disease as well as accommodate to its impact and plan for either the best or worst (21). Although extensive research evidence does not yet exist, early indications are that ACP can help improve quality of life by allowing patients who wish to openly discuss their different and often seemingly contradictory attitudes towards their illness and its impact on their life.

Death as a taboo

Discussing death and dying requires confronting deeply held social taboos. Such discussions are assumed to be fraught and emotionally draining for all concerned. Patients report being reluctant to initiate such conversations for fear of upsetting their GP or simply because they don't know which questions to ask, while GPs fear upsetting their patients by bringing up the issue before the patient is ready. The result is that such conversations often don't take place and, if they do, often take place only when events force them. Meanwhile, it falls upon the primary care team to become more proactive in offering to initiate such conversations at an earlier point in a patient's illness journey. GPs and their teams are, however, unlikely to be persuaded to do this unless they can be convinced that patients really are open to these conversations.

The current 'national conversation' to encourage the general public to talk more about death and dying should greatly facilitate ACP. This will take time to change despite current efforts to raise public awareness such as the NCPC Dying Matters Campaign.

GP inexperience

Research has shown that junior GPs, salaried GPs, and GPs who work relatively few clinical hours are all relatively inexperienced in palliative care provision. This leads to something of a chicken-and-egg situation where inexperienced professionals are less likely to become involved in palliative care and, therefore, remain inexperienced. At the same time, changes in professional working and employment practices in primary care may reduce the number of professionals who feel practised enough to undertake palliative care. It is important to note that continuity of care and pre-existing doctor-patient relationships appear to be the greatest facilitators of ACP, something that is challenged if only experienced GPs working many clinical hours feel competent to undertake ACP.

Reductionist thinking: box-ticking vs holistic care

There also appears to be a deep, professional distrust against some of the 'formal' or 'structured' Advance Care Planning among primary health care professionals. In particular, there is a concern about palliative care provision becoming a 'tick-box' activity. The common perception among primary health care professionals is that palliative care requires the kind of holistic care that they are best placed to provide. Therefore, using the suggested ACP tools to trigger open questions, rather than ticking boxes, but then communicating key factors to others can, in many cases, meet both the needs of holistic care but also systematic communication.

Time, resources, and coordination

The major concern that has been expressed to us by GPs is that GPs themselves will lack the time to be able to engage fully in ACP discussions. Some worry that ACP may be used by articulate, well-informed patients in a way that requires so much of the GPs time that their care for patients who are less able to ask for help may be compromised. Further inequalities of care might thus occur unless uptake is promoted especially in the relatively deprived and needy. Also if this information is not communicated to other relevant agencies, this may lead to a lack of coordination.

Taken as a whole, these barriers provide an inter-locking set of obstacles that tend to reinforce each other. Our experience is that addressing just one barrier will, therefore, not result in any increased uptake of ACP. Primary health care teams need to be convinced that ACP is something that patients want and that has a solid research evidence base. ACP itself needs to be reframed as a tool to help patients live well and, where possible, self-manage aspects of their life. Above all, for ACP to be conducted in the community it needs to be properly resourced and enabled, using a systematic approach to recording and communicating it, providing training to staff to improve their skills in communication, and supporting patients and their carers to feel that this is an issue they can discuss with their local family doctors or nurses.

Key areas for further development are therefore:

◆ triggers to identify the right time to discuss this area
◆ training in communication skills around difficult conversation (see case study)
◆ improved information transfer to appropriate others e.g. Locality Register, ePCS, summary care record
◆ self management tools for patients
◆ greater public awareness of the need to raise these issues early, and increased knowledge of ACP, ADRT, and LPoA.

Outcomes and benefits for patients, carers, and practitioners

ACP in the community was first mooted by some as a means of improving patients' chances of dying at home because if this preference is known it is more likely to be attained. However, a more nuanced understanding of ACP is that it should help a patient make choices and be enabled to live as well as possible. In this respect a better way of understanding the effects of ACP would be to understand various qualitative process as well as outcome measures, such as patient and carer perceptions of quality of life, resilience support, and a sense of control and self determination.

ACP in the community may share much with the controversial term 'survivorship planning.'(22) That is to say that planning ahead as a process is an activity that is as relevant to 'fighting' an illness as it is to dealing with that illness's effects on one's life. Understanding ACP in this way opens up the potential to start the process earlier and opens up the possibility for various members of the primary care team to take part in the process. From the practice perspective, ensuring that each patient who has been identified with supportive or palliative care needs has a palliative care summary can help ensure that no patient 'falls through the gaps.' Similarly, ensuring that each patient with a palliative care summary has been offered a care plan should help.

Case study 1

ACP performed by a community nurse specialist (CNS) as part of a research project with a 61 year old lady with metatstatic breast cancer (Mrs S).

Mrs S. lived alone having recently moved to a new area with a supportive family, but not living close by. Divorced; no contact with husband; seen by CNS approximately one month after being diagnosed.

Mrs S describes the ACP discussion, 'We just chatted and I felt better afterwards to know that somebody knew... I think it's probably that only when you start having these conversations that you sort of really decide and find out what options there are.'

The CNS reported that the ACP discussion was '... relatively straightforward because the patient herself was initiating the whole conversation right from the word go.'

Three months later Mrs S is more unwell and there is a clear physical deterioration. The CNS found it difficult to revisit the ACP discussion '... any time I've tried to go back down that route to revisit, there's a kind of stumbling block. I think it's fear. She hopes that she is probably not going towards that deterioration. She is struggling with that.'

This demonstrates the benefit of having early ACP discussion with patients when they are physically not so unwell, and build confidence for patients that their wishes are known by their care team. It also demonstrates the iterative, dynamic nature of the process; revisiting ACP can be complex and challenging as the illness progresses and the patients feels more frightened.

Practical Suggestions

1 Ensure that you have a supportive and palliative care register which is frequently discussed
2 Put into place a mechanism for sharing supportive and palliative care information with other service providers such as out of hours.

Case study 2

Training for palliative care conversations enhances GP/practice nurse confidence

Some conversations in palliative and end of life care can be difficult for clinicians. It seems likely that this is one factor explaining the fact that patients sometimes miss out on potentially helpful consultations. Examples include issues of worsening prognosis (especially in non cancer conditions) and the whole issue of planning in advance for care in the palliative phases of an illness.

Based on this insight, a half day seminar was developed by a team of clinicians interested in improving communication skills for those in primary care known as Effective Professional Interactions (EPI); for more information see EPI *www.effectivepi.co.uk*. This was titled 'Conversations in End-of-Life and Palliative Care'. The seminar was highly interactive and focused on practising difficult conversations with patients. All attendees were given a chance to rehearse clinical conversations and obtain feedback.

The seminar was piloted with two primary care teams in Cumbria. A total of 23 clinicians attended one of the two seminars—mostly GPs and practice/district nurses. 21 attendees gave written semi-structured feedback.

Overall evaluations were very positive (everyone rated the session as either 'good' or 'excellent'). All feedback forms mentioned one or more positive changes that participants were planning in their future clinical practice. In particular, most participants specified or implied increased confidence in broaching and conducting difficult conversations with patients:

e.g. 'Increased confidence with this very challenging topic. It is an interesting idea to see patients' questions as symptoms, rather than always needing immediate answers'.

'Gained increased confidence to have the conversations and a few key phrases (to do so).'

Based on these evaluations, some enhancements were made and this training is now on offer to primary care teams (contact EPI for more information about this seminar).

Case study 3
A GP's experience and the benefit of having an Advanced Care Planning discussion
A middle aged patient saw her GP regularly with a soft tissue tumour. Local excision had failed to cure her and the tumour was slowly progressive. She was a fit woman for her age and developing symptoms were actively managed. She eventually progressed to a tracheostomy and was fed via a PEG. She then started to develop distressful episodes of spontaneous bleeding from the tumour. These were managed by admission to hospital, cautery, and blood transfusions.

After the third such episode, her GP arranged to review her care in a planned consultation with the patient's husband present. She and her husband were asked about her wishes for future care, including her preferred response to further life-threatening bleeding.

She was clear that she did not wish CPR or aggressive intervention, but she did wish to have further transfusions if she recovered from an episode. She stated that her preferred place of death was at home. A number of other wishes for future care were discussed.

The GP wrote the plan in the patient's medical record and the district nursing notes. A letter was written to A and E and to the ambulance service. A letter was written by the GP for the patient to keep and show to any visiting paramedics.

At the next consultation, the patient mentioned her relief at having been able to have this discussion and to make these plans. She died a few weeks later at home having avoided further aggressive intervention. Her husband confirmed that the ACP discussion had been a source of relief to her at the time and that reflecting on it was helping him in his bereavement. (Malcolm Thomas)

Conclusion

This chapter has flagged many problems and offered some practical ways forward. At present, Advance Care Planning in the community is in an early stage of development, research evidence for its effectiveness is partial and successful implementations invariably small scale and, to date, have shown mixed results. In the UK, policy initiatives focused around the provision of higher quality end of life care have recommended ACP without necessarily defining its purpose. Although ACP is a central element of the DH End of Life Care Strategy in England, the Preferred Priorities of Care, and the Gold Standards Framework the barriers preventing its widespread, routine use are significant and mostly still to be overcome.

There are various aspects of ACP in the community though that point the way forwards. Most importantly, ACP can and should be used in the community for all progressive illness, not just cancer. To do this, however, requires practitioners to be aware of the different trajectories for each disease as ACP is not a 'one size fit alls' process (14). ACP also should be seen as an intervention which can be started as early as the patient wishes regardless of where the patient is currently receiving care. This requires community health workers to be aware of the potential for ACP and to understand it as a tool for living well. It also is the case that many people may begin the ACP process from within the community.

Despite its potential there are significant barriers to the widespread use of ACP in the community in the UK and less experience and evidence of effective use in the UK than in other countries (see Chapters 17, 19, and 20). The most successful interventions seem to be those that can identify a routine, regular trigger point to start ACP, as research on care homes indicated. However, making the process routine may draw resistance from some professionals who see the process as 'an art, not an algorithm.'(8) Despite this, it seems that the greatest facilitator to starting ACP is a pre-existing relationship between the patient and health care professionals and it seems also that ACP is a great device for facilitating that relationship; meaning that patients, family, carers, and professionals all stand to benefit. There are great prizes to be won but still much work to be done.

Further resources

National Gold Standards Framework Centre England. *Prognostic indicator guidance paper.* 2008. http://tinyurl.com/r7e3dn (accessed 7 September 2009.)

Primary Palliative Care Research Group, University of Edinburgh. http://www.homepages.ed.ac.uk/smurray1/ (accessed 7 September 2009.)

The Scottish Government. *Living and Dying Well: A national action plan for palliative and end of life care in Scotland.* 2008. http://www.scotland.gov.uk/Publications/2008/10/01091608/0 (accessed 7 September 2009.)

NHS. Advance Care Planning. http://www.endoflifecare.nhs.uk/eolc/acp.htm (accessed 7 September 2009.)

Effective Professional Interactions Training. http://www.effectivepi.co.uk (accessed 7 September 2009)

References

1 Royal college of physicians et al. (2009). *Advance care planning. Concise guidance to good practice.* Report 12. RCP, London.

2 Schickedanz AD, Schillinger D, Landefeld C et al. (2008). A clinical framework for improving advance care planning process: start with patients' self-identified barriers. *JAGS*, **57**:31–39.

3 Hebert RS, Schulz R, Copeland V, andArnold RM (2008). What questions do family caregivers want to discuss with health care providers in order to prepare for the death of a loved one? An ethnographic study of caregivers of patients at end of life. *Journal of Palliative Medicine*, **11**(3):476–83.

4 Norris K, Merriman MP, Curtis JR et al. (2007).Next of kin perspectives on the experience of end-of-life care in a community setting. *Journal of Palliative Medicine*, **10**(5):1101–1115.

5 Curtis JR, Engelberg R, Young JP et al. (2008). An approach to understanding the interaction of hope and desire for explicit prognostic information among individuals with severe chronic obstructive pulmonary disease or advanced cancer. *Journal of Palliative Medicine*, **11**(4):610–20.

6 Steinhauser AE, Christakis NA, Clipp EC et al. (2000). Factors considered important at the end of life by patients, family, physicians, and other care providers. *JAMA: Journal of the American Medical Association*, **284**(19):2476–82.

7 Johnstone MJ and Kanitsaki O (2009). Ethics and Advance Care Planning in a Culturally Diverse Society. *Journal of Transcultural Nursing*. epub. doi://10.1177/1043659609340803

8 Grossman D (2009). Advance care planning is an art, not an algorithm. Editorial. *Cleveland Clinic Journal of Medicine*, **76**(5):287–88.

9 Ceccarelli CM, Castner D, and Haras MS (2008). Advance care planning for patients with chronic kidney disease - why aren't nurses more involved? *Nephrology Nursing Journal*, **35**(6):553–57.

10 DesHarnais S, Carter RE, Hennessy W et al. (2007). Lack of concordance between physician and patient: Reports on end-of-life care discussions. *Journal of Palliative Medicine*, **10**(3):728–40.

11 Miyashita M, Sanjo M, Morita T et al. (2007). Barriers to providing palliative care and priorities for future actions to advance palliative care in Japan: A nationwide expert opinion survey. *Journal of Palliative Medicine*, **10**(2):390–99.

12 Murray S, Sheikh A, and Thomas K (2006). Advanced care planning in primary care. *BMJ*, **333**:868–69.

13 Lunney JR, Lynn J, Foley DS, Lipson S, and Guralnik JM (2003). Patterns of functional decline at the end of life. *JAMA: Journal of the American Medical Association*, **289**:2387–92.

14 Murray SA, Kendall M, Boyd K, and Sheikh A (2005). Illness trajectories and palliative care. Clinical Review. *BMJ*, **330**:1007–11.

15 Lynn J (2008). Reliable comfort and meaningfulness. Making a difference campaign. *BMJ*, **336**:958–59.

16 Davison SN and Simpson C (2006). Hope and advance care planning in patients with end stage renal disease: qualitative interview study. *BMJ*, doi: 10.1136/bmj.38965.626250.55

17 Murray SA, Boyd K, and Sheikh A (2005). Palliative care in chronic illnesses: we need to move from prognostic paralysis to active total care. *BMJ*, **330**:611–12.

18 Coventry PA, Grande GE, Richards DA, and Todd CJ (2005). Prediction of appropriate timing of palliative care for older adults with non-malignant life-threatening disease: a systematic review. *Age Ageing*, **34**:218–27.

19 Glare PA and Sinclair CT (2008). Palliative medicine review: prognostication. *Journal of Palliative Medicine*, **11**:84–103.

20 Monroe B and Oliviere D (2007). Resilience in Palliative Care. A Delivery in Adversity OUP, Oxford.

21 Murray SA, Boyd K, Kendall M, et al. (2002). Dying of lung cancer or cardiac failure: prospective qualitative interview study of patients and their carers in the community. *BMJ*, **325**:929–34.

22 National Coalition for Cancer Survivorship. *Survivorship Care Planning*. Website. Accessed 28 Aug 2009. http://www.canceradvocacy.org/resources/survivorship.html

Chapter 14

ACP in hospice and specialist palliative care

Simon Noble

'There is no second chance to improve the care of the dying patient.'
Hand written post-it note left by predecessor on hospice office wall.

This chapter includes:

An overview of ACP within the hospice or specialist palliative care inpatient setting

- The breadth of ACP amongst the inpatient population
- Barriers to ACP in the hospice
- Triggers for ACP discussions
- Communication issues
- ACP as death approaches.

Key points

- The breadth of ACP reflects the heterogeneous population served by hospices and specialist palliative care units
- ACP is a continuum and may change over several discussions or occur at unplanned moments
- The facilitation of ACP is everyone's responsibility
- Teams should develop a professional culture which recognizes ACP as an integral part of holistic patient assessment. Communication of ACP wishes between professionals within primary care and inpatient units is essential
- Successful ACP requires investment in training, specific communication skills development, and team debriefs.

Introduction

Hospices and specialist palliative care (SPC) inpatient units look after a relatively small proportion of patients with life limiting and terminal disease, yet by definition they are likely to have more complex needs. Likewise, community and acute hospital specialist palliative care teams will be involved in the care of many patients who do not require specialist admission yet have significant needs related to Advance Care Planning (ACP). Patients therefore may be in contact with specialist palliative care services at many key times throughout their illness creating opportunities for such ACP discussions. As the needs of individual patients will vary, so too do the services and resources offered by different palliative care teams. Some may take on a predominantly medical-ized model of care whilst others, especially within the community, may have a predominantly psychosocial focus. Some hospices may have a flourishing complementary therapies service, whilst others may not regard this as a core service. Regardless of the model of care offered by pal-liative care, ACP should be considered an essential and integral aspect of care for every team member. This chapter will focus on the challenges of ACP in the hospice and SPC environment. For the purpose of the chapter and use of space the term hospice shall be used to describe any inpatient unit designed to provide generic or specialist palliative care.

The challenges of ACP discussions in the hospice

In order to effectively facilitate ACP in any environment, one must first understand the barriers and potential obstacles that may prevent its successful execution. The introduction of the most comprehensive ACP policy is likely to be thwarted if such barriers are not considered beforehand and appropriately addressed.

Challenge: 'It's not my responsibility'

Some members of the team may not feel it is their role to be addressing ACP issues. Such views may be generated from a feeling of being unprepared or lacking the skills to discuss issues. They may feel that they are not sufficiently senior in the team hierarchy to be allowed to take on such as role.

Suggested solution

For it to be functional and successful, ACP must be considered to be an essential facet of care for every patient and the responsibility of every member of the team. Everyone needs to be empow-ered to respond to patients' opportunistic prompts for discussions related to their future care. Strong leadership to support the reticent members of the team and encourage their participation is essential. Ongoing references to patients' ACP wishes in team handovers and multidisciplinary meetings will engender a culture of ACP within the unit.

Challenge: 'We do this anyway; this is just introducing more paperwork'

One of the strengths of palliative care is the wealth of experience that healthcare professionals bring to the team which can be a benefit but can also be a barrier. People can sometimes be resist-ant to change especially if there is a perception that 'we have always done it this way'. Further resistance will occur if this change requires, what is seen to be, an increase in paperwork, which further removes practitioners from looking after patients.

Suggested solution

If, as the dissidents say, this is being done informally already then hopefully staff can see the advantages of formalizing the process and are willing to support a venture that improves patient choice and care. The reality is likely to reveal that it isn't in fact being done comprehensively and certainly not documented. Audit of case notes will identify whether ACP discussions are being recorded and also whether teams are able to deliver against the stated needs and preferences of the patient. Staff are more likely to cooperate with changes to documentation if they can see the ben-efits. Therefore, the paperwork (use of ACP tools or documentation) should be integrated into the clinical documentation and contain the most relevant information.

Challenge; paternalism and institutional thinking

Many of us are skilled in empathizing with patients but this can sometimes give us false reassurance that we know more about someone's wishes than we really do. Our experience may lead us to decide what is best for someone, having witnessed similar scenarios before. Whilst well intentioned these approaches can act as barriers to exploring patients' real wishes and enabling them to come to their own decisions. Rapid deterioration of a patient can act as a prompt to pull out all the stops, to get the person to their preferred place of death before it is too late, if we are aware of their preference in the first place.

Suggested solution

The key to addressing paternalism and institutional thinking is to encourage self awareness within the team that such firmly held beliefs may not be the most appropriate for all situations. Reflective practice, is a useful tool to address such behaviours though. This needs to be approached in a safe, non blaming environment and be led by an experienced facilitator. In addition to this approach, the benefits of ACP and the development of a shared understanding and ownership of the process is essential.

Case study 1

Paternalism prevailing: Jackie

Jackie was a 38 year old lady with advanced ovarian cancer and small bowel obstruction due to peritoneal metastases. With maximal pharmacological interventions her nausea was improved and her frequency of vomits limited to once a day. Her partner visited daily with their two young children and was clearly nervous about managing her at home.

Following the MDT meeting it was decided that it would be best for her to remain in the hospice for her final days. She died four days later.

Months following her death her partner shared his sustained feelings of guilt for not taking her home to die. He explained this had always been her wish, but neither of them had mentioned it since the team had told her she would be better remaining in the hospice.

Learning points:

◆ You cannot know a patient's wishes unless you ask

◆ These wishes should be documented and communicated to others within the MDT and to others beyond the team who may be involved at some stage

◆ The partner's expressions of fear of taking her home should be explored rather than taken at face value. Practical support and good liaison with community services might help reduce this understandable fear

◆ Despite our best intentions, we do not always know what is best for our patients, and we can sometimes inadvertently impose our own choices on our patients.

Timing of ACP discussions in the inpatient setting

As discussed earlier, a hospice admission may be for any number of reasons and involve a breadth of diagnoses and prognoses.

An appreciation of this heterogeneity helps us understand that patients may be at different places in their understanding of their prognosis and hence the potential difficulties of timing on ACP discussions. For example, someone who has lived for years with metastatic cancer such as breast or prostate cancer, receiving chemotherapy over several years, may be less inclined to confront their deterioration than someone with advanced lung cancer who has experienced limited active treatment and noticed rapid changes over a short space of time. Likewise, a patient with end stage heart failure or chronic obstructive pulmonary disease (COPD) will have experienced acute exacerbations which have responded to active therapies in the past, though with diminishing benefits, and may find it conceptually difficult to accept that they are deteriorating. While someone with motor neurone disease who has observed progressive deterioration in their respiration, nutrition, and motor function may identify these changes as a prompt for ACP discussions about their future care.

Practitioners need to be mindful that for many patients, this hospice admission will be their first and ACP discussions early on in the admission process may cause distress. We are yet to fully shake off the public perception that 'hospices are where you go to die' or 'once you go in, you are not coming home,' and an early conversation regarding such planning may cement such stereotypes. This is not to say such conversations are off limits; on the contrary, opportunities to explore patient's wishes for their future are at the heart of effective ACP. It is just important to be sensitive to cues that indicate whether discussing preference about future care is something the patient feels ready to address at that time (Box 14.1).

The initiation of ACP discussions is a balancing act between communicating a willingness to talk about wishes without being viewed as pushing the issue. A useful prompt for discussion will be to explore the patient's current understanding of their condition and their expectations of the admission to the hospice. Such questions can be extremely informative if time is given to listen to the responses and facilitate further dialogue. Professionals should resist the urge to 'strike whilst the iron is hot' and delve too deeply on the first conversation. Sometimes such interactions may lead the patient to contemplate issues they were not ready to face yet and cause them to withdraw from future ACP discussions.

It can be difficult for professionals to know when it is most appropriate to raise the issue of ACP. However it is important to be aware that some aspects of ACP may vary within the hospice setting. The patient agenda regarding ACP may extend beyond care in the final days (Box 14.2).

It is important that we respond to the patient's agenda and explore issues that are important to them at the time, and avoid pushing our own items we may feel eager to discuss. The process of ACP should be seen as a progressive and fluid one which can develop over time. Furthermore, the task of ACP may have been initiated in the community already and professionals should be mindful of any planning that is ongoing and to report back significant discussions. Patients may already have ACP discussions recorded with community and hospital or care home staff; if previous records are available this needs to be highlighted and used as a basis for further discussion. Likewise, on discharge, the recorded ACP tool can be sent home with the patient, and this should be communicated in the letter to the GP and hospital team involved with their care.

Box 14.1 An ACP discussion might include

- the individual's concerns and wishes
- their important values or personal goals for care
- their understanding about their illness and prognosis
- their preferences and wishes for types of care or treatment that may be beneficial in the future and the availability of these
- their preferences for place of care in the final stage and other related details.

Box 14.2 ACP discussions may also include

- ◆ Remaining personal goals
  - • Holiday planning
  - • Getting married/attending loved ones wedding
- ◆ Decisions whether to continue with oncological therapies
- ◆ Establishing guardianship of children
- ◆ Legacy work
  - • Memory boxes
  - • Writing wills/power of attorney
  - • Funeral planning

Triggers for discussion

Within primary care the trigger for ACP is likely to be one which signifies that someone's condition is progressing and prognosis less than 12 months. These may include:

- ◆ Worsening of symptoms or evidence of disease progression
- ◆ Significant shift in treatment focus e.g. disease progression despite active treatment
- ◆ Repeated hospital admissions.

These may likewise be triggers for discussions in the hospice setting but others may occur as well such as:

- ◆ The admission itself raising thoughts about the future
- ◆ Major life event e.g. the death of someone they know
- ◆ Following a new diagnosis e.g. new metastases
- ◆ Following a new intervention e.g. PEG feeding or non invasive ventilation in a motor neurone disease patient
- ◆ The news of a deterioration in their condition.

The above triggers are most likely to stimulate ACP discussions but practitioners may use these opportunities to explore remaining goals they wish to achieve. However, such goal planning and legacy work is more likely to arise (if cues are picked up) when discussing personal domains such as family and social issues.

Communication issues

Communication skills of staff

Hospice staff are likely to be skilled in communication issues such as breaking bad news, managing collusion, and handling distress and uncertainty, since these reflect the syllabus of most advanced communication skills training sessions. However, skills in ACP discussions are rarely covered as yet as a specific communication area and as such may be as challenging to hospice staff as to generalists.

Communication skills training is beyond the scope of this chapter but the importance of some focussed training in ACP is emphasized. This should be viewed as an ongoing skills programme involving all team members, with opportunities for reflection on significant ACP discussions as part of a team's education programme.

Various models of communication skills training are available and will be dependant on the local skills of facilitators and resources. Role play using team members as patients offers staff the opportunity to develop specific skills in a safe, controlled environment.

Particular scenarios that have been covered in such communication sessions by local units include:

◆ Identifying and responding to cues

◆ Handling uncertainty

◆ Establishing goals

◆ Discussing preferred place of death

◆ Introducing ACP documentation

◆ Responding to wishes for assisted suicide

◆ Identification of a proxy

◆ Identifying patient wishes through a proxy

Transferring information to others involved

Good communication is essential for ACP and is not limited to the skills of an individual to discuss patients' future wishes. The most able healthcare professional may be able to identify some of the most intricate and complex issues of a patient but this information is of no use unless it is communicated to the relevant teams who contribute to making such wishes a reality. Within the hospice setting, any significant ACP discussions should be documented in the notes or using the appropriate ACP tool or specific page in the notes, and raised at handover and team meetings.

These discussions should then be summarized at the time of a patient's discharge and communicated to the key professionals involved in care. This approach recognizes that for most patients, the hospice will not be the key worker in their illness journey; this will be the role of the primary care team led by the patient's general practitioner. Agreed methods of ACP communication should be established with primary care teams and this is best managed as part of the practice's Gold Standards Framework activities. Under this umbrella, hospice teams need to ensure they contact, where relevant, other stakeholders who may encounter the patient at some point. This list includes (but is not exhaustive):

◆ Primary care
  • General practitioner
  • District nurses
  • Community palliative care services
  • Social worker
  • Allied healthcare professional

◆ Acute sector
  • Hospital specialist e.g. oncologist, neurologist, cardiologists
  • Hospital specialist nurse
  • Hospital palliative care team

- ◆ Out of hours
  - Out of hours GP service register
  - Medical admissions or A andE team for patients with frequent admissions.

The key worker

Whilst hospices may benefit from the clinical leadership of the senior physician or nurse, the role of ACP will not necessarily fall to them. It is far more likely that opportunities to discuss ACP needs will arise during routine care or at more spontaneous moments with staff with whom they have developed a rapport. Hospice leaders should feel comfortable to empower the whole team to take responsibility for this whilst ensuring adequate support and clinical supervision where appropriate. Likewise the nominated 'key worker' may change with location and time and so leaders need to ensure the breadth of the team are sufficiently skilled to take on such roles. For one patient the key worker may be the ward nurse another, the occupational therapist, and another their district nurse at home. Patients whose admission has been primarily medical may find themselves engaging with the doctor whilst others who have explored spiritual domains of their life may prefer to have such planning with one of the pastoral care team.

ACP as death approaches

It is known that almost half the patients admitted to a hospice will remain there until death. For some patients and families, this will reflect their previously stated preferences for final place of care and bear testimony to effective ACP. However, not all patients who die in the hospice would wish to do so if given a choice, and likewise, other patients are unable to die in the hospice even when it is their preference. There are also those whose death was not anticipated; it is not uncommon to admit a patient for symptom control and then observe them to deteriorate. Also some patients, who have been ready for discharge home, may remain in the unit whilst funding and care arrangements are formalized, only to deteriorate before these plans are fulfilled.

Case study 2

Missed window of opportunity: Tom

Tom was a 75 year old man with metastatic carcinoma of the prostate, admitted from the Cancer Centre following radiotherapy for spinal cord compression. He was bed bound and his care needs were considerable. He was very keen to get home to die and the necessary care planning was initiated. The duty doctor was on leave and the locum did not feel he knew Tom well enough to complete the medical report, so this was delayed until the other doctor returned to work.

During this time Tom deteriorated and the team decided he was not likely to live long enough for the care package to be put in place. He died in the hospice six days later.

Learning points:

- ◆ Delays in putting a care package in place may lead to a missed opportunity to discharge a patient to their preferred place of care.
- ◆ It may have been appropriate to arrange a rapid discharge with a hospice at home team when signs of deterioration were noted rather than deciding to keep him in the hospice.
- ◆ Paper work is often put off until later since it is not considered the most pressing priority. Nevertheless, delays in such paperwork may prevent the delivery of a patient's expressed wishes.
- ◆ The wishes of the patient and their family must be held paramount, and processes developed to be able to ensure they are attained when time is short e.g. Rapid Discharge Policy to discharge patients within hours of their request to go home.

In order to address ACP in the end of life, one must first be able to identify whether someone is entering the terminal stages of their illness. Prognostication is recognized to be challenging with significant discordance between professionals as to how long someone has to live. However, the reliability of prognostication increases closer to death. It is tempting to see deterioration in condition as a trigger to keep a patient in the hospice and abandon discharge planning. If the patient's preferred place of care is the hospice, then such action would be appropriate, but a previously expressed preference to die at home should trigger the team into action to 'pull out all the stops' to get this person home; rather than slow or defer discharge planning. In short any deterioration in a patient's condition should be used as a trigger to identify their identified preferences for place of care to enable compliance with their wishes, where humanly possible.

One of the most challenging aspects of ACP is in the rapid discharge from the hospice to their home to die. This will involve coordination by a key worker and should include liaison with key people including:

◆ The family

◆ The patient's GP

◆ District nursing team

◆ Specialist nurses

◆ Social Services for carer visits/night sitters

◆ Pharmacy to ensure sufficient drugs are available

◆ Equipment loans e.g. for beds/hoists/commode

◆ Out of hours service to ensure desire to die at home is documented

◆ Ambulance control for discharge home and documentation of resuscitation status and desire for home death.

Some hospices and hospitals use formalized rapid discharge plans which can be kickstarted quickly to get patients home within a matter of hours if needed.

Practical suggestions

1 Build a culture of readiness to discuss ACP within the unit

2 Ensure ACP is a discussion point in team meetings and handovers

3 Develop communication between relevant health and social care professionals to ensure ACP wishes are known by all agencies

4 Deliver training for all staff involved in ACP including communication skills sessions focussed on ACP.

Conclusion

Meeting the needs and requests of patients is important to all, including hospice staff, whilst hospice staff may appear to have all the skills necessary to deliver effective ACP, it can still be an area of concern amongst the team. Such considerations are the responsibility of everyone and an integral and essential part of every patient's care. Teamwork, excellent communication, and ownership are the hallmarks of delivering good ACP. It must be recognized that such team work and communication extends beyond the walls of the inpatient unit and reaches out to include the care homes and hospital community where many professionals may have already begun such discussions addressing future needs and wishes. Advance Care Planning discussions are an intrinsic part of care for all hospice and specialist staff, respecting and honouring them a key part of planning good care, and in future it is likely that such formalized or opportunistic recording of ACP discussions will play a key role in determining the provision of best care for our patients nearing the end of their lives.

Chapter 15

Advanced Care Planning: thinking ahead for parents and children

Angela Thompson

This chapter includes:

+ The spectrum of conditions involved requiring ACP in paediatrics
+ The challenges of ACP in paediatrics
+ Drivers, evidence base, tools, and pathways to support paediatric ACP
+ Maintaining support for the family at the time of, and following death
+ Messages from special journeys.

Key points:

Families need care that:

+ is planned in partnership with them
+ is anticipatory
+ is regularly reviewed
+ takes account of the whole family's needs, including siblings, and especially the child/ young person
+ enables choice
+ encompasses parallel planning
+ provides access to 24/7 expertise in symptom control
+ engages in anticipatory bereavement care

Introduction

Planning for care at the end of life in paediatrics poses many challenges and stirs emotions. The range of possibilities to be encompassed is vast and is compounded by a lack of uniformity in approach and documentation of care plans (1). Yet despite the relative embryonic nature of Advanced Care Planning (ACP) in paediatrics, examples of good practice are emerging and coherent approaches are developing. The death of a child is any family's worst nightmare. Families facing these distressing days and years warrant the opportunity for care that is planned in partnership with them, facilitating choice and priority setting, and the best possible care, as the path ahead is anticipated and travelled along.

Which families are thinking ahead?

Which children need palliative care support and to whom does this thinking ahead apply? Paediatric palliative care covers a broad spectrum of conditions that cause families to live with the threat of death hanging over their child. It is helpful to offer these families both the opportunity and the support to think ahead, to plan to meet their needs from diagnosis through to care at the end of life. Palliative care for families with children with life limiting or life threatening conditions is offered to those who broadly sit within the following four groups (2). See Table 15.1.

The diversity of conditions, time scale, disease trajectory, and the impact upon daily life of both the condition and its management creates a breadth of issues for ACP in paediatrics. These challenges span across many care settings for each child—home, hospital, hospice, school, short breaks, and play venues.

It has long been recognized and clearly delineated by the Association for Children's Palliative Care (ACT) as outlined below (3), that children's palliative care differs from adult palliative care in several aspects:

- the number of children dying is relatively small
- many have rare conditions, some of which are familial, so more than one child within a family may be affected
- palliative care may last only a few days or extend over many years
- the whole family are affected
- ongoing cognitive development affects the child's understanding of their disease
- disease management and care provision, including educational provision, is complex.

The challenges that each of these points throws into the arena of advanced planning for care at the end of life are significant, not least because the children themselves are continuing to develop physically, emotionally, and cognitively. These ongoing changes lead to one of the key aspects of such planning; that of progressive, step by step planning, with the flexibility to change plans and reset priorities as circumstances change.

In addition there are some specific challenges in the implementation of ACP in paediatrics (see Box 15.1).

Table 15.1 Life limiting conditions categories

Category 1	Life-threatening conditions for which curative treatment may be feasible but can fail, where access to palliative care services may be necessary when treatment fails or during an acute crisis, irrespective of the duration of that threat to life. Examples: cancer, irreversible organ failures of heart, liver, kidney
Category 2	Conditions where premature death is inevitable, where there may be long periods of intensive treatment aimed at prolonging life and allowing participation in normal activities. Examples: cystic fibrosis, Duchenne muscular dystrophy
Category 3	Progressive conditions without curative treatment options, where treatment is exclusively palliative and may commonly extend over many years. Examples: Batten disease, mucopolysaccharidoses
Category 4	Irreversible but non-progressive conditions causing severe disability leading to susceptibility to health complications and likelihood of premature death. Examples: severe cerebral palsy, multiple disabilities such as following brain or spinal cord insult

Box 15.1 Challenges to ACP & its implementation in paediatrics

- Emotional aspects
- Breadth of conditions managed, many of which are long term
- Prognostic difficulties especially in neonates and in neurological conditions
- Advances in technological support developing ethical dilemmas
- Learning difficulties and developmental progression affecting competency and consent related issues
- Transition to adult services often occurs at a time of deteriorating health
- National uniform approach/format to documentation still under development
- Child Death Review Process requirements
- 24/7 access to CCN services variable limiting access to services out of hours

Securing a firm foundation

How then do we begin to secure a firm foundation upon which we can build good Advanced Care Planning? An early start is essential. Supporting the family along their journey by a multiagency coordinated care pathway approach brings opportunities for regular reviews, partnership planning, facing early anticipated and unexpected hurdles together, and builds trust between the family and the professionals (2). Opportunities for this foundation setting may be reduced where the disease progression is swift or a sudden onset of a severe complication occurs. Here the active help of 'in reach' of community palliative care services in hospital settings to consider with families and the hospital team their choices and wishes, set goals and priorities, and to establish appropriate support before potential discharge is essential.

Meeting the spectrum of challenges

Developing care plans for end of life care in paediatrics holds challenges in its implementation across a spectrum from premature neonates to young people transitioning to adult care. Catlin and Carter (4) developed a neonatal end of life care protocol in the USA, acknowledging that a newborn with a life-limiting condition may be recognized to have palliative care needs from a time early in the prenatal period through to a time following efforts in the neonatal intensive care unit (NICU). Significant emphasis within the protocol was paid to communicating palliative care needs to the family, as early as possible, in a sensitive and supportive manner, and to planning for and providing appropriate end of life care for their child. Similar work is currently being undertaken in the UK with the launch of the Neonatal Palliative Care Pathway in November 2009.

Planning ahead whilst growing up

For those at the opposite end of the paediatric age spectrum, transitioning to adult services often coincides with their most vulnerable health state and end of life phase. Many of these young people and their families will have spent their lives involved in planning to meet their needs in their various care setting such as home, school, and short breaks, with a team they have come to know well (2,5). When their end of life phase coincides with transitioning towards adult services, it is crucial that parallel planning continues. Parallel planning looks ahead for the young person to continue to live and need to receive services to support them within the adult sector, whilst at the same time it acknowledges the possibility of death occurring and develops plans together for care at the end of life. Lack of accurate predictability necessitates this if both scenarios are to be well prepared for. The Transition Care Pathway (6) highlights important aspects of care planning for such individuals, emphasizing the need for planning to commence early and be regularly reviewed and updated. Box 15.2 illustrates some of the core elements of care at this stage (6).

Tools to engage the family, child, and young person in thinking ahead

Support tools are becoming available to enable these difficult and sensitive discussions with the child and family, as to their priorities and wishes. The Lifetime service, UK, developed a framework to aid such discussions (7). Based upon a 3x3 framework, it enables families, the child/young person, and extra familial others, e.g. school and friends, to discover together and with the professionals what their priorities are, to incorporate their views, and so to determine how best to holistically support the family, and to review these decisions. It considers three periods: 'before death', 'at death', and 'after death'. Staff can use the framework to structure discussion and to provide the opportunity for the child and family to be heard, enabling families to receive the help and support they need, when they need it, and in the place that they are most comfortable. The aim should be for a holistic approach to end of life care where all the pieces of the jigsaw are in place from everyone's perspective.

Research is underway at Bangor University in the use of the 'My Choices' booklets, which help children and young people to think through what their choices would be and where they would choose to be cared for in different health states. Three booklets have been produced with the

---

Box 15.2 Core elements of end of life care for young people

- Care in the place of their choice.
- Professionals should be open and honest with young people and families when the approach to end of life care is recognized, with timely and open communication and information.
- Joint planning with young people and their families and relevant professionals should take place, with choices/options in all aspects of care, including complementary therapies.
- Young people and families should be supported in their choices, and goals for quality of life issues should be respected.
- A written plan for care around the time of death should be agreed, taking account of acute or slow deterioration. It is important that all professionals who may be involved are informed, including emergency services.
- Coordination of services at home where this is a chosen place of care, including provision of specialist equipment, should be in place.
- Expert symptom management, including access to 24 hour specialist symptom management advice and expertise by those suitably qualified and experienced, including access to out of hours medication.
- Emotional, spiritual, and practical support should be available for all family members.
- Short break care should be available with medical and nursing input when required.
- Care plans and plans for care at the end of life should be reviewed and altered to take into account ongoing changes.

input of children and young people with life limiting conditions; these cover the developmental ages of childhood.

Such tools support the discussions and enable written confirmation of the child's and family's wishes, at that point in time. These records are produced in a non threatening way, step by step, at the families pace, when they are ready, in partnership between the family and professionals and can be used to revisit and reprioritize wishes and plans as circumstances change.

Putting plans into action

Frameworks have been available to guide end of life care for adults, for example the Gold Standards Framework (8) and the Liverpool Care Pathway (9). These guidelines have been used in paediatrics and research continues around the adaptation of the Liverpool Care Pathway (10) and Gold Standards Framework for children (8). The GSF looks at applying questions used in adults such as 'would you be surprised if this child died within the next six months?' This would be anticipated to then trigger and enable appropriate and timely action planning with the family.

ACT has developed comprehensive multiagency pathway guidance (2) specifically for children and young people, encompassing all stages from diagnosis, through living with the condition, to moving into end of life care and bereavement. ACT's pathway work (2) acknowledges the need to respond to the recognition of the move into the end of life phase in a child or young person. This will include open and honest discussion with the family, reviewing their needs and goals and drawing up a plan for this new phase. Holding a multidisciplinary meeting with the involvement of the young person and family where possible, especially where death is likely to occur at home, is central to comprehensive care at the end of life.

Important aspects of this meeting are:

◆ to establish and communicate the revised care plans

◆ to set out clear guidelines for roles and responsibilities of those involved.

Holding such meetings at the GP's often enables their participation and provides opportunities to bridge build between professionals.

It also helps to:

◆ develop a unified approach to management

◆ provide visible evidence of support for the primary care team from the specialist palliative care services

◆ provide a forum in which to discuss clinical, social, and psychological issues etc.

◆ enable the primary care team to become familiar with the 'just in case medicines' placed in the home and the documentation used for symptom management

◆ allow joint consideration of anticipated complications, based upon:

  • the literature evidence for the underlying condition

  • the knowledge of the complications already experienced specific to the individual's unique disease progression

◆ consider the management of related potential complications/scenarios

◆ plan availability of the families 'virtual team' in and out of hours

◆ clarify the families initial single point of contact.

It consequently provides peace of mind to the family that the various teams involved in their child's care are communicating and working together with them at this crucial stage. Anticipation is the central cogwheel in this planning, around which all will need to be planned if care is to be effectively delivered.

A template can be used to assist planning at this stage; outlining key, essential information. The meeting will enable a definitive plan for contact in and out of hours, both for family and for front line staff who will require access to 24 hour specialist symptom control support. The template will then be forwarded for information to the out of hours services for primary care (Table 15.2).

This template sits alongside and does not replace documentation around resuscitation and symptom control issues at the end of life. The clear and concise documentation relating to these issues should be provided in relation to the possibilities of both acute, sudden deteriorations and also gradual demise. This in turn should be supplemented by a more detailed care plan of the child's and family's wishes, for example some families wish to confirm who needs to be there at the time of death, which music is to be played, songs to be sung and/or stories of happy memories to be retold as the time of death approaches.

Effective documentation of the wishes of the child/young person and their family for care around the time of death has been developed by Wolff (11), and has been successfully implemented within local authority/social care settings as well as health care settings. Many similar documentation templates are now in operation, based upon it, and ACT is seeking to draw together a standardized format. Its principle is to outline the decisions reached at that point in time for care in the face of either an acute deterioration or a gradual demise in the end of life phase. It empowers families in their decision making, allowing as much choice and control as possible, is flexible to accommodate changing circumstances and assists clear communication between families and professionals. It clarifies decisions with detailed practical instructions around the extent of resuscitation, and enables those dealing with an emergency situation to respond appropriately.

What are young people's views on planning for care at the end of life? A study examining adolescent's wishes around end of life care (12) explored whether differences existed between chronically ill and healthy adolescents with regard to their attitudes about end of life issues. 96% of chronically ill and 88% of healthy teens were found to want to share in decision-making if they were very ill. At times, conflicts of opinions will exist within families, and between families and staff.

Table 15.2 Template for end of life care multidisciplinary care meeting

Private and Confidential Medical Information

Planning Meeting re: Name: DoB:

        Address:

Meeting held at GP Practice:

Date:

Background Diagnosis:

Medications:

Known and suspected allergies:

Professionals involved:

Name	Role	Address	Contact number	Availability hours

Initial point of contact for family:

    In hours (8.30am–5.30pm):

    Out of hours (5.30pm–8.30 am and weekends):

Some high profile cases have required the court's intervention, as the ultimate arbiters, to assist in such situations where conflicting opinions exist, so that the best interests of the child can be served (14,15). Good care aims to avoid these traumatic conflicts, by families and staff walking the journey together over time, developing respect and understanding, crossing barriers together at earlier stages so that care at the end of life can be jointly planned to provide good quality, symptom managed days and weeks where life can be lived as fully and preciously as possible.

When death comes: planning to maintain the care

It is essential that care around the time of and after death is as thorough and professional as before death. Care needs to be taken to think ahead to address the issues that will arise, some of which are outlined below (6):

- There should be good care of the child's body and the family at the time of death
  - respecting the need for privacy, time and space, and sensitivity of the family's spiritual needs, religious beliefs, and cultural practices
- Parents should retain their parenting role after the death of their child
  - respecting their need to retain control of what happens to their child's body, to ensure they have mementoes and memories, and that all staff dealing with their child's body treat it with dignity
- Siblings should be supported and included in all decisions
  - respecting their need to be supported in decisions around seeing their siblings body, attending the funeral, making a special contribution to the service etc
- Parents should be asked if they want to take their child's body home or keep it at home after death, if appropriate
  - respecting the needs of some families to remain close to their child until the funeral either at home or in a special bedroom at the hospice
- All professionals/agencies should be informed of the death with parents consent
  - respecting parents need to give consent but then utilizing the up to date list kept in the child's records of contacts to be made following the child's death
- Families should receive appropriate written information
  - respecting that grief exacerbates the need for information about registering the death etc to be in written format
- Plans for after death should be revisited.

All these aspects are more likely to be addressed if a bereavement policy is held with a handbook readily available to guide those who manage such situations less frequently.

Supporting the family through grief

When a child dies, it is likely that there will be grandparents and siblings who will be deeply affected besides the parents and other close family members. Siblings warrant particular attention and care, and many children's palliative care services place an emphasis upon caring for the siblings, with access to professional support where grief appears complex. Clinical psychology and bereavement services are often closely associated with children's palliative care services. Where grief is less complex, the palliative care team will often provide the main ongoing support to the sibling(s) both in pre-bereavement and post-bereavement work, using tools such as memory

Box 15.3 Winston's Wish: primary clinical objectives (16)

To provide increased opportunities for:

◆ Support, information and education: supporting children and families to understand death and what it means to them

◆ Understanding and expressing grief: encouraging children and families to share and understand the feelings, thoughts, and individual ways of coping with loss

◆ Remembering: helping families to find ways of remembering the person who has died

◆ Communication: encouraging family members to talk openly to each other

◆ Meeting needs: providing opportunities to meet other families with similar experiences

boxes, which can be planned for and begun before the death, helping the child to prepare for the anticipated death and to gather items to cement their memories.

Winston's Wish is one organization which supports children when a significant individual in their life dies. Its primary clinical aims are outlined in Box 15.3, (16) and are principles that should be borne in mind when planning for any family's bereavement care. Its role in terms of providing support in relation to the realities for grieving children is outlined in Box 15.4, (13) and covers those aspects which should be uppermost in our minds when considering how families are coping.

Messages from special journeys

To be able to walk with a family along part of their journey at such a difficult time in their life is a privilege. Each such special journey deserves that we reflect upon it afterwards. Several key aspects are raised time and time again in discussions with families after their child's death in relation to aspects which they valued. These include:

◆ Being listened to and heard by professionals, as partners

◆ Being respected and not judged, but gently helped to think and work through their difficulties

Box 15.4 Realities for grieving children (16)

◆ All children and young people grieve.

◆ Grieving is a long term process.

◆ Children and young people revisit their grief and frequently construct a changing relationship with the person who has died.

◆ Younger children will need help in retaining memories which facilitate a continuing bond.

◆ Children express their grief differently to adults.

◆ Children cannot be protected from death.

◆ There are clear developmental differences between children and young people in the understanding, experience and expression of grief.

◆ A child's grief occurs within a family and community context and will be influenced by significant adults.

◆ Experiencing high quality responsive and timely care, as the family move from one stepping stone to another on the journey, so that life can be lived to its full

◆ Being treated with openness and honesty when the end of life phase approaches so that priorities can be re-established and plans developed so that families do not feel cheated of opportunities for special times together.

Perhaps the keys to these can be summed up as good communication and attention to detail within high quality, timely, responsive care. With this combination we can take a significant step towards providing families with the best quality of life possible for as long as possible, reassured in the knowledge that anticipatory thinking has put plans into place to endeavour to meet their needs and provide high quality best practice care. Our children and young people with palliative care needs, and their families, deserve nothing less.

Further resources

The Association for Children's Palliative Care: http://www.act.org.uk

Children's Hospices UK: http://www.childhospice.org.uk

Winston's Wish: http://www.winstonswish.org

Compassionate Friends: http://www.compassionatefriends.org

Child Bereavement Network: http://www.childhoodbereavementnetwork.org.uk/publications_suggestedReading.htm

Royal College of Paediatrics and Child Health: http://www.rcpch.ac.uk

British Association of Perinatal Medicine: http://www.bapm.org

References

1 Brook L (2008). A plan for living and a plan for dying: advanced care planning for children. *Archives of Disease in Childhood*, **93**(suppl):A61–66.

2 ACT (2004). *A framework for the development of integrated multi-agency care pathways for children with life-threatening and life-limiting conditions.* ACT, Bristol.

3 ACT (2009). *A guide to the development of children's palliative care services.* ACT, Bristol.

4 Catlin A and Carter B (2002). Creation of a neonatal end of life palliative care. protocol. *Journal of Perinatology*, **22**(3):184–95.

5 Weidner NJ (2005). Developing an interdisciplinary palliative care plan for the patient with muscular dystrophy, *Pediatric Annals*, **34**(7):546–52.

6 ACT (2007).*A framework for the development of integrated multi-agency care pathways for young people with life-threatening and life-limiting conditions: the transition care pathway.* ACT, Bristol.

7 Finlay F, Lewis M, Lenton S, and Poon M (2008). Planning for the end of children's lives–the Lifetime framework. *Child: Care, Health and Development*, **34**(4):542–44.

8 *Gold Standards Framework.* Available at http://www.goldstandardsframework.nhs.uk

9 *Liverpool Care Pathway.* Available at http://www.mpcil.org.uk/liverpool-care-pathway

10 Matthews K, Gambles M, Ellershaw JE, et al. (2006). Developing the Liverpool Care Pathway for the dying child. *Paediatric Nursing*, **18**(1):18–21.

11 Wolff A, Browne J, Whitehouse WP (2005). Personal resuscitation plans: the death of DNAR's? Abstract RCPCH Ethics and Law and Palliative Care Joint Session, G202. *Archives of Disease in Childhood*, **90**:A77–A81.

12 Lyon ME, McCabe MA, Patel KM, and Angelo LJ (2004). What do adolescents want? An exploratory study regarding end-of-life decision-making. *Journal of Adolescent Health*, **35**(6):529.

13 Dyer C (2008). Trust decides against legal action to force girl to receive heart transplant. *BMJ*, **337**:a2659.

14 Larcher V (2006). Ethics. In Goldman A, Hain R, and Liben S (eds) *Oxford Textbook of Palliative Care for Children*, 42–62. Oxford University Press, Oxford.

15 RCPCH (2004). *Withholding or withdrawing life sustaining treatment in children: a framework for practice*, 2nd ed. RCPCH, London.

16 Stokes J (2004). *Then, Now and Always*, 1st edition. Calouste Gulbenkian Foundation, Cheltenham.

Chapter 16

Issues around capacity

Lynn Gibson, Dorothy Matthews, and Claud Regnard

'Care begins when difference is recognised.'
Frank 1991

This chapter includes:

◆ Whose role is it to discuss future care?

◆ When does a person lack capacity?

◆ Which conditions may affect a person's capacity?

◆ Who should be involved?

◆ How can information be given?

◆ Have we developed a plan?

Key points

◆ The importance of true partnership working and open communication

◆ An individual must be assumed to have capacity unless proved otherwise

◆ Capacity assessments must be decision specific

◆ ACP is an on-going process that should be regularly reviewed

◆ This is something that is 'done with' the patient and not 'done to'.

Introduction

This chapter will explore and explain some of the issues that surround decision making for people who lack capacity for the decision being made. The concepts explained in this chapter should support the professional care team to apply the principles of ACP to those people who lack capacity.

Hattie's story

Background

Hattie is a 47 lady with a moderate learning disability and a diagnosis of bi-polar disorder. She has also been diagnosed with advanced breast cancer due to late reporting of symptoms and a delay in accessing investigations.

Social history

Hattie still lives independently in the family home in a small community, where she has lived for many years with her late mother and father. She has paid carers who visit her twice daily but she also has enablers who three times a week spend the day with her helping her access social outings within the community. Hattie's mother died of metastatic breast cancer 15 years ago. Hattie's mother had a radical mastectomy followed by radiotherapy and Hattie has vivid memories of her mother's illness and states that the radiotherapy, 'burnt her black'. Hattie has a brother who lives in America and a close family friend Brenda who has helped support her since her mother died. Hattie has been known to 'sack' the carers explaining that Brenda will look after her.

Medical history

Hattie has had numerous admissions to a mental health hospital in the past as a consequence of her bipolar disorder and, for a short time following diagnosis and subsequent surgery, she was admitted again as she could not cope. Hattie's disease was treated with an appropriate regime of chemotherapy, radiotherapy, and hormone therapy, but unfortunately owing to the advanced state of her disease at the point of diagnosis, Hattie developed metastatic disease and was been referred to a Macmillan nurse.

Challenges

Hattie's experience of her mother's disease and subsequent treatment has left her with lasting memories and preformed ideas of what may happen to her. Consequently, she initially refused radiotherapy for fear of being 'burnt', and will not consider reconstruction and/or wearing a prosthesis post surgery. Hattie does not fully comprehend the seriousness of the situation and has told everyone that she will be fine when she gets home, refusing to have any more 'strangers' in her house. Due to this and the many other complicated aspects of the situation an Advance Care Plan is thought to be the best way forward to reflect Hattie's wishes so that care can be coordinated and proactive.

Issue

When Hattie decides that she wants an ACP to inform people of her wishes, Brenda immediately feels it is her right and duty to take control of the situation. Hattie wants to go home, but Brenda wants her to stay in hospital because she is 'no longer capable' and she needs to be 'looked after'. Hattie's brother is in America and states he does not want to be involved, as he will not be returning to the UK in the near future.

Resolution

Everyone acknowledges the very important role Brenda has in Hattie's life. However, it is recognized that Brenda has no legal right to make decisions on Hattie's behalf. In the small community where Hattie lives, she is very well known. Her GP has known her for many years as do the district nurses, community learning disability nurses, and psychiatrist, however the person Hattie is relating well to in the current situation is the Macmillan nurse. The multidisciplinary team (MDT) decides that she is the best placed person to facilitate the conversation regarding an ACP as she has the clinical medical knowledge that is required and the experience of initiating difficult conversations. The Macmillan nurse also has an understanding of all the different facets of Hattie's life and in addition, Hattie likes her and relates well to her input. The decision has been made for the Macmillan nurse to facilitate the ACP, however she includes Brenda at every step of the process and informs the rest of the care team of the ACP discussions and decisions, Hattie agrees with this arrangement.

Clinical decisions: are you the right person to do this?

ACP is a process where there is discussion between an individual and any of their care providers irrespective of profession or role. To initiate such a discussion regarding how and where an individual would wish to receive care at the end of their life can be very daunting in the best of circumstances. However, this can be perceived as an impossible task when considering ACP with someone that you think may not have capacity.

If an individual wishes, their family and/or friends may be included in the development of their ACP although they cannot make decisions on the patient's behalf unless they were legally appointed to do so (e.g. Personal Welfare Lasting Power of Attorney in England and Wales). If a person does not have capacity then the decision must be made in the patient's best interests.

If you are unsure of a person's capacity or how to act in their best interests it is even more important to ask yourself the question, 'Am I the right person to do this?' When someone does not have capacity, it is impossible to plan on their behalf without knowing something about their background, likes, dislikes, abilities, methods of doing things, and generally 'what makes them tick'. Usually it is family members, friends, and/or paid carers who hold most of this information and they should be considered as possible instigators of the conversation of 'what happens if . . .' However, these individuals may be too emotionally attached or not have sufficient clinical knowledge or appropriate communication skills to steer the conversation and may therefore need a person who can facilitate the process and bring a degree of objectivity. That person may be you.

Is there an impairment of mind or brain preventing discussion of future plans?

One of the principles of the Mental Capacity Act (MCA) 2005 (England and Wales) is the assumption that an individual has the capacity to make the decision required (1). However, the MCA also recognizes that this capacity may be compromised by an impairment of mind or brain:

> For the purpose of this act, a person lacks capacity in relation to a matter if at the material time; he is unable to make a decision for himself in relation to the matter because of impairment or a disturbance in the functioning of, the mind or brain . . . Whenever the term, a person who lacks capacity is used, it means a person who lacks capacity to make a particular decision or take a particular action for them at the time the decision or action needs to be taken

An important consequence of this definition is that, although people may lack capacity to make a decision about one issue, they may be able to decide quite ably about another. For example, an individual may not have the capacity to decide to remain in the family home at the end of their life, however, they could make a decision to go out for the day. It also follows that other people may be uncomfortable with the decision or consider it unwise. However, the MCA is clear that, if a person has capacity for that decision, an apparently unwise decision does not imply a lack of capacity.

There are various reasons why a person may have an impairment of their mind or brain that will result in an individual not having capacity, this impairment may be permanent, temporary, or even change over time. Some examples where people may lack capacity are individuals who:

- never had capacity, e.g. significant learning disabilities
- have suddenly lost capacity, e.g. acquired brain injury
- gradually lose capacity, e.g. dementia
- have fluctuating capacity, e.g. delirium

If such impairment is suspected then capacity must be tested:

1 Can they understand the information? This must be imparted in a way the patient can understand

2 Can they retain the information? This only needs to be long enough to use and weigh the information

3 Can they use or weigh up that information? They must be able to show that they are able to consider the benefits and burdens of the alternatives to the proposed treatment

4 Can they communicate their decision? The carers must try every method possible to enable this.

In all situations it is important to ensure that all efforts are made to give information to the individual in a format that is the most appropriate for them. This may be audiotape, verbally, in picture format, via a DVD, using symbols, actually practically going through the proposed event, and in fact using any method with which the person will engage.

In Hattie's case it is very important to ensure that she has the required information at the right time delivered in a format and at a level that she can understand. For some people they may permanently lack capacity to make the decision that is required. In the absence of any nominated proxy e.g. Lasting Power of Attorney or Advance Decision to Refuse Treatment (ADRT) the professional must make a decision in the patient's best interests. This process of Best Interest Assessment is clearly described in the MCA and involves an interdisciplinary team discussion which should:

- encourage the participation of the patient
- identify all the relevant circumstances
- find out the person's views (i.e. wishes, preferences, beliefs, and values): these may have been expressed verbally previously, or exist in an ADRT, or Advance Statement made when the patient had capacity)
- avoid discrimination and avoid making assumptions about the person's quality of life
- assess whether the person might regain capacity
- if the decision concerns life-sustaining treatment, not be motivated in any way by a desire to bring about the person's death
- consult others (within the limits of confidentiality): this may include an Lasting Power of Attorney, IMCA, or Court Appointed Deputy
- avoid restricting the person's rights
- take all of this into account, i.e. Weigh up all of these factors in order to work out the person's best interests
- Record the decisions, agree review dates, and review regularly.

Hattie's story continued

Issues

1 Hattie does not want to wear a prosthetic breast.

2 Hattie does not want radiotherapy and is unwell due to an exacerbation of her bipolar disorder.

3 Hattie wants to go home with Brenda providing care for her with no strangers i.e. professional carers, entering her house.

Resolution

These are three very different decisions requiring three different levels of understanding and ability to weigh up the options; we already know that Hattie has potential challenges to her capacity due to both her learning disability and mental heath problems. Her bipolar disorder complicates the situation as Hattie's capacity fluctuates dependent on how well or unwell she is at the time of the decision to be made; however even if her mental health is stable she still has a learning disability to consider. In all three issues the Macmillan nurse in conjunction with the learning disabilities community nurse facilitates the process.

1 Hattie is given the prosthesis to handle and to show her friends. She is also given pictures of a lady with one and then the same lady without one. She is encouraged to look for the difference between the two pictures and to discuss. She is told there is no rush and she can decide what to do. She still decides not to wear one, wants her decision documented, and it is considered that she has the capacity to make that decision.

2 Hattie is again given information regarding radiotherapy in picture format accompanied by simple text; she is shown a video of the radiotherapy suite at her local hospital and then taken to visit. While there the

Macmillan nurse arranges for her to talk to a patient who is having a regime of radiotherapy similar to that which is being considered for Hattie. Hattie still is concerned about getting burnt and tells everyone that she does not need the treatment as she is now cured. It is decided that Hattie does not have the capacity at the time to make the decision regarding radiotherapy as her mental health is impairing her decision making processes. Although the MDT could make the decision to proceed with the radiotherapy in her best interests it is decided to wait a while until her mental health improves. A little while later the decision is revisited using the same process and Hattie decides to have the treatment. After that regime of radiotherapy Hattie decides that she wants it documented on her ACP that if the doctors think it will help her she will have further radiotherapy, but only if her mental health is not an issue.

3 This is the most difficult decision as it is the one where there are the most variables and for someone with compromised capacity 'the future' can be an abstract concept. This situation needs excellent communication skills, Hattie needs many people to help her to have the information she requires whilst making her decision. This scenario also requires advance decision making about financial matters as well as health and social care. In this instance a meeting was convened to give Hattie the information she required. All stakeholders were invited and on large pieces of paper Hattie's likes, dislikes, wishes, things she considered she was good at and things she considered she wasn't as good at etc. were charted. The people in attendance (including Brenda) then discussed what they could do to help and how often, out of this fell a plan for the future. It demonstrates to Hattie that she does need people to help her live in her family home, it verifies to Brenda that she is not alone in undertaking the total care package and a compromise was reached. Hattie will go back to her house as she wishes and the information gained from the meeting will help to inform the ACP.

Is this the patient's first discussion of their future plans?

It is always important to ascertain whether or not the individual has already made an ACP or has expressed in other ways their wishes regarding their future. If they have, it is important to ask them if it is possible to view it, and clarify whether their wishes have changed.

Hattie's story continued

In Hattie's case she has no previous ACP as she has never considered that she might have a life limiting condition that will affect where she will live and the support she may require. However, she does have a person centred plan (PCP) as advocated by the Department of Health (2) which documents her strengths, likes, and dislikes as well as her aspirations, dreams, and personal goals for the future. This PCP should be considered as a statement of her wishes and preferences, be considered carefully when assessing Hattie's best interests for a particular decision and when developing her ACP. When it was decided to get everyone together to discuss her ACP she was happy to present her PCP which informed the process.

Issue
Although Hattie has held discussions regarding her future care in the past none constituted an ACP and the care providers are unsure of how this will be achieved.

Resolution
In keeping with the MCA and good practice Hattie was involved centrally in the process of developing an ACP using her previous statement of wishes and preferences (her person centred plan). It is important for everyone involved to be familiar with the principles of the MCA, especially in this instance principle four where 'if a decision is made under the Act for or on behalf of a person who lacks capacity it must be done or made in his/her best interest'. In Hattie's case it has already been discussed and understood what can influence her capacity.

Does the patient want to discuss their future care?

It is very important to ascertain very early in the process who actually wants the ACP. The definition states that it 'is a process of discussion between an individual and their care providers' and the fact that the individual comes first should never be forgotten, even when working with people with potentially impaired capacity.

It is preferable for the discussion to have been initiated by the person with capacity, but sometimes professionals have to introduce and facilitate the planning process for future needs if the person with capacity gives permission to do so. However, this is dependent on them understanding the concept of their illness and the anticipated deterioration of their condition. As when receiving any difficult news it is not always possible to fully comprehend all aspects of the situation and people deal with this in different ways. The key principle of breaking difficult news is to always allow the individual to be in control of the flow of information as well as the conversation. This premise is suggested when discussing ACP, which helps to prevent the process becoming a 'tick-box' exercise. It is also important to realize that planning future care in people who lack capacity for a particular decision in a person's best interests can only be made if a problem currently exists, or there is a current risk of a problem.

Hattie's story continued

In Hattie's case it is very important to ensure that she has an understanding of the information she has already been given before undertaking the ACP process. It is also very important for everyone else involved, especially Brenda, that they understand that the impetus has to come from Hattie and that the ACP is not being developed to record and confirm their own wishes for Hattie's future care.

Issue
Is it Hattie who wants to discuss her future care or is it the professionals involved with her?

Resolution
The Macmillan nurse clarifies with Hattie over several visits, what she already knows, her understanding of the information already conveyed, and what else she wants to know, as well as her understanding of the ACP process. It is reiterated to her that she is in control of what is discussed and documented and that it is her wishes that are being acknowledged and acted upon. It is also explained to Hattie that she will keep her ACP and she can decide who else (if anyone) can have a copy for safekeeping. It is also explained that ACP is a voluntary process and Hattie can change her mind at any time. This might mean amending or even withdrawing the ACP either on agreed review dates or otherwise.

Is the patient ready to discuss end of life care?

Some people are happy to discuss what care they want at the end of their life even before having any life limiting illness diagnosed, planning categorically what treatments they will and will not consider as well the obvious arrangements such as their funeral. Other people, even when a confirmed diagnosis of a life limiting illness has been given, prefer 'the one step at a time' approach. Occasionally people, despite facing the need to make decisions (which is obvious to other observers) will withdraw from the decision making processes altogether. Some more unexpected behaviours/attitudes must not be a cause to discriminate against the decision maker, everyone (with capacity) is allowed to make unwise decisions.

Death and all the associated rituals can be a difficult concept for people with capacity, let alone those where capacity might be impaired or lost. In some instances where capacity has been lost over a period of time, e.g. dementia, the individual may have already informally made their views known through a series of general conversations over the years, for example expressing their wish 'to be cremated with family and friends attending all wearing red'. This individual may not have made any formal record of what treatment options they possibly would or would not have; however, it is important for family and friends to adhere to known wishes and use the information available of what the individual's beliefs were and their background to inform such decisions.

For someone who has never had capacity for more complex decisions, this concept becomes more difficult to deal with. The impact of social, cultural, and generational differences on death and bereavement might be considered as 'off limit' topics. This was often because of the paternalistic assumption that such individuals would never understand and that the whole subject was too upsetting for them to be included in any aspect related to death and bereavement. That approach is now discouraged and people with learning disabilities are often involved in discussing and even to some extent planning their own funerals.

Hattie's story continued

Hattie has experience of both her father's and in particular her mother's death, therefore does understand the concept and has very particular views on what she wants for herself. Hattie was not present at her mother's death in the hospital. Her mother was reported to be in a great deal of pain. Hattie is very concerned that she will be in pain and be on her own 'at the end' and is also worried about what will happen to her house. Sensitively exploring these issues, often over several meetings, may allow her to share her feelings. This underlines the need for an ongoing dialogue, and the inherent risks of a seeing ACP as a single task.

Issue

1 Hattie does not want to be on her own 'at the end' so wants to stay at home in her own bed

2 Hattie does not want to be in pain

3 Hattie is worried about her house

Resolution

1 It has been explained to Hattie that her wishes to remain at home will be documented in her ACP, however, the circumstances of her going into hospital for further treatment need to be considered. The possibility of her refusing treatment has been discussed. A plan is developed using information gathered previously to inform its content.

2 Provision for the diagnosis and management of pain has been explored and discussed. Although Hattie at the moment has the ability to verbally report (although not accurately) her pain, this may not be possible in the future due to either an exacerbation of her mental health and/or a deterioration in her physical health. It is decided to use an observational tool, such as the Disability Distress assessment Tool (DisDAT) (3),) which will be used to document her content and distressed states. This can be completed prior to its probable use in conjunction with friends and family. Using this method it is less likely for the professionals involved to 'miss' any symptom that relies on verbal reporting and thus appropriate symptom control can be delivered and monitored.

3 This issue is tricky to resolve in that it involves Hattie's brother who is her next of kin but who has stated that he does not want to be involved at the moment.

As it has already been decided that Hattie has the capacity to make some decisions but not others, everyone agrees that she can inform the process however she does not have the capacity to draw up a LPA for personal welfare.

In her discussions with the Macmillan nurse it becomes clear that her greatest worry is that if she wasn't living in the house it will be broken into and vandalized. To resolve these worries it is agreed that Brenda can look after the house in the short term if Hattie is re-admitted to a hospital (or hospice) for treatment of symptoms. However, if this becomes a long term arrangement Brenda could not commit to this responsibility. In the event of this happening Hattie's brother will come from the USA and take over the practical and financial responsibilities of looking after the house. Hattie is happy for her brother to manage her financial affairs even though he is not her official LPA. All of this information has been documented in her ACP

Does the patient want to refuse treatment?

Hattie's ACP is not a document that includes a record of any decisions to refuse treatment. There is legal right for a person with capacity to complete an Advance Decision to Refuse Treatment (ADRT) that meets the requirements of the MCA. An excellent template for such a document exists. (National End of Life Care Programme and National Hospice Council (4)). Advance Decisions are discussed in Chapter 9.

An Independent Mental Capacity Advocate (IMCA) (see Chapter 8) is to support the decision making process for people who lack capacity to make important decisions about serious medical treatment and/or changes of living accommodation, and who have no family or friends that with whom it would be appropriate to consult.

Hattie's story continued

In Hattie's case she is extremely clear that she does not want to have further radiotherapy due to the experience she had with her mother.

Issue

Hattie does not want to receive further radiotherapy; however, she does not have the capacity to make an ADRT.

Resolution

At the moment Hattie has discussed this with her Macmillan nurse who has documented Hattie's wishes in her ACP. In the future if there is a clinical indication for further radiotherapy this will be discussed with Hattie utilising all reasonable methods to maximize capacity and established communication techniques. If Hattie either lacks capacity to make this decision or is unbefriended an IMCA can be appointed to support the decision making process.

Does the patient want this discussion documented?

There is no legal requirement for any discussion relating to a person's wishes; neither for their future care to be documented nor for any particular method to be used to record the discussion between the individual and their care providers. Therefore, when developing an ACP, there is often no formal 'tool' used across localities or within organizations. However the National End of Life Programme (5) provided the opportunity for documentation intended for many aspects of care to be developed, with examples of an Advance Statement such as the Preferred Priorities of Care (PPC) and many organizations either use this and/or an adapted version of the tool (6).

An ACP can be a hand held document which can accompany the individual between different care settings. It is owned by that person and their permission is required for it to be shared. If the person does not want their wishes formally documented, the facilitator of the discussion must abide by this, documenting only that a discussion has taken place. As previously described an ACP should be regularly reviewed and communicated to key individuals involved in the care of the person, therefore it is a contemporaneous and active document.

Hattie's story continued

Hattie is happy to have her wishes documented, however, there is some concern that she will either lose the ACP or in periods when her mental health deteriorates she may destroy it. There is also the possibility that in times of crisis her wishes will not be considered because of a lack of knowledge about its existence.

Issue

Hattie's ACP will not be acknowledged, and/or reviewed appropriately in the future.

Resolution

Hattie is happy that other key people involved in her care have duplicate copies of her ACP. She agrees that as part of her regular care review meeting her ACP will become an agenda item and she will have the opportunity to reconsider her decisions if indicated. Hattie also wants her care manager to be the person who is responsible for updating the ACP when required and ensuring that the people who need to know about it are informed of its existence.

Summary

ACP should always be seen as an ongoing process, reviewed at regular intervals. When facilitating plans with people who may have impaired or fluctuating capacity it is essential to adhere to this principle. There are opportunities and challenges in planning for future care with anyone including people who may lack capacity. It is crucial to maximize capacity ensuring the discussion is at their pace and in a format they understand. ACP is something that is 'done with' the person rather than something that is 'done to'—a principle that most care providers would say is central to any process but often but difficult to adhere to.

For effective ACP with people who lack capacity, families, carers, and professionals, need to listen to, and learn from each other, always keeping the individual at the heart of discussion and focus for the plan, using the Best Interests process as described in the MCA. Working in partnership with people and professionals also offers the opportunity for more supportive working practices. This chapter has identified that ACP can be complex, require considerable patience and resilience, and test all concerned. This includes professionals and experts who also require the support through clinical supervision to maintain their effectiveness and professional longevity.

References

1 Mental Capacity Act (2005). In Mental Capacity Act *Code of Practice* (2007), Sec 2(1)42. The Stationary Office, London.

2 Department of Health (2001). *Valuing People: A New Strategy for Learning Disability for the 21st Century.* The Stationary Office, London.

3 Regnard C, Reynolds J, Watson B, Matthews D, Gibson L, and Clarke C (2007). Understanding distress in people with severe communication difficulties: developing and assessing the Disability Distress Assessment Tool (DisDAT), *Journal of Intellectual Disability Research,* **51**(4):277–92.

4 The National End of Life Care Programme and the National Hospice Council for Palliative Care (2008). *Advance Decisions to Refuse Treatment,* A Guide For Health and Social Care Professionals. Gateway ref: 10350. Department of Health, London.

5 Department of Health (2003). *End of Life Programme.* The Stationary Office, London.

6 Regnard C, Matthews D, and Gibson L (2009). Discussing preferred priorities of care (advance care planning). In Regnard C and Dean M (eds), *A Guide to Symptom Relief in Palliative Care,* 6th ed. Radcliffe Medical, Oxford.

International experience of ACP: what can we learn from other countries?

Chapter 17

Advance directives and Advance Care Planning: the US experience

Anne M Wilkinson

'Everyone is ambivalent about death: both the family members who confront this most singular and terrifying event, and the physicians, nurses, and others who regularly witness it.'
N Dubler (1)

'Patients are at most risk of receiving care inconsistent with their preferences when they cannot participate in decision making . . .'

This chapter includes:
- Introduction: the challenges of end of life
- The ethical and legal foundations of advance directives (ADs) and Advance Care Planning (ACP) in the United States
- The evidence base regarding the application of ADs and ACP in clinical settings in the USA
- Lessons learnt from the failure of the AD process in the US and the future of ACP
- The history of the development of ACPs in USA began with refusals of treatment and ADs but has now moved towards a greater emphasis on statements of preferences and wishes.

Key points
- ACP is more than documenting life-sustaining treatment choices or identifying a surrogate decision-maker; it is a comprehensive, continuing communication and 'shared decision-making' process between the patient, family, and providers designed to elicit patient values and health-related quality of life goals for treatment.
- ACPs should be targeted to appropriate patients (e.g. age, medical condition); tailored to the patient's current and future disease states and life circumstances; flexible to address changing circumstances or patient preferences; and reviewed regularly (e.g. at each serious exacerbation of disease).
- Plans could also include 'time-limited trials' of invasive medical treatments with clear parameters for stopping if ineffective or poor response.
- If the patient chooses to forego aggressive, curative treatment or wishes to die at home, then palliative and supportive care services for patient and family quality of life, such as 24/7 crisis response to the home, caregiver respite services, or terminal sedation, must be available and reliably provided.

> - ACP interventions should use consistent documentation; systematic implementation processes; provide appropriate training across all relevant providers, region-wide; and build in systematic accountability to ensure patient wishes are honoured and that quality improvement activities ensure continuous performance improvement in the systems of ACP.
> - The US model of ACP encourages the full integration of palliative or hospice care into the care plans early in the disease trajectory to complement active, disease-modifying treatments, and to facilitate the transition to in the final stages.

Advance Directives (ADs) were promoted as a way of giving seriously ill individuals and their loved ones more control over their care, a 'voice' in medical decision-making, and to ensure that the individual's wishes about refusal of treatment were known, even if they were unable to communicate those wishes. However, a large body of evidence has accumulated, showing that ADs, as embodied in the Patient Self-Determination Act of 1991, failed in accomplishing these goals. The literature suggests that most people would prefer not to stare death in the face—at least not their own (2), and few want to 'micro-manage' their own death (3). However, the failure of ADs led to the development of the Advance Care Planning (ACP) process in the USA, and has resulted in several examples of excellent practice, acceptance by patients and families, and models of care that have much to teach others interested in successful program development in this area.

Time to move on from advanced directives

Advance directives promise much but deliver little, writes one doctor from Texas. They were developed more than three decades ago to give patients a say in their future care, but the original concept was overoptimistic. Even the most thorough advanced directive can be derailed in the end by the complexities of modern care, the poor preparation of proxy decision makers, the ambiguity of the patient's wishes, or the strong will of other parties, he writes. Complete control over the manner of death is an unattainable goal.

Despite decades of encouragement, most people fail to complete advanced directives, preferring instead to ignore the uncomfortable reality of death or leave end of life decisions for someone else or to fate. Even when an advance directive exists, it may not be accessible at a time of crisis. Some are signed once but never updated, leaving relatives unsure of the patient's current wishes.

Some kind of AD will always be important, writes the doctor, but advance directives don't work. Until we come up with something better, doctors should prepare patients and their families for the uncertainty that lies ahead and support them courageously through difficult decisions when they finally come (4). Advance Care Planning (ACP) is that 'something better'.

The challenges of end of life medical care

More effective public health measures and advances in biomedical technology during the latter half of the 20th century have substantially extended life expectancy around the world. In the United States, individuals reaching the age of 65 now have an average life expectancy of almost 19 years (17 years for males; 20 years for females) (4). However, a number of new challenges arise for populations living into late old age. For one thing, few of us die 'suddenly' anymore. The majority now live long and healthy lives, surviving illnesses and traumatic injury that, in the past, would have proved fatal. Chronic illnesses, including cancer, organ system failure (primarily heart, lung, liver, or kidney), dementia and stroke, are the leading causes of death for most Americans. These illnesses disproportionately affect the elderly and contribute to late life physical frailty and disability, diminished quality of life, and the receipt of complex medical technology that places substantial demands on the public health and social service systems.

As individuals approach the end of life, their disease process may create a number of immediate life-threatening emergencies. However, prognosis in non cancer patients has been shown to be persistently ambiguous, making it difficult for health care professionals to identify when a person is dying. In some cases, invasive interventions that were successful in the past may be, in the current crisis, less likely to provide benefit while carrying the same or greater risks (5). In addition, the individual may experience a loss of consciousness and be unable to express his/her wishes for medical care. Moreover, the difficulty of discontinuing life-prolonging treatment once started may mean aggressive therapy until the point of death, depriving the person of the opportunity for appropriate supportive or palliative care measures. Aggressive medical care under such circumstances may only serve to extend survival in very compromised states or prolong, and not necessarily improve, the dying process (3).

Advance directives (ADs) and, later, Advance Care Planning (ACP), were promoted as a way of giving seriously ill individuals and their loved ones more control over their care; a 'voice' in medical decision-making, and to ensure that the individual's wishes about a refusal of treatment are known, even if they are unable to communicate or have lost the ability to make decision at the time that the treatment they wish to refuse is under consideration.

There are three main types of health care directives utilized in the US, following a similar pattern in other countries (see Box 17.1):

* various forms of statements of preferences in what are known as a 'values history'
* the surrogate or proxy designation directive, often called a durable power of attorney for health care (DPOAHC)

Box 17.1 Definitions and terminology used in the USA: equivalence for other countries

Statement of wishes or preferences
* Values history: a document that aims to record a person's values, beliefs, and/or customs that are important to the person and which should be respected in end of life decision-making.

Refusal of treatment
* Instructional ADs (living wills): formal, legally endorsed written documents in which patients state their preferences (what is desired/not desired) for future treatment should they become incapacitated, usually involving choices about invasive treatments such as cardiopulmonary resuscitation, mechanical ventilation, artificial feeding and hydration, provision of blood and antibiotics, and surgical procedures.
* Life-sustaining treatment choices:
  * Cardiopulmonary resuscitation (CPR)
  * Mechanical ventilation
  * Artificial feeding and/or hydration
  * Medications, such as antibiotics
  * The use of blood products
  * Surgical procedures

Proxy designation
* Surrogate or proxy: an individual, other than a patient's legal guardian, authorized to make a health care decision for the patient and who becomes the substitute decision-maker in the event the advance directive is put into force.
* Durable power of attorney for health care (DPOAHC): the designation of a surrogate or proxy to make healthcare decisions for the individual granting the power.

◆ the instructional directive which may include some indication of preferences, often labelled a 'living will'.

Instructional ADs can vary widely in formality; ranging from brief, simple written (sometimes verbal) statements made to loved ones or physicians (e.g. no heroic or extraordinary measures) to very complex legal documents prepared with the help of an attorney using a standardized (often state-specific) form explicitly providing instructions regarding precise medical treatments to be used or withheld in particular medical situations or scenarios (7–9). Patients are most at risk of receiving care inconsistent with their preferences when they cannot participate in decision-making. Patients who lack capacity must rely either on written or verbal statements made prior to their incapacity or on surrogates, who are ethically and legally recognized to make decisions on the patient's behalf. Surrogates are encouraged to use a 'substituted judgement' standard when making decisions; that is, they should make decisions 'in the same way' that the patient would have if s/he were not incapacitated. In effect, this means that surrogates are expected to decipher how the patient, if able to fully understand his/her condition, would make treatment decisions (10). If the surrogate is unable to communicate confidently about the patient's preferences, then they are asked to make treatment decisions based on the patient's 'best interest' (11).

A brief history of the foundation of advance directives in the United States

The right to consent to or refuse treatment is grounded in the Western bioethical principles of autonomy and self-determination and is a widely accepted common-law right of all individuals who have full legal capacity (12,13). As far back as 1914, case law established the requirement that health professionals obtain a patient's consent for invasive medical procedures based on their right of self-determination. The court decision affirmed that 'every human being of adult years of sound mind has the right to determine what shall be done with his own body' (2). (See Box 17.2.) By the 1960s, medical professionals were using newly developed life-sustaining technologies (e.g. mechanical ventilators, cardiopulmonary resuscitation (CPR)) to prolong life, often in the face of dismal prognoses and with a quality of life so dreadful that many people preferred death to being kept alive under such circumstances.

The term 'living will' first appeared in the US in 1969, with the introduction of a testimony-type document designed to prevent or cease 'extraordinary' measures to prolong life and to allow a patient the legal right to a death with dignity, if and when they were unable to engage in independent decision-making (2).

Box 17.2 Legal cases and legislation in the USA

◆ Cardozo decision affirming patient autonomy and self-determination, 1914
◆ The term 'living will' first appears in the US, 1969
◆ Karen Ann Quinlan Supreme Court decision, 1975
◆ The Natural Death Act, California, 1976
◆ Advance directive legislation, Arkansas, 1977
◆ Durable power of attorney for health care (DPoAHC), Pennsylvania, 1983
◆ Nancy Cruzan, Supreme Court decision, 1990
◆ Patient Self Determination Act (PSDA), US Congress, 1991

States began passing various forms of living will legislation by the mid-1970s in response to consumer rights and hospice advocate's demands for legal protections against unwanted treatment at the end of life: California passed the Natural Death Act, the first giving legal force to living wills, in 1976. In 1977, Arkansas became one of the first states to pass legislation recognizing advance directives and, in 1983, Pennsylvania became the first state to enact legislation establishing the legal basis for the durable power of attorney for health care (DPoAHC). Today, all fifty states and the District of Columbia have statutes legalizing the use of living wills, health care proxies and/or the durable power of attorney (2).

A critical question concerning advance directives is whether the right of autonomy/self-determination can be assured if the individual lacks capacity (14). Two high-profile court decisions in the 1970s and 1980s epitomized the ethical and medical dilemmas concerning life-sustaining treatment and patient preferences for end of life care. The first case, in 1975, involved Karen Ann Quinlan, who, at the age of 21, was left in a persistent vegetative state after a cardiac arrest and without an advance directive. In 1976, the New Jersey Supreme Court granted her parents the right to withdraw her from life-support. The Court held, based on the principle of autonomous choice, that the onset of incapacity did not eliminate a patient's right to refuse medical treatment and that an individual's constitutional right to privacy outweighs the state's interest in preserving life (14–18).

In the second case, Nancy Cruzan had been left in a persistent vegetative state after an automobile accident in 1983 and had no living will or other advance directive. After a number of years, her parents concluded that she would not want to be kept alive in her current state and wanted to withdraw her artificial life support (a feeding tube). The hospital caring for her, fearing legal repercussions, refused to do so without a court order. Although local courts affirmed the parent's right to withdraw life support, the Missouri State Supreme Court reversed the decision on the grounds that Ms Cruzan's parents lacked 'clear and convincing evidence' that this choice reflected her wishes. In 1990, the US Supreme Court affirmed Cruzan's right to refuse life support but also affirmed a state's constitutional right to set high barriers (e.g. clear and convincing evidence) for decisions withdrawing food and water from patients where they have not spoken clearly for themselves as a procedural safeguard of surrogate decision-makers (14–18).

As a direct result of the Nancy Cruzan case, Senator John Danforth of Missouri sponsored, and the US Congress passed, the Patient Self Determination Act (PSDA) in 1991, providing a national legal basis for living wills and with the aim of encouraging competent adults to complete advance directives (19). The PSDA requires health care facilities receiving Medicare and Medicaid funding to ask incoming patients whether they have an advance directive and, if not, to provide written information on treatment options, right-to-die information, and AD forms to adult patients (20).

The evidence on end of life planning in the US: has the process failed?

Advance Directives: with the passage of the PSDA, advance directives received tremendous public and health care provider support, although there had been little research conducted to determine whether written advance directives would be able to achieve the goal of preserving patients' self-determination and autonomy rights (21). Almost 20 years after the adoption of the PSDA, we now have a large, though varied, body of evidence on the clinical application and effectiveness of advance directives (22–28). Advance directives require three steps for implementation in order to have an impact on medical care:

1 the completion of an AD

2 the physician's and surrogate decision-maker's recognition of the AD

3 the physician's honouring of the person's choices for medical care (20).

The accumulated evidence suggests that, despite the codification of advance directives in state and federal law and widespread public support for them in healthy and ill populations as well as the medical community, few people complete ADs. In addition, ADs are often not available when needed and the treatment that people would choose at the end of life is often very different from the treatment they receive.

Adoption of advance directives remains low, ranging from 5 to 25 per cent of Americans completing an AD (22–24). What is more, acutely ill individuals, for whom ADs are particularly relevant, complete advance directives at rates only slightly higher than the healthy or chronically ill (29–31). The evidence regarding the completion of advance directives by differing racial or ethnic groups is mixed, with most studies finding African Americans and Hispanics less likely than whites to complete an AD and less likely to specify that life-sustaining treatments be withheld or withdrawn (22,32).

One of the most anticipated outcomes of the PSDA and its explicit support of advance directives was that it would stimulate and improve the quality of end of life discussions among patients and their providers. Although patients want to have end of life discussions, it appears that these discussions still rarely occur, and when they do, the content of the discussions focuses on completion of AD forms rather than on the patient's values, end of life care goals, or desired health-related quality of life outcomes from treatment, all of which would be of substantial use in end of life decision-making. Moreover, the patient's surrogate decision-maker or family is rarely included in these discussions, an omission that can lead to errors and family conflict at times of crisis (23). In addition, research has shown that the context of AD discussions, the way these discussions are undertaken, as well as clinician specific and other system factors, have been shown to significantly influence what decisions are made (33). For example, a number of studies have found that hospital bed availability profoundly influences the likelihood of dying in a hospital, irrespective of patient preferences (28,34).

A further goal of ADs was to improve the understanding of patient treatment preferences by the surrogate decision-maker. Nevertheless, surrogates consistently err in predicting patient preferences; that is, surrogates tend to choose interventions that the patient would refuse rather than withhold care desired by the patient. Conversely, physicians continue to predict less care than the patient would want (35,36). Further, it has been shown that many surrogates rely on factors other than the legal formula of 'what the patient would have wanted', such as the surrogate's own best interests or the mutual interests of themselves and the patient or that they base their judgements on documents with which they have little familiarity (37).

Simple educational efforts aimed at clinicians and consumers to increase AD completion rates have not been effective. More comprehensive educational interventions, such as multi-faceted, longitudinal interactive patient-centred programmes (e.g. person-to-person counselling or education, training in AD form completion, printed educational materials, and multiple direct interactions between patients and clinicians over many visits) have been found to moderately increase completion rates. Those who do complete ADs tend to be older, married, white, have greater disease burden, have higher income and education, have prior knowledge about advance directives, hold a positive attitude about end of life discussions, have had a long-standing relationship with their primary care physician, or their physician has an AD themselves (22,23).

Although the passage of the PSDA appears to have resulted in an increase in the number of Do Not Resuscitate (DNR) orders in hospitals and reductions in feeding tube use and better documentation of ADs in nursing homes; there is conflicting evidence on their impact on care at the end of life. ADs appear to have the weakest effect in intensive care units, where the most aggressive care is provided and where the majority of deaths involve difficult decisions about resuscitation, or withholding or withdrawing life-sustaining treatment (38,39). ADs are completed most often in nursing home and hospice settings, with reported completion rates of up to 70% in nursing homes and up to 94% in hospices (40). However, the comprehensiveness and applicability of nursing home ADs vary substantially (41). (Box 17.3 summarizes barriers to AD completion)

ADs are narrowly focused on the patient's right to refuse unwanted life sustaining treatment (LST); they are often physically unavailable when needed, too vague to be useful in decision-making, or are at odds with the patient's current clinical circumstances. Indeed, ADs can even impede effective decision-making. Once completed, ADs are rarely reviewed to reflect changes in patient conditions, preferences, or new medical treatments and AD discussions rarely include surrogates or family members (42). (See Box 17.4.)

What patients do want is honest information about prognosis and the likely course of their illness earlier in the disease trajectory; an opportunity to express general preferences, including their values, beliefs, and goals for care; and to not have to make decisions on their own (43–45). What is more, many people do not want their surrogate to rigidly follow a static, written document. Rather, they want their loved ones to have flexibility in decision-making to adapt to changing circumstances and for their surrogate and physician to exercise judgement in determining the current course of care when insufficient information is available or when there are extenuating circumstances (42).

Box 17.3 Patient and physician barriers to advance directive completion (22,23)

Patient barriers to advance directive discussions:

1 General anxiety regarding death and the reluctance on the part of patients, families, and providers to broach the subject of 'death' and end of life care planning

2 The patient's view that ADs are important for others but 'irrelevant' to them or that they are 'unnecessary' because their family and physician will 'know what to do'

3 Lack of knowledge or confusion by the patient or caregiver about advance directives and/or how to complete one

4 The perception that advance directives are complex, hard to execute, and once completed, cannot be changed

5 The perception that even if an AD is completed, the advance directive statement will not be followed by clinicians

6 Checklists of consent for specific treatments do not meet patient changing wishes or needs

7 Past negative experience with dying friends or family members influences willingness to complete

8 Ethnic and racial minority cultural and health literacy barriers limit completion in non-white populations

Physician barriers to advance directive discussions

1 Lack of time

2 Lack of necessary communication skills and expertise

3 Perceived low health literacy of patients

4 Perception that their patient's are not 'sick enough'.

Box 17.4 Patient and family wishes at end of life (43–45)

- To receive adequate pain and symptom management and comfort care
- Avoid inappropriate prolongation of dying
- Good patient-physician communication
- Clear patient-centred decision making processes and to retain some control over end of life decisions
- Preparation for what to expect
- Strengthening relationships with loved ones
- Achieving a sense of completion in life
- Being treated as a 'whole person'
- Continuity of care
- Emotional, practical, and spiritual support
- Relieving burdens that their dying would impose on loved ones.

Advance Care Planning

Advance Care Planning (ACP) emerged in the mid-1990s as the evidence on the limitations of ADs began accumulating. ACP attempts to fill the gaps in ADs by using a more comprehensive, process-oriented method of end of life planning. ACP is a multistage and multilayered education and communication process between a patient, their family, and their physician involving discussion, education, and reflection to achieve a shared understanding of the individual's current state of health, their goals for care, their values and preferences for future treatment. Once a plan is established, ACP ensures the documentation of these preferences in the patient's medical record, the communication of these decisions to family and friends, and the periodic review of the decisions as circumstances change.

The emerging evidence on ACP suggests that it has been far more successful than advance directives in enhancing patient/provider communication and reduces unnecessary hospitalizations, aggressive treatments at the end of life, and care that is inconsistent with patient goals (22,46). Recent research on a number of successful ACP programmes, including the most well known of them (Respecting Choices; Five Wishes; POLST; and Let Me Decide), identified five programme elements that these newer, more successful ACP programmes share (15):

- a facilitated, clinician initiated discussion process to develop individualized plans
- standardized documentation and forms
- proactive but appropriately staged timing of discussions
- systems and processes that ensure planning occurs
- ongoing evaluation of the programme and quality improvement.

Other elements showing promise for facilitating ACP include the use of easy-to-understand ACP educational materials and multimedia instructional tools, systematic clinician training in communication skills, and extensive clinician-led discussions over time about patient values (22,23). (See Box 17.5 for goals and content of ACP discussions.)

Box 17.5 Goals and content of ACP discussions

Advance Care Planning should:

♦ Enhance patient/family understanding about their illness, including prognosis and likely outcomes of alternative care plans and determine how the patient and family's values may influence decision-making.

♦ Define the key priorities in end of life care, develop consensus regarding the desired short and long-term goals of care, and develop a care plan that reflects these priorities.

♦ Shape future clinical care to fit the patient's preferences and values and adapt it to changes in the patient's clinical situation or preferences.

♦ Assess patients for psycho-social and spiritual needs and help patients/family find hope and meaning in life, and achieve a sense of spiritual peace.

♦ Strengthen relationships with loved ones.

♦ Offer valid and reliable treatment alternatives to life-sustaining treatment choices, such as 'time-limited trials' of invasive technology or 24/7 crisis interventions at home to enhance quality of life.

♦ Develop and support a well-defined and meaningful role for the family in the 'shared' decision-making process of ACP.

♦ ACP should include considerations of illness burden, both on the family but also in terms of the financial burden that the illness may incur.

♦ Offer and deliver bereavement services to surviving family members.

Examples of good practice

Five Wishes

The Five Wishes is a 12 page 'living will', developed in 1997 by the Aging with Dignity organization to increase advance directive completion. It incorporates written, verbal, and video components to guide adults through the advance directive completion process in a group setting and includes five components of end of life treatment decisions: an advance directive, a healthcare proxy, specific comfort and treatment, and personal information for loved ones. Five Wishes is written in plain English and covers a range of issues typically not found in statutory living wills or health care power of attorney documents, such as how comfortable a person wants to be and a range of wishes about medical, personal, spiritual, and emotional needs. Five Wishes meets the legal requirements for advance directives in 40 states and the District of Columbia (47). However, only anecdotal evidence of the programme's effectiveness is available.

Five Wishes *http://www.agingwithdignity.org/5wishes.html*

My wish for:

1 The person I want to make care decisions for me when I can't (Healthcare agent or LPOA)

2 The kind of medical treatment I want or don't want (include DNAR life support treatment etc)

3 How comfortable I want to be (related to pain, depression, mouthcare, bathing, music, readings, hospice)

4 How I want people to treat me (to be accompanied, prayers, pictures, die at home etc)

5 What I want my loved one to know (love, forgiveness, fears, funeral arrangements etc)

Let Me Decide

A Canadian ACP programme for nursing facilities, involves structured health care provider, consumer, and family education about advance directives and utilizes a step by step guided process for competent individuals or the next-of-kin of incapacitated patients to state preferences for treatment for life threatening illnesses across a range of health care choices, including cardiac arrest and nutrition. Unlike the Five Wishes programme, Let Me Decide has substantial empirical data to support its effectiveness. One randomized, controlled trial (RCT) of the programme for 1,292 nursing home residents in Ontario between 1994 and 1998 found that the intervention resulted in significantly higher prevalence of planning, and reductions in hospitalizations, aggressive care, and resources used in the intervention group. Intervention residents were less likely to die in the hospital and families were more satisfied with the process than in control facilities (48). Another RCT found reductions in emergency calls from the intervention nursing homes to the ambulance service and reductions in hospital length of stay (49). Similar results were found for the use of Let Me Decide in the elderly living in the community (50–52).

The Respecting Choices programme

The Respecting Choices programme (*www.gundersenlutheran.com/eolprograms*) began in 1991 as part of a community-wide, integrated 'systems' approach to end of life planning in La Crosse, Wisconsin. Respecting Choices programme components include:

1 community outreach and education

2 non-professional training as programme facilitators

3 standards of practice and documentation adopted community-wide.

The initial evaluation of the programme reported that 85% of patients in the intervention had written advance directives at the time of death and these ADs had been executed an average of 1.2 years prior to death. Of these directives, 96% were found in the medical record where the person died; and treatment decisions made in the last weeks of life were consistent with written instructions in 98% of the deaths where an advance directive existed (53). Extensive subsequent research has shown this patient-centred ACP programme to be effective in promoting shared decision-making and greater satisfaction with the decision-making process (54–56). Respecting Choices is now being implemented in communities across the United States, Canada, and Australia.

The Physician Orders for Life-Sustaining Treatment (POLST)

The Physician Orders for Life-Sustaining Treatment (POLST) form, developed in 1998 (*www. polst.org*), is a standardized, one-page, brightly coloured pre-printed document designed to travel across treatment settings to ensure continuity of care. It is completed by a physician based on conversations with the patient and/or appropriate surrogate decision-maker, and provides specific treatment orders for cardiopulmonary resuscitation, medical interventions, artificial nutrition, and antibiotics. The POLST form has been shown to accurately represent patient treatment preferences in the majority of cases and that treatments at the end of life tend to match orders (57–61). Most hospitals, nursing homes, emergency services, and hospices in Oregon now use the POLST and thirteen states have adapted versions of the form. In 2004, a National POLST Paradigm Task Force was formed to support national growth of the programme (62). (Table 17.1 summarizes some of AD and ACP successes and failures in the US.)

Table 17.1 A summary of AD and ACP use in the US

Successes and failures in the US Process Advance Directive

Successes	Failures

◆ PDSA: 1991
  • Enshrined in law the right to have an AD, and if Medicare/Mediaid funded, health providers must ask the patient if they have an AD and if not, provide them with information and forms to complete
◆ Uptake of AD by some but they were:
  • older, married, white, high disease burden, higher income and education, prior knowledge of AD, had a positive attitude about end of life discussion, long standing relationship with primary care physician or their physician had an AD themselves
◆ Increased number of DNAR orders and decreased feeding tubes
◆ Better documentation of AD in nursing homes and hospices
◆ People want honest information about prognosis, and the likely course of illness earlier in the disease trajectory, an opportunity to express general preferences including values, beliefs, and goals for care and to not have to make decisions on their own (42–44) they want their surrogate and health provider to have flexibility in decision making and exercise appropriate judgement (41)
	◆ Uptake has been shown to be poor 5–25%
	◆ Varies with racial and ethnic groups
	◆ Has not stimulated quality of life discussions at end of life
	◆ Focused on completion of AD form
	◆ Surrogate rarely included (22,23)
	◆ The way discussion is handled affects decisions (33)
	◆ Does not improve understanding by surrogate and sometimes conflicts with patient choice
	◆ Education measures not very effective
	◆ Weak effect of ADs and DNARs in intensive care units where urgently needed
	◆ Applicability of ADs in nursing home varies (41)
	◆ Too focused on right to refuse treatment
	◆ Rarely reviewed

Examples of successful Advance Care Planning models

Five Wishes

◆ Little published evidence, though anecdotally well received

Let Me Decide

◆ RCT shows increased planning and reduced hospitalization, aggressive care, and resources used for nursing home residents (46)

◆ Reductions in ambulance emergency calls and reduced length of stay for nursing home residents and community-dwelling elderly (49–52)

Respecting Choices

◆ 85% had ADs at death, written on average 1.2 years earlier

◆ 98% treatment decisions consistent with plans

◆ Greater satisfaction with shared decision making (53–56)

POLST

◆ Accurately represents patient treatment preferences in majority

◆ Treatment at end of life tend to match order (57–61)

◆ National POLST Paradigm Task Force Development (62)

Lessons learnt from the failure of the AD process in the US and the future of ACP

Attention to understanding and honouring the patient's wishes for care at the end of life may be one of the more important goals in healthcare and requires active, ongoing, and directed communication between a patient and their healthcare provider. Advance directives were intended as simple statements designed to retain the patient's voice in medical decision-making should they become incapacitated. Instead, they evolved into complex, legalistic, yet ineffective documents too simplistic to be useful in most end of life clinical situations. In contrast, ACP interventions that focus on the patient and family values and goals of care rather than on completing statutory forms, and that use a comprehensive, systematic, and community-wide approach to implementation, have consistently demonstrated positive results on patient, caregiver, and provider satisfaction with care and on resource use.

In some ways the main objective of ACP has moved from a dialogue between the patient and the medical professional, to an ongoing conversation between the patient and their caregiver/family enabling and empowering this relationship, enhancing surrogate decision-making, and effecting the preferences and choices of the person approaching the end of life.

There is, as yet, no national or international policy or framework to guide consistency of application of ACP or to encourage continuity or transferability across states (16). In addition, although the successful ACP programmes have similar components, there is little consensus on what constitutes ACP (e.g. best practices) or on a uniform method of conducting ACP and, most importantly, for whom and when ACP should be done. The evidence suggests that nurses and specially trained lay people can successfully conduct ACP, yet patients continue to state that they expect their primary care physician to initiate such conversations (22,23).

It is not clear how ACP fits into established health care management, delivery, and reimbursement mechanisms. There is no Medicare reimbursement mechanism to pay for the practitioner's time to conduct ACP, which makes it difficult to establish these programmes into routine care. Obtaining a values history and participating in shared decision-making, two clearly preferred modes of ACP, requires physician expertise in end of life communication skills, which are sorely lacking today. Can ACP, which by its very nature requires time, commitment, and specialized training for health professionals, be done in a valid manner and still be efficiently incorporated into daily practice? Can our fragmented health care system reliably ensure the application of a patient's wishes and plans over time and across settings? Moreover, although the literature has identified fairly consistent patient/family identified elements of a good death (see Box 17.4); it is not clear how well or in what ways ACP contributes to achieving these desired ends. ACP has been shown to be successful primarily in specific populations, how and in what ways can ACP be more responsive for all populations (e.g. the intellectually or physically disabled)? Finally, ACP has few well defined and valid quality indicators to measure performance (e.g. documentation; number of family conferences; a reliance on life-sustaining treatment decisions) (63).

ACP, at its most basic, is a process of ongoing communication and thinking ahead to future health states and treatment choices, shared decision-making in the identification of the goals of care for that future, choosing another trusted person to speak for oneself in the future, and the need for flexibility of judgement and interpretation in order to make the most appropriate treatment choices in real time with real people. While ACP has enormous potential to improve end of life care, the goals of ACP will be hard to accomplish in the US without changes in current systems of care delivery and payment and established routines of care. Significant progress has been made in the US over the past 30 years, and the valuable lessons learnt have been successfully spread to other countries. The process of ACP must be viewed as an important tool for shared decision making; and though complex, hard to measure, and time-consuming to implement, has been shown to be of considerable value in meeting the needs and requests of people facing the end of their life.

Further resources

Aging With Dignity Organization—Five Wishes - http://www.agingwithdignity.org/5wishes.html

New Grange Press. Let Me Decide: booklets, videos available at: http://www.stpetes.ca/newgrangepresss/let_me_decide_series_books_videos.html

Respecting Choices program www.gundersenlutheran.com/eolprograms

The Physician Orders for Life-Sustaining Treatment (POLST): www.polst.org

References

1 Dubler N (2005). Conflict and Consensus at the End of Life. In Jennings B, Kaebnick G, and Murray T (eds), *Improving End of Life Care: Why Has It Been So Difficult? Hastings Center Report Special Report,* **35**(6):S19.

2 Brown BA (2003). The history of advance directives: a literature review. *Journal of Gerontological Nursing,* **29**(9):4–14.

3 Lynn J and Goldstein N (2003). Advance care planning for fatal chronic illness: avoiding commonplace errors and unwanted suffering. *Annals of Internal Medicine,* **13**(8):812–816.

4 Perkins HS (2007). Controlling death: the false promise of advance directives. *Annals of Internal Medicine,* **147**:51–7.

5 Center for Disease Control (2003). Deaths: Public health and aging: trends in aging—United States and Worldwide. *MMWR Weekly,* **52**(06)101–106. Available at www.cdc.gov/mmwr/preview/mmwrhtml/mm5206a.htm (accessed 12 March 2009)

6 Weissman DE (2004). Decision making at a time of crisis near the end of life. *JAMA: Journal of the American Medical Association,* **292**(14):1738–44.

7 Simón-Lorda P, Barrio-Cantalejo IM, Garcia-Gutierrez JF et al. (2009). Interventions for promoting the use of advance directives for end-of-life decisions in adults. *Cochrane Database of Systematic Reviews,* **1**:1–12.

8 Doukas D and McCullough L (1991). The values history: the evaluation of the patient's values and advance directives. *Journal of Family Practice,* **32**(2):145–53.

9 Van Asselt D (2006). Advance directives: prerequisites and usefulness. *Zeitschrift fur Gerontologie und Geriatrie,* **39**(5):271–375.

10 Collins LG, Parks SM, and Winter L (2006). The state of advance care planning: one decade after SUPPORT. *American Journal of Hospice and Palliative Medicine,* **23**(5):378–84.

11 Rich BA (2002). The ethics of surrogate decision making. *The Western Journal of Medicine,* **176**:127–29.

12 Beauchamp TE and Childress JF (2001). *Principles of Biomedical Ethics,* 5th Ed. Oxford University Press, Oxford.

13 Jennings B (2005). Preface. In Jennings B, Kaebnick GE, and Murray TH (eds) *Improving End of Life Care: Why Has It Been So Difficult? Hastings Center Report Special Report,* **35**(6):S2–S4.

14 Fagerlin A, Ditto PH, Hawkins NA, Schneider CE, and Smucker WD (2002). The use of advance directives in end-of-life decision making. *American Behavioral Scientist,* **46**(2):268–83.

15 Hickman S, Hammes B, Moss A, and Tolle S (2005). Hope for the Future: Achieving the original intent of advance directives. In Jennings B, Kaebnick G, and Murray T (eds) *Improving End of Life Care: Why Has It Been So Difficult? Hastings Center Special Report,* **35**(6):S26–30.

16 Chiarella M (2008). Practical legal issues in end of life care. *Australian Nursing Journal,* 2008;**15**(8):21.

17 Murray TH and Jennings B (2005). The Quest to Reform End of Life Care: Rethinking Assumptions and Setting New Directions. In Jennings B, Kaebnick G, and Murray T (eds), *Improving End of Life Care: Why Has It Been So Difficult? Hastings Center Report Special Report,* **35**(6): S52–S57.

18 Prendergast TJ (2001). Advance care planning: pitfalls, progress, promise. *Critical Care Medicine*, **29**(2):N34–39.

19 U.S. Congress (1991). Patient Self-Determination Act. Omnibus Budget Reconciliation Act (OBRA), Pub L 101–508, 1990.

20 Galambos CM (1998). Preserving end-of-life autonomy: The Patient Self-Determination Act and the Uniform Health Care Decisions Act. *Health and Social Work*, **23**(4):275–81.

21 Fagerlin A and Schneider CE (2004). Enough: the failure of the living will. *Hastings Center Report*, **34**(2):30–42.

22 Wilkinson AM, Wenger N, and Shugarman LR (2007). Literature review on advance directives. U.S. Department of Health and Human Services, Assistant Secretary for Planning and Evaluation, Office of Disability, Aging and Long-Term Care Policy. Available at: http://aspe.hhs.gov/daltcp/reports/2007/advdirlr.pdf

23 Lorenz KA, Lynn J, Morton SC, et al. (2004). End-of-Life Care and Outcomes, AHRQ Evidence Report/Technology Assessment. 110, Publication. 05-E004-1, Rockville MD. Available at: www.ahrq.gov/clinic/epcsums/eolsum.htm.

24 Ramsaroop SD, Reid MC, and Adelman RD (2007) Completing an advance directive in the primary care setting: what do we need for success. *Journal of the American Geriatrics Society*, **55**:277–83.

25 Jezewski MA and Meeker MA (2005). Constituting advance directives from the perspective of people with chronic illnesses. *Journal of Hospice Palliative Nursing*, **7**(6):319–27.

26 Guo B and Harstall C (2004). *Advance directives for End-of-Life Care in the Elderly: Effectiveness of Delivery Modes*.: Alberta Heritage Foundation for Medical Research (AHFMR), Alberta, Canada.

27 Patel VR, Sinuff T, Cook DJ. Influencing advance directive completion rates in non-terminally ill patients: a systematic review. *Journal of Critical Care*, **19**(1):1–9.

28 Hanson LC, Tulsky JA, and Danis M (1997). Can clinical interventions change care at the end of life? *Annals of Internal Medicine*, **126**(5):381–88.

29 Kish SK, Martin CG, and Price KJ (2000). Advance directives in critically ill cancer patients. *Critical care nursing clinics of North America*, **12**(3):373–83.

30 Knauft E, Nielsen EL, Engelberg RA, Patrick DL, and Curtis JR (2005). Barriers and facilitators to end-of-life care communication for patients with COPD. *Chest*, **127**(6):2188–96.

31 Wu P, Lorenz KA, and Chodosh J (2008). Advance care planning among the oldest old. *Journal of Palliative Medicine*, 2008;**11**(2):152–57.

32 Bullock K (2006). Promoting advance directives among African Americans: a faith-based model. *Palliative Medicine*, **9**(1):183–95.

33 Song, MK (2004). Effects of end-of-life discussions on patients affective outcomes. *Nursing Outlook*, **52**:118–25.

34 Hansen SM, Tolle SW, and Martin DP (2002). Factors associated with lower rates of in-hospital death. *Journal of Palliative Medicine*, **5**(5):677–85.

35 Shalowitz DI, Garrett-Mayer E, and Wendler D (2006). The accuracy of surrogate decision makers: a systematic review. *Archives of Internal Medicine*, **166**(5):493–97.

36 Meeker MA (2004). Family surrogate decision making at the end of life: Seeing them through with care and respect. *Qualitative Health Research*, **14**(2):204–25.

37 Vig EK, Taylor JS, Starks H, Hopley EK, and Fryer-Edwards K (2006). Beyond substituted judgment: how surrogates navigate end-of-life decision-making. *Journal of American Geriatrics Society*, **54**(11):1688–93.

38 Thelen M (2005). End-of-life decision making in intensive care. *Critical Care Nurse*, **25**(6):28–37; quiz 38.

39 Lilly CM, Sonna LA, Haley KJ, and Massaro AF (2003). Intensive communication: four-year follow-up from a clinical practice study. *Critical Care Medicine*, **35**:S394–9.

40 Resnick HE, Schuur JD, Heineman J, Stone R, and Weissman JS (2008). Advance directives in nursing home residents aged 65 or older: United States 2004. *American Journal of Hospice and Palliative Care*, **25**(6):476–82.

41 Teno JM (2000). Advance directives for nursing home residents: Achieving compassionate, competent, cost-effective care. *JAMA: Journal of American Medical Association*, **283**(11):1481–82.

42 Ayers Hawkins N, Ditto PH, Danks JH, and Smucker WE (2005). Micromanaging death: process preferences, values, and goals in end-of-life medical decision making. *The Gerontologist*, **45**(1):107–117.

43 Steinhauser KE, Christakis NA, Clipp EC, McNeilly M, McIntyre L, and Tulsky JA (2000). Factors considered important at the end of life by patients, family, physicians, and other care providers. *JAMA: Journal of American Medical Association*, **284**(19):2476–82.

44 Clark EB (2003). Quality indicators for end-of-life care in the intensive care unit. *Critical Care Medicine*, **31**:2255–62.

45 Singer PA, Martin DK, and Kelner M (1999). Quality end-of-life care: patients' perspectives. *JAMA: Journal of American Medical Association*, **281**(2):163–8.

46 Lorenz KA, Lynn J, Morton SC, et al. (2008). Evidence for improving palliative care at the end of life: a systematic review. *Annals of Internal Medicine*, **148**(2):147–59.

47 Aging with Dignity. Available at:http://www.agingwithdignity.org/5wishes.html accessed 23 January 2009.

48 Molloy DW, Guyatt GH, Russo R et al. (2000). Systematic implementation of an advance directive program in nursing homes: a randomized controlled trial. *JAMA: Journal of American Medical Association*, **283**(11):1437–44.

49 Caplan GA, Meller A, Squires B, Chan S, and Willett W (2006). Advance care planning and hospital in the nursing home. *Age and Ageing*, **35**(6):581–85.

50 Molloy DW, Russo R, Pedlar D, and Bedard M. (2000). Implementation of advance directives among community-dwelling veterans. *The Gerontologist*, **40**(2):213–217.

51 Reinders M and Singer PA (1994). Which advance directive do patients prefer? *Journal of General Internal Medicine*, **9**(1):49–51.

52 Molloy DW, Silberfeld M, Darzins, P et al. (1996). Measuring capacity to complete an advance directives. *Journal of American Geriatrics Society*, **44**(6):660–64.

53 Hammes BJ and Rooney BL (1998). Death and end-of-life planning in one midwestern community. *Archives of Internal Medicine*, **158**:383–90.

54 Song MK, Kirchhoff KT, Douglas J, Ward S, and Hammes B (2005). A randomized, controlled trial to improve advance care planning among patients undergoing cardiac surgery. *Medical Care*, **43**(10):1049–53.

55 Schwartz CE and Hammes B (2004). Measuring patient treatment preferences in end-of-life care between patients and their health care agents helps define and document the patient's wishes for both patient and agent. *Journal of Palliative Medicine*, **7**(2):233–45.

56 Romer AL and Hammes BJ (2004). Communication, trust, and making choices: advance care planning four years on. *Journal of Palliative Medicine*, **7**(2):335–40.

57 Tolle SW, Tilden VP, Nelson CA, Dunn PM (1998). A prospective study of the efficacy of the physician order form for life-sustaining treatment. *Journal of the American Geriatrics Society*, **46**(9):1097–102.

58 Hickman SE, Nelson CA, Moss AH et al. (2009). Use of the physician orders for life sustaining treatment (POLST) paradigm program in the hospice setting. *Journal of Palliative Medicine*, **12**(2):133–41.

59 Hickman SE, Tolle SW, Brummel-Smith K, and Carley MM (2004). Use of the physician orders for life-sustaining treatment program in Oregon nursing facilities: beyond resuscitation status. *Journal of American Geriatrics Society*, **52**(9):1424–29.

60 Schmidt TA, Hickman SE, Tolle SW, and Brooks HS (2004). The physician orders for life-sustaining treatment program: Oregon emergency medical technicians' practical experiences and attitudes. *Journal of American Geriatrics Society*, **52**(9):1430–40.

61 Schmidt TA, Hickman SE, and Tolle SW (2004). Honoring treatment preferences near end of life: the oregon physician orders for life-sustaining treatment (POLST) program. *Advances in Experimental Medicine and Biology*, **550**:255–562.

62 National POLST Paradigm Initiative Task Force. Getting Endorsed. Available at : http://www.ohsu.edu/polst/about/task-force.htm.

63 Lorenz K, Lynn J, Dy S, Shugarman LM, et al. (2006). *Cancer Care Quality Measures: Symptoms and End-of-Life Care*; Evidence Report/Technology Assessment No. 137; (Prepared by the SCEPC under Contract No. 290-02-003); AHRQ Publication No. 06-E001; Rockville MD).

Chapter 18

A common sense guide to improving Advance Care Planning: from theory to practice

Anne M Wilkinson and Joanne Lynn

'The improvement of any system requires three elements: will, ideas and execution.'
Tom Nolan, Senior Fellow Institute for Healthcare Improvement

This chapter provides guidance on implementing ACP practices in a local area, utilizing the Plan-Do-Study-Act (PDSA) Quality Improvement model, based on extensive experience from the USA and is adapted from the Common Sense Guide to Improving Palliative Care, Oxford University Press, 2007.

This chapter includes:

- Introduction, definition of ACP and 'doing' Advance Care Planning
- The Plan-Do-Study-Act (PDSA) quality improvement process
- The three fundamental questions and necessary steps to improvement
- How to accelerate improvement and spread the gains
- Illustrative case example: 'Team Delta'
- Telling your story: time series run charts
- Examples of ACP, changes to try and common barriers to ACP
- Getting 'started' on improving ACP: give them something to talk about
- Frequently asked questions
- Communication strategies to initiate and target Advance Care Planning.

Key points

- Ensuring the centrality of the patient and family's voice in treatment decision-making is one of the most important goals for achieving patient and family-centred late life care.
- While challenging to do in busy healthcare settings, numerous healthcare professionals have been able to regularly conduct effective Advance Care Planning (ACP) and change their 'usual' health care culture by using the Plan-Do-Study-Act (PDSA) quality improvement cycle.
- By answering the 'three fundamental questions' (What are the AIMS? What are the CHANGES? What are the MEASURES?); establishing an effective team committed to

> making changes in 'usual' practice in their settings; and targeting the appropriate patients, reliable ACP can be embedded in everyday healthcare practice, regardless of setting.
>
> ◆ Once systematic gains have been achieved, teams can work on spreading the improvements to other professionals and settings.
>
> ◆ Advice and resources are provided to help teams begin to 'do' Advance Care Planning and to 'tell their story' showing off their successes.

Introduction

Ensuring the centrality of the patient and family's voice in treatment decision-making is one of the most important goals for achieving patient and family-centred late life care (1,2). Many factors influence treatment decisions near the end of life: How old is the patient? How sick? Will treatment enhance life or mostly prolong suffering? What does the patient want? What does the family want? In the best-case scenario, the patient, family, and healthcare providers have discussed treatment options and preferences and documented these wishes in the form of an Advance Care Plan. This way, everyone is prepared for eventual crises because they have agreed on a clear care plan that reflects the patient's values.

Advance Care Planning is a multi-stage and multi-layered process of communication and discussion between an individual, their healthcare providers, and those close to them concerning future health care. ACP is a 'process' that can be undertaken by a team in a variety of settings: a hospital, community setting or care home, or in a primary care physician's office and can be instigated and conducted by a medical practitioner, a nurse, a social worker, or other relevant health or social service professional. ACP involves education, information, communication, discussion, reflection, and review of the individual's current situation and the available treatments and procedures related to the individual's condition.

Although the issue of end of life planning has increasingly been in the public eye, few patients have had these discussions with their physician or family; and, even when they have, decisions may not be documented in the patient's medical record. Without plans, a crisis situation can escalate quickly, especially if the patient cannot communicate or if the family's preferences conflict with the clinician's. In these cases, treatment decisions are not made, they simply happen, and usually based on habits that are presumed to reflect what patients generally want.

ACP can be challenging for a variety of reasons, including:

◆ Everyone is reluctant to talk about the patient's declining health and approaching death.

◆ Clinicians find it easier to offer hope, comfort, and medical technology rather than 'let people die.'

◆ Clinician's lack of necessary communication skills and expertise.

◆ Patients and families find it hard to believe that treatments such as resuscitation will not restore health.

◆ Clinicians and family may not accept the patient's treatment priorities and values.

However, these barriers can be addressed. One method that has shown results has been the application of quality improvement techniques to the development and implementation of Advance Care Planning processes and plans.

The Plan-Do-Study Act (PDSA) quality improvement process

Quality improvement in healthcare is designed to bridge the chasm between the best available evidence and knowledge about clinical care and actual, everyday practice. Developed by the

Institute for Healthcare improvement (IHI) and Associates in Process Improvement in the US in the 1990s, quality improvement techniques allow the testing of creative ideas and solutions with small groups of patients, and then look to build on these successes to achieve even more improvement. The model for improvement is called the Plan-Do-Study-Act (PDSA) quality improvement process; a practical, proven quality improvement tool. With this approach, teams can start at virtually any point in the clinical routine and make changes for the better. The PDSA quality improvement process is not meant to replace change models that organizations may already be using. Rather, it is designed to accelerate improvement; that is, to take good ideas, test them quickly on small samples of patients and, if beneficial, incorporate them into daily routine. This model has been used very successfully by hundreds of health care organizations in many countries to improve many different health care processes and outcomes.

The model has two parts: the first part requires asking (and answering) three fundamental questions, which can be addressed in any order but which guide all subsequent improvement activities:

◆ What are we trying to accomplish? (the AIM)

◆ How will we know that a change is an improvement? (MEASURES)

◆ What changes can we make that will result in improvement? (CHANGES).

Although the questions are simple and straightforward, answering them takes thought and analysis and the healthcare team's answers to these questions form the basis for the improvement efforts.

The second part of the model requires taking action using the Plan-Do-Study-Act (PDSA) cycle to test and implement changes in real work settings (Fig. 18.1). The PDSA cycle thrives on trial and error and more is often learned from failure than success. Take an idea—then test it—that is, plan the test, do the test on a small sample of patients, observe the consequences, and then act on what is learned from the test.

The aim

An aim is a written statement of the accomplishments expected from the improvement effort. Improvement requires setting specific aims because unguided actions rarely yield improvement. Aims must be clear, have a numerical goal, a timeframe for completion, and must be able to be measured.

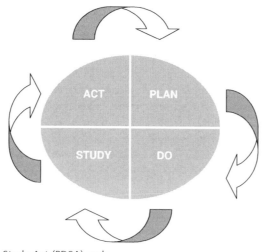

Fig. 18.1 The Plan-Do-Study-Act (PDSA) cycle.

By specifying a clear aim, teams avoid 'aim drift' and keep on focus. For example, a team might aim for the following:

By 15 June 75% of patients entering the ICU will have their advance care wishes identified and documented in their medical record within four hours of admission.

This example aim clearly states a quantifiable, and therefore measurable, goal (75% of patients), identifies which patients are to be included (ICU patients on admission), identifies what is to be accomplished (patient advance care wishes elicited and documented in their medical record within four hours of admission to the unit), and a timeframe for the accomplishment of the goal (by 15 June). It is important to set aims that will matter to patients and families; such aims are most likely to motivate professional caregivers to want to improve practice if there is a clear link to the patients they serve.

The team

Once the aim has been identified organizations wanting to make improvement need to provide appropriate staff, sufficient time, and adequate resources to accomplish the task. Improvement usually requires interdisciplinary action; therefore, an interdisciplinary team made up of physicians, nurses, social workers, chaplains, pharmacists, administrators, quality assurance personnel, and even data managers may be important to achieving the aim. Selecting the right team is an important first step in improvement and usually requires from five to eight people from many disciplines to share the work. A team will also require administrative support to encourage system-wide acceptance of the endeavour.

The changes

It is important to note that while all improvement requires change, but not all changes are an improvement. Change ideas can come from anywhere: 'best practices,' 'brainstorming' on the problem, good hunches based in experience, models or programs tried elsewhere, critical thinking about the current system, or even from the patients and families being served to understand more about what is needed. Ask frontline staff members to help identify 'bottlenecks' and suggest ways to fix what isn't working. Teams should focus on changes that are most likely to result in improvement.

Testing the change

People are more willing to try out a change when they know that along the way, they can quickly modify it if needed and that it is 'only a test' to see if the idea works better than what is being done now. Tests allow teams to gain confidence in the change being tested as more patients in different settings are exposed to the change and the results are consistently positive. Tests can be run on as few as one patient, but to have credible evidence that the change really is an improvement, multiple small samples over a few weeks or months of time are important. Ongoing data collection allows a team to determine whether they reached their numerical goal as stated in their aim. Convincing indicators are often those documented in a 'time-series' such as, percentage of clinic patients each month who have had an Advance Care Planning discussion or the average response time for pain relief on the oncology unit each week. Data plotted over time show the temporal relationship between changes made and the results, making a convincing case that specific changes lead to improvement. Sometimes it is enough to measure 'before' and 'after,' but this doesn't allow for the evaluation of whether it was a specific intervention or series of interventions that had the desired effect.

Measuring the change

Measurement is an important part of the improvement process, allowing teams to determine whether or not a change tested actually leads to an improvement in care. Improvement efforts require at least one or two key indicators (measures) that can be documented over time (over PSDA cycle 'tests') and over different small samples of patients. Teams need only 'just enough data' to convince a benevolent sceptic—someone who wishes the project well but who isn't gullible—that the data and measurement are credible, on target, and demonstrate a viable improvement outcome. Quality improvement measurement should provide answers to specific questions. For example: Did instituting a new pain assessment and response protocol reduce the incidence of pain? Did establishing a set of Advance Care Planning progress notes and procedures increase the percentage of patients who had a discussion of their treatment preferences by the healthcare team? Did the provision of clearly written information and reminders prevent families from making unnecessary emergency room visits?

Teams need to be committed to doing all the steps of the cycle:

Step 1: Plan a change

- State the objective of the change: develop an AIM statement
- Make predictions about what will happen and why
- Develop a plan to test the change: What will the team do? Who will do what? When? Where? What data must be collected?

Step 2: Do a change

- Carry out the test
- Document problems and unexpected observations
- Collect and assess data.

Step 3: Study a change

- Analyse the data
- Compare the data with the team's predictions
- Summarize what was learned and plot the data on a 'run chart' to show progress.

Step 4: Act on the next change

- Modify plans for the next change and/or modify the change based on what was learned
- Identify new 'problem' areas and develop change plans to address them
- Push work into a new area, new patient population, or institutionalize the changes that resulted in improvement
- Prepare plans for the next cycle(s).

The smallest informative change you can make by next Tuesday

Accelerating improvement means acting quickly. Most improvement efforts fail because so much time is spent considering, studying, and meeting that nothing ever happens. Begin small tests right away! Running small scale tests sooner improves patient care much more surely and quickly than waiting until everything is 'perfect'. Even big changes can be tested on a small scale—for example, with only one or two physicians, with the next five patients, for the next three days. In general, make the strongest change that the team can do quickly, on the smallest sample that will be inform- ative. When the change shows an improvement, then expand the scope. Each properly completed PDSA cycle provides valuable information and forms the basis for further improvement.

Spreading the gains

Teams find that when they improve care for one group of patients or in one unit, the entire organization is likely to want to spread the change further: from cancer to cardiac patients, from one unit to another, or even from one hospital to another within the system. The opportunity to use the PSDA model in multiple areas is compelling. Therefore, teams need to promote their improvement efforts—sharing them within the organization, with other health care groups, and with the community to gain community support and spread the gains. Teams show what they have learned by using a storyboard that tracks progress in the key areas. Storyboards tell the story of the work of the project, how it was done, and what it accomplished using simple graphs to demonstrate the change and improvement. Storyboards should be quick to read and easy to understand, include only critical information, and make the aim and results of the project clear and apparent. Innovation can become a 'way of life' for an organization, even though, at first glance, it may seem daunting. As the example and guidance in this chapter show, Advance Care Planning (ACP) is ripe for improvement. In addition, to be truly effective, ACP needs to be standardized, incorporated into daily practice, and spread across healthcare providers and healthcare delivery settings.

This section will help you meet challenges by describing quality improvement (QI) projects that work. The story of Team Delta's project to improve ACP is based on a composite of several successful teams.

About 'Team Delta'

Team Delta is in a long-term care facility in a major city. About 20% of residents die each year. The facility had many ongoing QI programmes, but nothing aimed at medical decision-making at the end of life. Team members had seen too many dying patients whose families insisted on tube feeding and hydration, even when doctors explained why these treatments would not be beneficial. Family members and staff agonized over what to do, especially when the resident could not communicate. Families and physicians were left trying to puzzle out what would be best. The team wanted a better way to prepare patient, families, and staff for these situations. They wanted to try a more organized approach to medical decision-making and ACP, including ways to update records as treatment preferences changed.

Identifying the problem and setting an aim

You may know that most of your seriously ill patients do not have good Advance Care Planning, but you are not exactly sure where to start an improvement project. Do families always just want 'everything done?' Are staff 'afraid' to have these conversations earlier in the resident's stay because they 'don't know what to say' or are afraid that they might 'upset' the resident or family? Do patients really want to avoid these discussions? Before you act on your hunches, be sure that you know the problem well. Others on your team need to agree about what the problem really is. Your team might ask staff about their perceptions or ask residents' survivors. Do you have data that can clarify which are the most important areas or resident populations to start with? Even asking a few of your team members such questions can help identify the problem.

Team Delta

After a few brainstorming sessions, Team Delta talked to a few family members whose loved ones had recently been hospitalized or had died in the facility. They identified the following problem areas:

- Residents, family, and staff were not aware of the need for ACP or the content of ACP discussions
- Even residents at high risk of dying did not routinely have a current ACP documented in their medical record, nor were they invited to participate in ACP discussions
- For residents who had ACP discussions, completed ACPs often were not documented.

Once Team Delta identified key problem areas, the team needed to develop and set one or more aim statements that it could measure and work towards. Team Delta developed the following aim statements to reflect its broad sequential goals:

Aim 1: Within six months, 80% of the facility's professional caregivers will have participated in an educational seminar on ACP, treatment choices, and disease progression.

Aim 2: Within three months, 95% of new and 'at risk of death' residents will have an ACP discussion documented in their medical records.

Aim 3: Within six months, 95% of new and 'at risk of death' residents who have had an ACP discussion will have a completed Advance Care Plan documented in their charts.

The team then came up with this overarching aim statement:

Aim statement: Within six months, 90% of new and 'at risk of death' residents will have a completed ACP documented in their record (95% with discussion, and 95% of those discussions documented = 90% overall completion rate).

Thus, team delta identified:

What will improve: Documented ACPs

By when: Within six months

By how much: Ninety per cent (instead of the current occasional)

For whom: New and 'at risk of death' residents.

How to have comprehensive discussions with patients and families, how to document the patients' decisions and later changes in those decisions, and how to transfer patients' information to other healthcare settings are all part of a good ACP programme. Common problems related to ACP include the following:

♦ Patients who are vulnerable and close to death end up getting inappropriate and undesired aggressive treatment because there is no other plan

♦ Your healthcare system claims that ACPs are a priority, but no one knows how they are tracked, who is responsible for having them completed, or what is included in the discussions

♦ Your practices encourage legal forms for advance directives (or ADs) but not more comprehensive and useful care planning (ACP statements of preference)

♦ Your system documents many patients' decisions, but the care plan does not travel with the patients when they transfer to another unit or facility

♦ Your protocol uses only a checklist of yes or no questions around the use of advanced technology with little regard for the social, psychological, or spiritual aspects of care planning

♦ Your organization wants to make ACP a routine part of care, but only for patients very near death

♦ Providers are reluctant to bring up ACP because they do not feel confident that they will know what to say or how to respond.

Choosing a team

You have already identified the problem and created an aim statement. Now you need to invite other people who can help you reach your goals to join your team. Together, identify opportunities for improvement. For each patient population, try to recruit clinicians and others who are closest to them, such as physicians, nurses, social workers, and chaplains. Think beyond the obvious people, however, and you will discover others who can help make your programme work. An admissions clerk, for instance, can help some projects by asking patients about whether they have an advance directive and where it is filed. If community adoption of a routine Advance Care Planning process is part of the goal, your team can enlist colleagues who work in other settings to assist with procedures that assure that Advance Care Plans transfer with the patient or to recruit key players in your community.

Team Delta

The original force behind Team Delta was a unit nurse who had experienced too many over-whelmed families faced with complex medical treatment decisions for loved ones who were near death and could not communicate. She recruited a few of her co-workers, including a social worker, and sought advice and ideas from the facility's medical director. In order to raise aware-ness of the problem, Team Delta decided to focus on the team leader's unit as a starting point and involve the rest of the facility over time. In addition, they focused on new admissions, unstable patients, and severely demented residents as the first set of residents (and their families) to target. The team quickly realized that they would need help from a number of others in the facility, including the director of nursing, the staff educator, certified nursing assistants (CNAs) on the floor, and families. In addition, they would need help from the information specialists to flag charts electronically and to help measure their progress.

Measuring success

Team Delta

To get a baseline, Team Delta reviewed 10 charts for residents who had died recently. No discus-sion of prognosis or treatment preferences had been documented, and no decisions had been made regarding life sustaining treatments. Moreover, of the 10, six had died after being trans-ferred to the hospital. The team decided to set a standard of having started a discussion with a resident and/or family member and documented existing decisions in the medical record within 72 hours of admission. The team started identifying 'at risk of death' patients and severely cogni-tively impaired residents. Based on their aims, team members identified which measures they needed to track to best monitor their progress. Over the next few weeks, the team began to imple-ment its changes, tracking whether the patient and family engaged in ACP; educating the facility staff on ACP and documentation of patient wishes; and assuring that their decisions were recorded.

A list of some of the measures that other teams have tracked to follow their progress in ACP follows. The measures may be actual numbers or percentages. The percentages must have a denominator (e.g. patients eligible for ACP) and a numerator (e.g. patients who complete advance directives).

Process measures

- New admissions or targeted patients on a unit or floor who have an advance directive (AD) (e.g. DNR, healthcare proxy, living will)
- Providers using checklists of ACP topics and a 'script' for discussions with patients
- Patients and/or family caregivers who have completed an educational session on ACP
- Healthcare providers can quickly find the patient's ACP
- Targeted patients who have discussions with an ACP 'SWAT' team within 48 hours of admission.

Outcome measures

- Targeted patients who had an ACP discussion and decisions documented in their medical record within 48 hours of admission
- Targeted patients whose documented treatment decisions were followed during serious illness
- New admissions or targeted patients with discussions of ACP
- Families saying that the discussion and decision-making were helpful or very helpful.

Adverse-effect measures

- Family members of patients who complain about the 'focus on things going badly'
- Family members who say that ACP discussions are 'too formal' or 'too impersonal'
- Families who have some family members disagree with the patient's AD
- Patients who insist upon a generally unwise course of care, rather than opting for a trial of treatment or allowing for later decisions by a proxy.

Telling your story: time series charts

Time series charts are an effective way to quickly tell the story of your results. Below are two of Team Delta's time series charts. The changes they tested as part of their quality improvement project for ACP are noted on the following graphs and explained below (Fig. 18.2 a and b).

Identifying and testing changes

Team Delta

Once Team Delta finalized its aims and how to track them, it looked at best practices to identify good ideas to try on the study unit in order to improve ACP. The team decided to try the following ideas:

1 Invite residents and families to attend a class that provides information on various options and helps them to complete ACP forms.

2 Offer mandatory classes for clinicians to help them understand and initiate ACP discussions, including role playing.

3 Involve frontline staff, such as admissions clerks, to get the advance directive forms completed and entered into the system.

4 Develop a staff education and public awareness campaign within the facility to raise awareness, understanding, and recognition of the importance of ACP.

5 Make ACP review part of the routine quarterly interdisciplinary team (IDT) meetings.

6 Reach out to hospital partners to settle on standardized and adequate documentation and 'transfer' procedures for ACP.

With the help and dedication of team members, Team Delta tried one change at a time. Once a strategy showed better results, they implemented it on a larger scale.

There are a number of ways that you can improve ACP for your patients. Some interventions that QI teams have tried and that have proven successful follow.

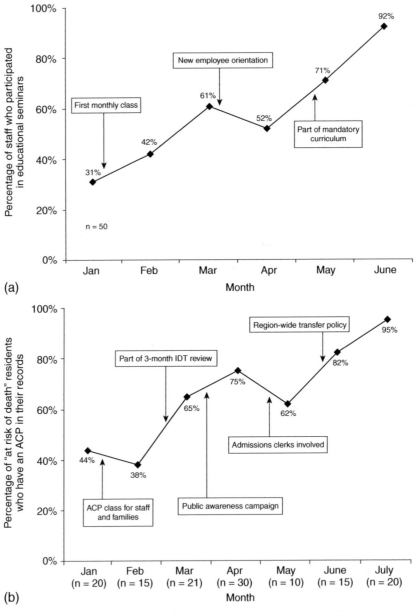

Fig. 18.2 (a) and (b) Time series charts for Advance Care Planning project. (a) Within six months, 80% of the facilities' direct caregivers will have participated in an educational seminar on ACP, treatment choices, and disease progression. (b) Within six months, 90% of new and 'at risk of death' patients will have a completed Advance Care Plan documented.

Reproduced from Lynn, J. et al. The Common Sense Guide to Improving Palliative Care. Oxford University Press USA, 2007, with permission.

Change ideas to improve ACP

- Develop a systematic approach and designate providers to initiate, document, and complete ACPs (e.g. list of topics to cover, who is responsible for each item, where the documents will be kept).

- Add a pop-up box about the patient's ACP availability on the computer order screen (e.g. when DNR order is written, at admission, or at discharge from the hospital).

- Conduct automatic ACP review at quarterly IDT conferences in long-term care institutions.

- Incorporate questions about the patient's proxy and DNR orders into admission forms with more comprehensive follow-up by clinicians (e.g. ACP 'SWAT' team) while in the hospital or nursing home.

- Encourage time-limited trials for invasive technology or treatments with agreement about when to stop.

- Be clear about DNR and proxy orders at admission; use community follow-up (with primary care physicians, community social workers, home health providers, and other providers in the system) to continue and complete ACP documents and periodically review them with the patient and family.

- Standardize ACP procedures, to be completed in a set time frame (e.g. 72 hours after admission; within one week of admission).

- Develop standardized 'scripts' for starting ACP discussions. One of the best openings: 'At this time in your life, what is it that makes you happy?' Then, ask the same question regarding what makes you 'sad' or 'anxious.' Then discuss prognosis and other difficult issues (see Physician Orders for Life-Sustaining Treatment (POLST) in the Resources section at the end of this chapter).

- Implement a standardized healthcare proxy form for use throughout the institution.

- Train clinicians to conduct family meetings, help patients and families to express wishes and make decisions, and document the settled plan of care.

- Develop posters, brochures, and similar materials with the patient and family members. For example, staff can wear buttons that ask, 'I Have an Advance Care Plan, Do You?' or 'Ask Me about Advance Care Planning.'

- Monitor the process of ACP and patient and family reaction to it, as well as the accuracy of documentation of patient wishes on transfer.

- Make plans about the patient's preferred place to die.

As you think about changes you would like to make, plan for obstacles. QI teams frequently encounter similar barriers, regardless of the setting in which they are working. Below is a list of common barriers; remember that others have overcome them—and you can, too.

Common barriers to ACP

- Not being able to offer key treatment options, such as palliative sedation or clinician visits in the home for symptom exacerbation, really limits how much you can improve things for your patients.

- 'The big lie' that all will be well and that we do not need to deal with this. For example, during inpatient rehabilitation for older people, it is tempting to communicate a sense that the patient is not really up against a serious, chronic condition but is just a little off course and on the verge of recovery. That lie means not only that death comes as a shock to the family but also that no useful care planning can take place.

- Patients may express a desire to die at home, but the caregiver may fear being unable to manage worsening health at home. In this case, you need to think about what you can really offer in terms of support (on-call physicians, hospice, oxygen, etc.) and what the family can manage.

- Multiple physicians and other providers, with no real communication among them, leave the patient and family with the sense that no one is in charge or responsible, that no one grasps the situation accurately, and that no one can really ensure that the ACP is followed.

- Providers may be reluctant to 'bring up bad news' (e.g. they may be uncomfortable with the conversation; they do not know how to start such a talk). In this case, groups find that providing physicians and nurses with a script to follow helps them overcome their anxieties.

- Providers fear that patients do not want to have these discussions.

Give them something to talk about

To give them something to talk about, get started! Here are a few key points to remember about Advance Care Planning (ACP):

1 Get started on the project, and do not wait for everything to be perfect.

2 Do not carry a lot of baggage from limited interpretations of your state's laws. This may require challenging overly restrictive institutional procedures.

3 Get feedback from patients and families to find out how you are doing and to get the boost that you may need to continue your efforts.

4 Do not just focus on cardiopulmonary resuscitation (CPR); instead, build ACP discussions around a good life, right up to the end.

5 Address the practical issues that your patients face, such as whom to call in time of need, which medication to take, and how symptoms will progress.

6 Use every crisis situation survived as an opportunity for rehearsing preferred options. Ask the patient and family (and professional care givers) what should have been done, and what can be done differently next time.

7 Avoid using medical jargon. Tailor your language to your setting and patients. 'Artificial hydration' may not mean much to a 75 year old spouse.

Frequently asked questions

What should we discuss when deciding ACPs?

- Present the clinical situation, now and in the future, and options for the care plan in more than one way so as to ensure comprehension.

- Discuss the patient's health status and quality of life following treatment.

- When using medical technology, offer the use of time-limited trials rather than forcing a choice between 'never' and 'forever.'

- Promise reassessment on a scheduled basis, and promise to stop if treatment is not helping.

- Listen to the patient, allowing time for him or her to respond and express wishes, fears, and concerns.

- Honour the search for meaning, treat symptoms, and ensure continuity.

- Set reasonable expectations for prognosis and treatments: what can your system promise the patient in the last years and weeks of life?

- Support families through all phases of illness, and plan for bereavement issues after death.

- Be capable of and willing to provide sedation for those near death if that is what the patient needs.

Communication strategies to initiate Advance Care Planning

The following table summarizes some useful communication strategies to initiate Advance Care Planning depending on the health status of the person you are talking with (Table 18.1).

Table 18.1 Summary of some useful communication strategies to initiate Advance Care Planning

With healthy people

Content of discussions	Action items	Suggested communication strategy
◆ Identification and notification of surrogate/proxy decision-maker. ◆ Identification of preferences about undesirable outcome states (e.g. persistent vegetative state). ◆ Note atypical beliefs or preferences (e.g. Jehovah's Witness).	◆ May complete durable power of attorney. ◆ Discuss proxy appointment and values with surrogate. ◆ Write down preferences.	◆ 'There are many drugs that we can use to treat your hypertension; one is less expensive, but you must take it twice a day. A second must be taken only once a day, but it costs more.' ◆ 'If you become too sick to speak with me about your healthcare preferences, who should I turn to to help me make decisions?' ◆ 'Do you have any specific concerns that you would like to share with me?' ◆ 'In some states, your preference to forgo a feeding tube if you are terminally ill or in a prolonged coma is only honoured if it is written down in your advance directive.'

With people diagnosed with a serious illness

Content of discussions	Action items	Suggested communication strategy
◆ Same as above. ◆ What is important for you now (values, beliefs, psychosocial needs)? ◆ Discuss treatment burden and potential adverse-outcome states. ◆ Discuss time-limited trials of treatments (not 'never' vs. 'always') ◆ Discuss likely course with proposed treatments and likely outcomes. ◆ Discuss what the next steps could be in the follow-up and management of the patient's condition.	◆ Same as above. ◆ MD discusses prognoses and outcomes, with and without recommended treatments. ◆ MD/RN talks to surrogate. ◆ MD/RN offers spiritual support.	◆ 'I anticipate that you will have a good recovery from this stroke. We are going to treat you with a blood thinner that will substantially reduce your risk of a further stroke. However, the risk is not zero. It is important that you plan ahead. Do you have any concerns or thoughts about your medical care if you do not have a good recovery?' ◆ 'Unlike TV shows, resuscitation is rarely effective when your mother has a serious illness like a stroke that produces unconsciousness.' ◆ 'What do you know about what is likely to happen?'

(Continued)

Table 18.1 (*contd*) Summary of some useful communication strategies to initiate Advance Care Planning

With people diagnosed with a serious illness that will limit life expectancy, or coming to the end of a long life

Content of discussions	Action items	Suggested communication strategy
◆ Same as above. ◆ Explicit discussion about courses of potential treatments, likely outcomes, individual economic consequences. ◆ Discussion of time-limited trials of treatments. ◆ What is important for you to accomplish in the time you have left? ◆ How can I help you achieve this?	◆ Same as above. ◆ State specific preferences and formulate contingency plans. ◆ Be sure that key decisions are written down and transferred with the patient.	◆ 'Mrs X, your breathing is really a problem for you almost all the time now. Tell me a little about your thoughts. In this part of your life, what makes you truly happy? What makes you worried or upset? What do you think will happen? What do you hope for? What do you hope to avoid? What do you expect the end to be like?' ◆ 'You said that you want medical care to focus on comfort. Even if you get more short of breath, you want to stay home. Is that correct? If you do get short of breath, and it does not respond to usual treatments, we will use morphine and your family can call...'

The PDSA model of improvement (3)

◆ What are we trying to accomplish? = the AIM

◆ How will we know that a change is an improvement? = the MEASURES

◆ What changes can we make that will result in an improvement? = CHANGES

Further resources

Handbook for Mortals. http://www.medicaring.org

Caring Connections. http://www.caringinfo.org

POLST. http://www.ohsu.edu/ethics/polst/

Respecting Patient Choices Program, Gunderson Lutheran, La Crosse, Wisconsin. http://www.gundluth.org/eolprograms

Five Wishes. http://www.agingwithdignity.org

Vermont Ethics Network. http://www.vtethicsnetwork.org

Gold Standard Framework for Palliative Care. http://www.goldstandardsframework.nhs.uk

Institute for Healthcare Improvement. http://www.ihi.org

References

1 Steinhauser KE, Christakis NA, Clipp EC, McNeilly M, McIntyre L, and Tulsky JA (2000). Factors considered important at the end of life by patients, family, physicians, and other care providers. *JAMA: Journal of American Medical Association*, **284**(19):2476–82.

2 Singer PA, Martin DK, Lavery JV et al. (1998). Reconceptualizing advance care planning from the patient's perspective. *Archives of Internal Medicine*, **158**:825–832.

3 Lynn J, Schuster JL, Wilkinson AM, and Noyes Simon L (2007). *Improving Care for the End of Life: A Sourcebook for Health Care Managers and Clinicians*, 2nd Ed. Oxford University Press, Oxford.

Chapter 19

Advance Care Planning in Canada: past experience and current strategies

AnnMarie Nielsen and Sharon Baxter

'We plan in advance for all kinds of events; events such as birthday parties, anniversary celebrations, and vacations. We plan for our education and we plan for our retirement. In spite of the fact that planning in advance is something we do everyday, we often don't plan in advance for healthcare.'
Planning in Advance for Your Future Healthcare Choices, Fraser Health (1)

This chapter includes:

◆ Overview, introduction, and definition of ACP

◆ The Canadian landscape and current legislation

◆ Professional recognition for Advance Care Plans/directives

◆ Professional education

◆ Public awareness and education

◆ Other national activities

◆ Adaptations and specialized Advance Care Planning.

Key points

◆ Canada's multiple jurisdictions with differing health care services and laws create an extra layer of challenge in creating portable Advance Care Plans, and in educating Canadians about them.

◆ Within the past decade, a number of health care professional organizations have recognized the value of Advance Care Planning, and have given direction to their members on what is expected of them in terms of professional ethics.

◆ Professional education initiatives have led to the inclusion of end of life care competencies into medical school curriculum and licensing and certification exams, as well as to the creation of resources for the education of currently practicing professionals.

◆ Public awareness has been growing from the grass-roots level up to the national level, with a new national awareness strategy planned for within the next few years.

◆ Growing recognition of specialized Advance Care Plans has led to adaptations for cultural groups, specific diseases, and paediatrics.

Overview

A common irony with social issues that affect everyone is that often, there is no one to take the lead in its development. Such may have been the case with Canada over a decade ago. However, Canada has had the good fortune in recent years to have a number of organizations provide a strong leadership role in further developing Advance Care Planning competencies, resources, and awareness.

It is an exciting time to be a part of Advance Care Planning (ACP) in Canada; the recent conclusion of some noteworthy projects, combined with the ongoing efforts of newly created projects, is building significant momentum in the development of ACP in Canada. The next decade promises to bring considerably improved competencies among health care professionals, as well as higher levels of awareness among Canadians of all ages.

Introduction

Advance Care Planning in Canada is a rapidly evolving issue. From terminology clarification to recent and pending legislation, activity is bubbling up from the local and provincial/territorial level and coalescing into broader national initiatives. This chapter will detail key past initiatives in Canada and look at the strategies that are currently in progress, as well as what those strategies hope to accomplish.

This chapter will describe the social and cultural backdrop against which ACP developments are taking place. It will examine the Canadian health care and legal systems, and how they impact on the progression of ACP. It will explore the issue of ACP in Canada, and trace the development of professional education and public awareness initiatives. Finally, it will provide some information about emerging areas of specialization in ACP.

Definition

Many definitions of Advance Care Planning or ACP exist. For the purposes of this chapter, the definition that we will use is: a process whereby a capable (mentally competent) adult engages in a plan for making personal health care decisions in the event that this person becomes incapable (legally incompetent) to personally direct his or her own health care (Box 19.1).

The Canadian landscape

Before beginning any discussion of developments in Canada, it is first necessary to become familiar with the landscape—that is to understand the health care system and social, cultural, and legal context within which ACP laws, mores, and resources are developed.

Canada is one nation, but in many respects, it operates more like a coalition of smaller nations with its 13 provincial and territorial jurisdictions and locally developed health care systems.

Box 19.1 Equivalence with other international terminology in ACP of three common themes

1 Statement of wishes and preferences
2 Refusal of treatment
3 Proxy designation of power of attorney.

Canada's health care system is explained succinctly in a booklet from the Living Lessons® (2) programme, *Influencing Change: A Patient and Caregiver Advocacy Guide* (3):

> Canada's health care system is a number of insurance plans that provide coverage to Canadians. It is publicly funded and administered, meaning that each system is managed by each province or territory within guidelines and principles set out by the federal government in the Canada Health Act . . . The provinces and territories are responsible for the administration of healthcare delivery. Many provinces and territories have established structures within their borders to deliver healthcare services that are based on what their communities need. These are often referred to as district health authorities (DHAs), local integrated health networks (LIHNs), or centres de santé et de services sociaux (CLSCs) depending on the province or territory. Their purpose is to allow a community focus in the delivery of care.

Canada's legal system, too, is not homogeneous from one province or territory to another. While Canada's legal system is founded on the British common law system, Quebec adheres to a civil system for private law; yet both legal systems are subject to the Constitution of Canada. The federal legal system governs criminal law, leaving matters related to Advance Care Planning to the provincial and territorial level legal systems, of which there are thirteen—ten provincial and three territorial.

The coalition of smaller nations analogy extends to Canada's culture. It is impossible to define Canada's culture, other than to say that it is multicultural. A wide variety of ethnicities and nationalities of origin are represented in Canada's citizenry, some having been Canadians for generations and others having only recently arrived from their land of birth. This brings a rich variety of values and cultural norms to every aspect of Canadian life, including health care and ACP, but can also create frustrations and misunderstandings, all the more so in the emotionally charged arena of end of life care.

Despite its multiculturalism, Canada is, as with many industrialized nations, predominantly a death-denying culture. Many Canadians, whether as health care consumers or health care providers, are uncomfortable and unwilling to discuss the topic of Advance Care Planning. Many assume that it is a subject to consider only when the need arises, as in the case of a terminal diagnosis.

Geographically, Canada is the second largest landmass in the world, but with a population of only 33 million, its population density is low. While most of Canada's population reside in more urbanized areas, a significant portion of its population lives in rural and remote settings. Communication can be difficult in these areas, limiting the opportunities for public awareness and education.

Current legislation

No overarching national federal law exists that governs advance care directives; it is a locally developed provincial and territorial area of responsibility. However, not every province and territory has enacted laws regarding advance care directives. Of the 13 provincial and territorial jurisdictions, 11 have advance directive legislation; New Brunswick and Nunavut (Inuit homeland) do not, although New Brunswick is in the process of developing *Advanced Health-Care Directives (Living Wills) Legislation*. British Columbia and Alberta have recently participated in legislative reviews of advance directive legislation, resulting in several proposed amendments.

In relation to ACP/advance directive legislation, Canada again functions as three smaller nations, with varying legislations in each area. Some provinces and territories allow for instructional advance directives, while others allow only for the appointment of a proxy decision-maker, in the event of incapacity. Table 19.1(4) provides a synopsis of which jurisdictions have advance care directive legislation, and which elements are addressed in their legislation: instructional, proxy or both.

Table 19.1 Canadian provinces and territories with Advance Care Planning legislation (4)

Province	Instruction	Proxy
Alberta	✓	✓
British Columbia	✓	✓
Manitoba	✓	✓
New Brunswick	No legislation	
Newfoundland and Labrador	✓	✓
Northwest Territories	✓	✓
Nova Scotia	-	✓
Nunavut	No legislation	
Ontario	✓	✓
Prince Edward Island	✓	✓
Quebec	-	✓
Saskatchewan	✓	✓
Yukon	✓	✓

Because each province and territory operates independently of one another in developing advance directive legislation, and at diverse points in time, dissimilar terminology has evolved. For example, in Alberta, the term used for advance directives is 'personal directive', Manitoba uses the term 'health care directive'; Nova Scotia uses 'medical consent'; and Newfoundland and Labrador and Prince Edward Island both use 'advance health care directive'. This can create confusion when Canadians move between jurisdictions.

In addition to the different terminology used, the independent development of legislation also creates some problems with recognizing an advance directive in one jurisdiction that was created in another. An ACP document that is legally binding in one province or territory may not necessarily be recognized in another. Reciprocity protocols—statements indicating that a province will accept an advance directive written in another province—have been established in seven provinces but three provinces do not recognize those created elsewhere. See Table 19.2 for a synopsis.

Professional recognition for Advance Care Plans/directives

In addition to the steps taken by federal, provincial, and territorial governments, a number of professional associations have recognized the need for its membership to be aware of their legal and ethical responsibilities. In 1999, the Boards of Directors of the Canadian Medical Association (CMA), the Canadian Nursing Association (CNA) and the Catholic Health Association of Canada (CHAC) approved a joint statement on *Preventing and Resolving Ethical Conflicts Involving Health Care Providers and Persons Receiving Care*, which supports that the 'needs, values, and preferences of the person receiving care should be the primary consideration in the provision of quality care' (5).

Individual nursing and medical associations have included recognizing advance care choices in their *Codes of Ethics*. In the Canadian Medical Association's *Code of Ethics* (updated 2004), physicians are advised to 'Ascertain wherever possible and recognize your patient's wishes about the initiation, continuation, or cessation of life-sustaining treatment' (Section 27), and 'Respect the intentions of an incompetent patient as they were expressed (e.g. through a valid advance directive or proxy designation) before the patient became incompetent' (Section 28).

Table 19.2 Advance Care Plan reciprocity protocols among Canadian provinces and territories

Province/Territory	Reciprocity status
Alberta	X–possible legislation currently under consideration
British Columbia	✓ - if the advance directive complies with local requirements
Manitoba	✓ - if the advance directive complies with local requirements
New Brunswick	X
Newfoundland and Labrador	X–not recognized in other provinces/territories
Northwest Territories	✓ - if the advance directive complies with local requirements
Nova Scotia	X–not recognized in other provinces/territories
Nunavut	X
Ontario	✓ - if the advance directive complies with local requirements
Prince Edward Island	✓ - if the advance directive complies with local requirements
Quebec	X–not recognized in other provinces/territories
Saskatchewan	✓ - if the advance directive complies with local requirements
Yukon	✓ - if the advance directive complies with local requirements

In 2008, the Canadian Nurses Association released a position statement on 'Providing Nursing Care at the End of Life', which includes a section on ACP recognizing the importance for individuals, healthy or ill, to make informed choices related to end of life care.

Professional education

A key element in ACP is the advice and guidance that individuals receive from appropriately educated professionals. However, prior to 2003, end of life and ACP issues were not a part of the curriculum in any of Canada's seventeen faculties of medicine. A number of initiatives have been undertaken to address this gap in education of health care professionals.

The earliest ACP education available to health care professionals in Canada in 1999–2007, was through the *Ian Anderson Continuing Education Program in End-of-Life Care* (Ian Anderson Program), a joint project based at the University of Toronto, with funding from Mrs Margaret Anderson, in memory of her late husband. During its seven years in operation, this programme provided both generalist and specialist physicians with the opportunity to earn continuing educations credits accredited by the college for family physicians, physicians, and surgeons.

The programme consisted of thirteen modules, each written by an expert in the field on topics related to Advance Care Planning, as well as pre- and post-test materials. While the Ian Anderson Program has been discontinued, its resources remain available on its website (see Box 19.2).

Box 19.2 Where to find Advance Care Planning resources for professionals

Ian Anderson Continuing Education Program in End-of-Life Care

http://www.cme.utoronto.ca/EndOfLife

Educating Future Physicians in Palliative and End-of-Life Care

http://www.peolc-sp.ca/efppec/english

A larger, more nationally encompassing initiative commenced in 2003 with the launch of the Educating Future Physicians in Palliative and End-of-Life Care project (EFPPEC), a joint project of the Canadian Hospice Palliative Care Association (CHPCA) and the Association of Faculties of Medicine of Canada (AFMC). The overall goal of the EFPPEC project was for every medical student and resident to graduate with knowledge, skills, and appropriate attitudes in end of life care, necessitating a number of steps.

EFPPEC first developed national consensus on undergraduate competencies in medical education. Then, working with the Ontario Palliative Undergraduate Network (OPUN) and the Réseau Universitaire Québécois en soins palliatifs (RUQSP), EFPPEC developed an undergraduate curriculum in palliative and end of life care based on the EFPPEC competencies and their own work. A final review was conducted by the Undergraduate Committee of the Canadian Society of Palliative Care Physicians, before pan-Canadian consensus was reached on this curriculum through a survey process involving all 17 faculties of medicine in Canada. A final step in the project accomplished the integration of palliative and end of life questions in licensing and certification examinations, in consultation/collaboration with the major professional associations in Canada.

Resources developed by EFPPEC over the course of the project include not only the Undergraduate Medical Education Curriculum, but also Advance Care Planning Curriculum Material and Teacher's Guide, an interprofessional education module intended for formal caregivers and undergraduate and postgraduate students in the health professions. It has been produced in an interprofessional approach for an audience which includes health care professionals such as physicians, nurses, social workers, spiritual advisors, and trained volunteers for palliative care services.

The EFPPEC project completed its work in 2008, but all EFPPEC documents are now available on the Palliative Learning Commons housed on the website of the Canadian Hospice Palliative Care Association (see Box 19.2).

Other national activities

As previously noted in this chapter, health care services and legislation regarding Advance Care Planning vary with differing terminology and reciprocity arrangements among the 13 jurisdictions in Canada, making it difficult to accomplish cross-boundary national initiatives.

One such initiative, however, was 'Advance care planning: the Glossary project', in 2006, an initiative of the Public Information and Awareness Working Group of the Canadian Strategy on Palliative and End-of-Life Care. The objective of the report was to 'bring clarity to the concepts and terms used in ACP in Canadian provinces and territories and in the health, social and legal sectors in order to facilitate pan-Canadian dialogue about Advance Care Planning'(6).

In May 2007, Fraser Health and the Calgary Health Region, two health authorities leading the country in ACP resource and policy development, co-sponsored the Inaugural Canadian Symposium on Advance Care Planning. It offered an opportunity never before available in Canada to showcase innovative programs, foster policy discussion and networking, and share research findings. Over 90 representative healthcare providers and organizations, policy makers, and others identified emerging practices for supporting ACP and explored ways to both introduce and refine strategies for ACP.

In 2008, Health Canada provided the funding for the British Columbia Cancer Agency and Canada Institute of Health Research 'Cross-Cultural Considerations in promoting Advance Care Planning in Canada', 'to provide insight into how diverse cultural and Aboriginal groups in Canada might respond to advance care planning (ACP) becoming a part of the health care system'(7).

Public awareness and education

Canada's health professional community has come to recognize the value of Advance Care Planning. However, the Canadian public has not been as swift in becoming aware of ACP or accepting that it is applicable to them. A 2004 Ipsos-Reid survey indicated that 49% of respondents felt it was important for them to discuss end of life care with their physicians, yet only 9% said they had actually done so (8). Beginning in 2007, the CHPCA began distributing information pamphlets in large urban centres across Canada, designed to introduce the topic to Canadians. Reaction to the pamphlets was telling. The CHPCA received requests for more information; however, it also received numerous requests to discontinue sending any more information, since, as the caller would say, the recipient was not ill and therefore was not in need of information about ACP. Clearly, more education is needed. Several initiatives have been undertaken or are in progress, to address this concern.

Many provincial governments have created information pamphlets and fact sheets regarding their own legislation, making the information available in plain language. Organizations such as hospice palliative care programmes and public legal education organizations have also developed information brochures and flyers.

In addition to the professional education resources it developed, the Ian Anderson Program also developed a number of resources to help educate the public about ACP. Resources include a video targeting caregivers, produced with the ALS (or Motor Neurone Disease) Society of Canada in 2001—*Making Hard Decisions: the Essence of Being Human*, now available through the ALS Society of Canada from their website. Most recently, in 2007, an *Advance Care Planning DVD* was created that provides an introductory look at some of the basic concepts involved in ACP. Using a storied approach, the DVD highlights a number of common health care scenarios and their impact on individuals, families, and health care professionals.

Each year, the CHPCA launches a week-long awareness campaign, National Hospice Palliative Care Week, focusing on hospice palliative care-related issues. For three consecutive years, from 2006 to 2008 inclusive, the campaign theme focused on Advance Care Planning (Fig. 19.1). The 2006 theme, 'My Living, My Dying: Informed, Involved and In-Charge… Right to the End', was aimed at the public and captured the pressing need for Canadians to discuss their end of life wishes with their loved ones, friends, family, and doctor. In 2007, the theme, 'Advance Care

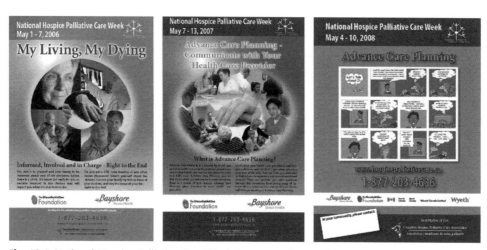

Fig. 19.1 National Hospice Palliative Care Week Awareness Posters 2006–2008.
© Canadian Hospice Palliative Care Association. Used with permission.

Planning—Communicate with Your Health Care Provider', focused on the role of primary health care providers in end of life care planning. Finally, the theme in 2008, 'Advance Care Planning: Let's Talk About It', highlighted the importance of individuals and health care providers working together to create the most appropriate Advance Care Plan for each individual. In each of the three years, resources were developed in support of the theme. Many of these resources continue to be available on the CHPCA website.

Two examples of good practice can be seen in Box 19.3.

The latest professional education initiative, a five-year project, began in late 2008, and is part of a larger ACP project coordinated by the Canadian Hospice Palliative Care Association 'Advance Care Planning in Canada: A Framework and Implementation' (ACP in Canada). The overall goal of this project is to raise the awareness of Canadians about the importance of ACP and to equip them with the tools they need to effectively engage in the process. The secondary goal of the ACP

Box 19.3 Two examples of good practice in Advance Care Planning public awareness and education from British Columbia and Alberta

Two health authorities have recently emerged as early leaders in the development of public education tools: Calgary Health Region, Alberta, and Fraser Health, British Columbia.

In 2004, Fraser Health hired one full-time staff person to develop ACP resources for the public. Since then, it has developed a number of resources, including a workbook, several information pamphlets/booklets and a DVD. Its resources are available for only the shipping charges to any person or organization that makes a request, and it often receives requests from the public, community groups, faith groups, and banks. The project had been intended to be a short-term one-time initiative, but proved to be so popular that it has continued.

Calgary Health followed suit in 2005, launching an ACP initiative to create resources. Drawing on the successes of Fraser Health, it modified the workbook and DVD, re-branding it for Calgary Health. It also created an on-line educational module to familiarize the public with ACP issues such as what an advance care directive is and what is included in Alberta's advance care legislation. It works closely with Emergency Medical Services, cancer groups, long-term care facilities, and family physicians to ensure that information is readily available to the health care professionals who work directly with patients, as well as through them, to ensure that information is available to patients.

Both make their resource materials widely available within their province. As well, both organizations have tailored material to suit their specific situation. For example, Calgary Health worked with the ALS Society to create a module specific to the concerns of those with ALS (MND). Fraser Health has ensured that its materials are available in Cantonese and Punjabi, as well as English, due to the high immigrant population that it serves.

Most of the resources developed by these two organizations are available on their websites:

Fraser Health Care Advance Care Planning Information and Resources *http://www.fraser-health.ca/SERVICES/HOMEANDCOMMUNITYCARE/ADVANCECAREPLANNING/Pages/default.aspx*

Calgary Health Advance Care Planning Information and Resources
http://www.calgaryhealthregion.ca/programs/advancecareplanning/index.htm

in Canada project is to prepare professionals/health care providers with the tools they need so they can facilitate and engage in the process of ACP with their clients.

Project managers have determined that it is necessary to first accomplish the secondary goal, in order that professionals/health care providers have the resources they need to answer questions and work most effectively with individuals who approach them about ACP. Work is currently under way that will lead to the creation of these resources; once they are available, the final two years of the project will focus on creating and implementing a large-scale public awareness campaign.

With the variety and scope of public awareness measures in place, it is to be hoped that within five to ten years, the trend to avoid discussing ACP will begin to turn, and more Canadians will have effective health care directives in place.

Adaptations and specialized Advance Care Planning

Most of the educational programmes and public awareness initiatives and resources in Canada are aimed at adults of mostly European heritage. However, there is growing recognition that Advance Care Planning resources and information must be adapted to a number of groups.

Culturally adapted resources range from simply translating resources into specific target languages, depending on the community; to modifying the content of information, language used, and the mode of presentation. As well, *Cross-Cultural Considerations in Promoting Advance Care Planning in Canada* examined several different ethnic cultures and the deaf community, to identify key issues for adaptation in ACP.

Advance Care Planning for paediatrics is beginning to garner attention as well. The Canadian Pediatric Society recently released a position statement, in which it recognizes the importance of supporting health service providers in initiating ACP conversations with families and children dealing with life-threatening illness.

Finally, small steps are also being taken in the direction of focusing on disease-specific ACP such as that for ALS (MND) in Calgary.

Conclusion

A strong body of work has emerged in Canada through the efforts of individual initiatives. Although the majority of these initiatives have been short-term and have been unable to take on awareness at a national level, the work that has been completed to date, especially that of education for professionals is sure to make the next steps more productive. Recent projects, such as the CHPCA's nationally-aimed 'Advance Care Planning in Canada: A Framework and Implementation', are building on the accomplishments of their predecessors; early successes have enabled current projects to attack the issues on a broader basis, speeding the rate at which Canadians become willing to talk about—and create their own—Advance Care Plans.

Further resources

Canadian Hospice Palliative Care Association (2009). Advance Care Planning in Canada Project including Environmental Scan. Available at: http://www.chpca.net/projects/advance_care_planning.html (accessed 30 April 2009)

Canadian Medical Association (2002). *Code of Ethics*. Available at: http://www.cma.ca/index.cfm/ci_id/53556/la_id/1.htm (accessed 30 April 2009)

Canadian Pediatric Society: Advance care planning for paediatric patients. *Paediatric Child Health*, 2008;**13**(9):791–796.

Dunbrack J et al (2008). Implementation Guide to Advance Care Planning in Canada: A Case Study of Two Health Authorities (unpublished), Health Canada, March. http://www.fraserhealth.ca/News/NewsReleases/Documents/ACPImplementationGuide.pdf

End of Life Project, Health Law Institute, Dalhousie University. A Summary of Canadian Legislation Concerning Advance Directives. http://as01.ucis.dal.ca/dhli/cmp_advdirectives

Educating Future Physicians in Palliative and End-of-Life Care (2007). Facilitating Advance Care Planning: An Interprofessional Educational Program: Curriculum Material. http://www.afmc.ca/efppec/docs/pdf_2008_advance_care_planning_curriculum_module_final.pdf

Educating Future Physicians in Palliative and End-of-Life Care Palliative Learning Commons. http://www.peolc-sp.ca/efppec/english/

Chapter 20

The evolution of Advance Care Planning in Australia with a focus on hospital care

William Silvester and Karen M Detering

'A coordinated, systematic model of patient-centred advance care planning using non-medical advance care planning facilitators, assists in identifying and respecting patient's end of life care wishes, improves end of life care from the perspective of the patient and the family and diminishes the likelihood of stress, anxiety and depression in the surviving relatives (1).'

This chapter includes:

- Synopsis of evolution of Advance Care Planning in Australia
- Results of a randomized controlled trial of Advance Care Planning in elderly inpatients
- The key elements to successful Advance Care Planning.

Key points

- Despite the intentions of good legislation, the provision of good end of life care is still inadequate.
- Advance Care Planning improves end of life care and patient and family satisfaction and reduces stress, anxiety, and depression in surviving relatives.
- Advance Care Planning only occurs if health professionals are trained to facilitate it with patients and their families and if system changes are made to support and authorize a change in clinical practice.

Synopsis of evolution of Advance Care Planning in Australia

The importance of respecting patient autonomy in the setting of end of life care was first recognized in Australia in 1987 by the Dying with Dignity Inquiry of the Victorian Parliament (2). A conclusion from the report stated:

> The Committee is in agreement with the views of witnesses that a decision to allow hopelessly ill, suffering human beings to die naturally is a profound act of compassion. Such decisions are morally appropriate with the deepest respect for life. The Committee finds that good medical practice not only encompasses a duty of care, but also requires ongoing discussions with the patient and/or family in the formulation and implementation of clear not-for-resuscitation policies and guidelines, whenever possible.

As a result legislation was passed in the state of Victoria in 1988. Called the Medical Treatment Act (3), it enabled people to appoint a medical enduring power of attorney and to refuse unwanted medical treatment. It also recognized the importance of providing legal protection to doctors who, acting in good faith, withheld treatment that they believed was not in the patient's best interests.

Over the next decade similar legislation, to respect the right of patients to refuse treatment in the setting of terminal conditions or poor neurological outcome, was passed in most states and territories. This statutory law, however, appeared to have little impact on medical practice and the overall awareness of, and respect for, patients' rights regarding the choice of treatment near the end of life by health practitioners remained abysmally poor.

Results of a randomized controlled trial of Advance Care Planning in elderly inpatients

In 2002 the Austin Hospital in Melbourne received a grant from the National Institute of Clinical Studies, to trial the introduction of the Wisconsin-based Respecting Choices® programme (4) of Advance Care Planning (ACP) over a one year period. This programme was trialled with success, when other programmes had failed, e.g. SUPPORT Study (5).This was due to its methodology of:

◆ training non-medical staff to discuss ACP

◆ supporting patients to document their wishes

◆ putting organizational system changes in place (e.g. ensuring that the documents were filed prominently)

◆ educating medical and other key staff (6).

Due to the successful implementation at the Austin Hospital, the Australian Federal and Victorian State Governments funded the expansion of the newly named Respecting Patient Choices® (RPC) programme to other health services within the state of Victoria, to other Australian states and territories and to be trialled in aged care facilities. This further expansion was also successful and has resulted in the establishment of the RPC model of Advance Care Planning in multiple hospitals, health services and aged care homes across Australia.

One important aspect of the RPC expansion has been the extensive modification of the Wisconsin Respecting Choices® programme to Australian conditions, taking into account the difference between the health systems in the USA and Australia.

The second aspect of the RPC evolution has been the importance placed upon evaluation and research in order to improve the model of Advance Care Planning. When introduced in residential care homes, more than half of the elderly, or their families, underwent ACP discussions and, of these more than half completed Advance Care Plans. More than 90% of requests were for comfort care in the event of a deterioration and not to be transferred to hospital (7).

The outstanding result of the trial was that the residents' or families' wishes were respected and that the likelihood of being transferred to hospital to die, instead of being kept comfortable in the nursing home, was reduced from 46% in those not introduced to ACP to 18% in those who did have a discussion (P < 0.001). The introduction of ACP was received enthusiastically by residents, families, staff, and general practitioners.

More rigorous research has been conducted in the hospital setting in the form of a randomized, controlled trial of ACP for patients aged 80 or over admitted under the care of cardiologists, respiratory, and internal medicine physicians. This study, published in the BMJ (1), was conducted in a large university hospital at the behest of the medical 'doubters' who kept on saying 'where is the randomized controlled trial. Following randomization 309 English speaking elderly patients, all legally competent, were followed for 6 months (Box 20.1).

The study demonstrated that 125 (81%) of the 154 patients randomized to Advance Care Planning underwent a discussion facilitated by a non-medical staff member trained in the RPC model. In the intervention group there was a higher level of satisfaction about the care received in hospital from both patients and family members. Of the 56 patients who died by six months, end of life wishes were much more likely to be known and followed in the intervention group (25/29, 86%) compared with control group (8/27, 30%; P < 0.001).

Furthermore, in the intervention group, family members of patients who died had significantly less stress (P < 0.001), anxiety (P = 0.02), and depression (P = 0.002) than those of the control patients.

The key elements to successful Advance Care Planning

The key elements of success of this model are thought to be:

 * the use of trained non-medical staff to facilitate the discussion
 * ensuring that the discussions are patient-centred
 * involving the patient's family in the discussions
 * making sure that the completed documents are correctly filed in a prominent position within the patient records
 * implementing systematic education of doctors (8).

It is important to note that patients and their families welcome such discussions and very few refuse such interventions. By focusing on 'what it means to live well', their understanding of their illness and treatment options, and their values and beliefs, it ensures that the patients are listened to and that they have an opportunity to reflect on their views and to document their wishes. Then, when the time comes, the family are not burdened by the difficult decisions that need to be made and are not left later feeling anxious about whether they made the right decision or depressed that their loved one's dying phase was inappropriately prolonged (9,10).

This research, and the RPC model of Advance Care Planning, is generalizable to most health care settings and will continue to support the expansion of ACP to be a part of normal care in all health services in Australia. It has been derived from Respecting Choices, a programme that has been successfully implemented in multiple health services in the United States, as well as Canada, Germany, Spain, and Singapore.

Box 20.1 The Austin Hospital randomized controlled trial of hospital patients using ACP (1)

 * 154 of the 309 patients were randomized to Advance Care Planning
 * 125 (81%) received Advance Care Planning
 * 108 (84%) expressed wishes or appointed a surrogate, or both
 * Of the 56 patients who died by six months, end of life wishes were much more likely to be known and followed in the intervention group (25/29, 86%) compared with control group (8/27, 30%; P < 0.001).
 * In the intervention group, family members of patients who died had significantly less stress (P < 0.001), anxiety (P = 0.02), and depression (P = 0.002) than those of the control patients.

Advance Care Planning can deliver to patients the five factors known to be important for a 'good death':

◆ managing symptoms

◆ avoiding prolongation of dying

◆ achieving a sense of control

◆ relieving burdens placed on the family

◆ the strengthening of relationships.

Paradoxically, Advance Care Planning can be as relevant to the patient's 'now' as it is to their 'future'. This is because when they recognize their right to have a say about future care if they become incapacitated, they also start to exercise their right to be fully informed and express choices about their current treatment.

References

1 Detering KM, Hancock AD, Reade MC, and Silvester W (2010). The impact of advance care planning on end of life care in elderly patients: randomised controlled trial. *BMJ*, **340**:c1345.

2 Victorian Parliament: Social Development Committee (1987). *Inquiry into options for dying with dignity*. Government Printer, Melbourne. www.austlii.edu.au/au/legis/vic/consol_act/mta1988168 (accessed 25 March 2010)

3 http://www.austlii.edu.au/au/legis/vic/consol_act/mta1988168/ accessed on 5th Sept 2010

4 Hammes BJ and Rooney BL (1998). Death and end-of-life planning in one midwestern community. *Archives of Internal Medicine*, **158**:383–90.

5 The Support Investigators (1995). A controlled trial to improve care for seriously ill hospitalized patients. The study to understand prognoses and preferences for outcomes and risks of treatments (SUPPORT). *JAMA: Journal of American Medical Association*, **274**:1591–8.

6 Prendergast TJ (2001). Advance care planning: pitfalls, progress, promise. *Critical Care Medicine*, **29** (2 suppl):N34–9.

7 Silvester W **et al**. (January 2006) *Final evaluation of the Community Implementation of the Respecting Patient Choices Program*- Report to Australian Government Department of Health and Ageing. Austin Health.

8 Briggs LA, Kirchhoff KT, Hammes BJ, Song M-K, and Colvin ER (2004). Patient-centered advance care planning in special patient populations: a pilot study. *Journal of Professional Nursing*, **20**:47–58.

9 Lautrette A, Darmon M, Megarbane B, et al. (2007). A communication strategy and brochure for relatives of patients dying in the ICU. *The New England Journal of Medicine*, **356**:469–78.

10 Wright AA, Zhang B, Ray A, et al. (2008). Associations between end-of-life discussions, patient mental health, medical care near death, and caregiver bereavement adjustment. *JAMA: Journal of American Medical Association*, **300**:1665–73.

Chapter 21

Advance Care Planning discussions in Australia: the development of clinical practice guidelines

Josephine M Clayton

The most important component of Advance Care Planning discussions is an exploration of the person's understanding, values, goals and priorities in the context of their prognosis or health situation.

Australian National Guidelines published in 2007 helped to affirm the value of ACP discussions, promoted their use, and were disseminated widely in Australia through endorsing organizations.

This chapter includes:

◆ An overview of Advance Care Planning discussions (ACP) from an Australian perspective

◆ Australian policy and development of national ACP guidelines in 2007

◆ Consensus recommendations for clinical practice, including timing of ACP discussions, and ways to open the discussion

◆ Suggested means to improve communication using the PREPARED framework

◆ Dissemination of guidelines and next steps.

Key points

◆ Discussions about death and dying are difficult

◆ Sensitive discussions about end of life issues are a very important aspect of care for patients with advanced life limiting illnesses

◆ Consider the recommendations conveyed by the acronym PREPARED

◆ ACP discussions, including discussions about no CPR orders, should take place in the general context of a conversation about the persons values, goals etc

◆ Involving key proxy decision-makers in ACP discussions is a key factor.

Introduction

Optimal communication about prognosis and end of life issues has been identified by patients and their carers as one of the most important aspects of care at the end of life (1). As outlined in previous chapters of this textbook, end of life and Advanced Care Planning (ACP) discussions are important in order to:

- assist patients to die in accordance with their wishes
- give families time to prepare for the patient's death
- avoid inappropriate interventions at the end of life.

Clinicians need to provide information in a way that assists patients and their families to set goals and priorities, make appropriate decisions, be informed to the level that they wish, and cope with their situation. Yet this can be hard to achieve, as discussions about prognosis and end of life issues are difficult for health professionals, patients, and families. Deficiencies have been identified in communication between health professionals and patients about these topics (2). Many health professionals lack confidence and are uncomfortable about end of life and ACP discussions. One of the main reasons that have been identified for this is a perceived lack of training and clear guidance about these topics (3).

In 2007 Australian guidelines titled *Clinical practice guidelines for communicating prognosis and end of life issues with adults in the advanced stages of a life-limiting illness, and their caregivers* (4), were published to assist clinicians with this difficult but important task. This chapter describes the development of these guidelines, their key recommendations, and their more specific recommendations regarding ACP discussions, as well as discussions regarding 'No CPR orders'. At the start of this chapter there is a brief summary regarding policies for ACP in Australia.

ACP in Australia

Like other parts of the world Advance Care Planning in Australia refers to discussion of treatment decisions/choices and goals of care at the end of life and the patient's wishes for medical care in the future if they are no longer able to be involved in the discussion. The potential benefits and limitations of ACP have been well described in other chapters of this textbook. They are summarized from the author's perspective in an Australian context in Box 21.1.

The legal status of advanced directives in Australia is summarized in the guidelines (4) as follows:

> An advance directive is a statement (either made orally or in writing) by a person that outlines their wishes for future health and personal care. The directive generally becomes effective when the person is unable to make decisions for themselves. Advance directives (5) are legally binding in Australia, either at common law or under statutes. The Australian Capital Territory, Northern Territory, Queensland, South Australia and Victoria have statutory schemes for advance directives. In the other States the law of advance directives is governed by common law . . . In some jurisdictions a person can make an enduring medical power of attorney, (as in LPOA in the UK) or appoint someone an enduring guardian, whereby a family member or other trusted person is appointed to make health decisions on the person's behalf should they lose mental capacity to make their own decisions. Even in the absence of such an appointment, all Australian jurisdictions have guardianship arrangements that recognize the authority of persons close to the patient to make medical treatment decisions on that person's behalf in the event of lack of decision-making capacity . . . The status of advance directives and the status and responsibilities of representatives of incompetent patients is complex and varies from jurisdiction to jurisdiction in Australia.

Box 21.1 Potential limitations and benefits of ACP

Potential limitations of ACP:

- Patients' preferences may change over time (hence important to keep the dialogue open)
- There is confusion amongst health professionals regarding the best way to document ACP discussions due to multiple forms and different legislation in different States of Australia
- The limitations regarding documentation of ACP discussions, lack of electronic recording and fragmentation of care between primary and hospital settings in Australia may mean that the outcome of ACP discussions may not always be made available in emergencies and, hence, the patients wishes for end of life care may not always be honoured (e.g. patients may be resuscitated despite preference to the contrary)
- Many healthcare professionals (HPs) in Australia seem to lack confidence in having ACP discussions and there is concern regarding time constraints
- Some HPs in Australia seem to lack knowledge about ACP processes and medico-legal aspects of honouring advanced care directives in emerging clinical situations.

Potential benefits of ACP:

- May increase likelihood of patients being cared for at the end of life according to their wishes
- May reduce unnecessary and burdensome interventions at the end of life
- May improve patient's sense of completion and preparedness for dying, both of which have been identified as important to people with advanced life limiting illness (1)
- Likely to reduced decision making burden for families and may improve bereavement outcomes
- Likely to enhance open discussion of dying between patients and their families
- May improve quality of dying and satisfaction with care.

Some useful information about ACP policies in Australia is shown in further resources at the end of this chapter. Clear and easily identifiable documentation of ACP discussions is essential in order to ensure that patient's wishes are able to be recognized at the time that their condition deteriorates. Documentation of ACP discussions remains a challenge in Australia, as in other parts of the world. There is no single standardized document for reporting ACP discussions in Australia that is accepted across all health settings or in all parts of the country. Many health services in Australia do not yet have electronic medical records. Various health care services, individual GP practices, and residential aged care facilities have developed their own documentation for recording Advanced Care Planning discussions and/or for medical orders relating to end of life care. Ensuring that documentation is recognized and accompanies the patient when they transfer between care settings is another challenge. In depth discussions of documentation issues is beyond the scope of this chapter.

The main focus of this chapter is communication between health care providers and patients and their families about ACP and end of life issues. The development of guidelines on this topic will now be described.

Development of clinical practice guidelines

The communication guidelines (4) were developed using the following process:

- an extensive literature review including a systematic review and a review of previous related guidelines and expert opinions
- refining of the guidelines with an expert advisory

More details about this process are provided below.

Systematic review

A systematic review (6) was conducted in accordance with the principles and processes recommended by the Cochrane review. Eligible studies included those of any design published in the English language evaluating communication of prognostic/end of life (EOL) information to patients with advanced life limiting illnesses & their families (not including those currently in intensive care settings). The medical literature was searched, using various computerized databases, to identify relevant studies and reviews for the period between 1996 and November 2004. In addition, hand searching was conducted up until 2005. One hundred and twenty three articles met the inclusion criteria for the review out of a total of 4294 articles retrieved from searches. Reviewers extracted data from each study using a standardized format. Most of the studies in the review were descriptive in methodology, examining providing practices and patient and/or caregiver views, attitudes, knowledge, and behaviour. Such studies are considered low level evidence by rating scales for clinical guidelines (7). However, such rating scales are designed for research questions/methods which not readily applicable to the topic of these guidelines.

Review of consensus guidelines and expert opinion

Relevant consensus guidelines and published expert opinions were incorporated into the guidelines because of the lack of evidence for some topics.

Expert advisory panel

An expert panel was convened comprising 35 Australian and New Zealand health professionals and consumers (nine palliative care medical specialists, three medical oncologists, three palliative care nurses, three consumers (including two cancer patients and one caregiver), two general practitioners, two psychosocial experts, two ethicists, two linguists, one oncology nurse, one cardiology nurse, one aged care nurse, one research nurse, one geriatrician, one respiratory physician, one radiation oncologist, one intensive care specialist, and one lawyer. The panel members were chosen to reflect the multidisciplinary nature of care for patients with advanced, progressive, life-limiting illnesses. Representatives were selected based on their clinical expertise or a track record of publications on this topic. Consumer bodies provided consumer representation. The guidelines were refined with the assistance of the expert panel using consensus methods (modified nominal group technique/Delphi method (8)). Several rounds of feedback were obtained before consensus was reached on the final guidelines document.

Endorsing bodies

The final guidelines document was sent to various relevant consumer organizations for their endorsement. Box 21.2 shows the list of organizations who formally endorsed the guidelines.

> ## Box 21.2 Organizations who formally endorsed the MJA clinical ACP guidelines
>
> ◆ Australasian Society of HIV Medicine
> ◆ Australian and New Zealand Society of Palliative Medicine
> ◆ Australasian Chapter of Palliative Medicine, Royal Australasian College of Physicians
> ◆ Australian College of Rural and Remote Medicine
> ◆ Australian General Practice Network
> ◆ Australian Society of Geriatric Medicine
> ◆ Cancer Voices Australia
> ◆ Cardiac Society of Australia and New Zealand
> ◆ Clinical Oncological Society of Australia
> ◆ Motor Neurone Disease Association of Australia
> ◆ Palliative Care Australia
> ◆ Palliative Care Nurses Australia
> ◆ Royal Australian College of General Practitioners
> ◆ Royal College of Nursing, Australia
> ◆ Thoracic Society of Australia and New Zealand.

Limitations of the guidelines

The limitations of the guidelines (4) are acknowledged as follows:

> The systematic literature review which informed these guidelines was limited to studies of patients, and/or their caregivers, with a known progressive life limiting illness. The recommendations or suggested phrases may not be applicable to patients with debilitating chronic illnesses with a life expectancy of greater than two years, patients having treatment with curative intent, and those in whom intensive care treatment would still have a reasonable chance of being effective. Likewise end of life discussions with well elderly people and those in residential aged care facilities (known as care homes in the UK) with uncertain disease trajectories are beyond the scope of these guidelines. All of the articles included in the systematic review were written in English and most of the patient and/or caregiver participants in these studies were from Anglo-Saxon backgrounds. Hence, some caution is required in interpreting these guidelines for patients from non-Anglo-Saxon backgrounds.

Key recommendations

The key recommendations of these guidelines are for health professionals to consider the recommendations conveyed by the acronym PREPARED (Table 21.1). The recommendations are outlined in Chapter 24.

More specific recommendations

The guidelines cover a wide variety of topics relating to prognostic and end of life discussions. The recommendations are presented in tabular form, together with the level of evidence for that

Table 21.1 The PREPARED guidelines

P	Prepare for the discussion
R	Relate to the person
E	Elicit patient and caregiver preferences
P	Provide information tailored to individual needs
A	Acknowledge emotions & concerns
R	(foster) Realistic hope
E	Encourage questions and further discussions
D	Document

recommendation and useful phrases where applicable. Some topics covered by the guidelines are relevant to all prognostic and end of life discussions, including:

- timing of the discussion
- preparation for the discussion
- physical and social setting
- how to discuss prognosis and end of life issues
- general strategies to facilitate hope and coping.

Other topics covered by the guidelines refer to certain content areas or issues, including discussions about the following topics:

- commencing or changing disease specific treatments
- cessation of disease specific treatments
- introducing specialist palliative care services
- life expectancy
- future symptoms and symptom management
- Advance Care Planning
- 'No CPR' orders
- process of death and dying
- requests for with holding prognostic/EOL information
- dealing with conflicts (family/doctor/patient)
- dealing with denial/requests for medically futile treatments.

More specific recommendations relating to ACP discussions

More detailed recommendations from the guidelines relevant to ACP discussions will now be described, in particular recommendations regarding: timing of discussions, general ACP discussions, and specific discussions regarding 'no cardiopulmonary resuscitation orders' (no CPR).

Timing of discussions

Table 21.2 provides recommendations from the guidelines regarding the timing of discussions about end of life issues and ACP. That is when health professionals should consider raising the topic themselves, apart from when the patient initiates the discussions (e.g. by asking a question).

Table 21.2 Recommendations regarding the timing of ACP discussions

Recommendation	Evidence Level
All patients with advanced progressive life limiting illnesses should be given the opportunity to discuss prognosis (including life expectancy, how the illness may progress, future symptoms, and effect on function) and end of life issues.	DS
◆ Do not assume that the patient does not want to discuss the topic simply because he/she does not raise the issue, or because of cultural background.	
◆ Give the patient the option not to discuss it or defer the discussion to a later time.	
Consider raising/introducing the topic in the following circumstances:	
◆ With all patients and their caregivers once it is clear that the patient has a life limiting advanced progressive illness; or if the doctor would not be surprised if the patient died within 6–12 months.	DS
◆ When there is a change in condition, or a perception (by patients, caregivers or clinical staff) of change.	DS
◆ When a treatment decision needs to be made.	DS
◆ If there are requests or expectations that are inconsistent with clinical judgment.	DS
◆ If disease specific treatment is not working or there are complications from this treatment that limit its effectiveness.	DS
◆ At time of referring patient to specialist palliative care services.	DS

DS = Descriptive studies—for full reference list refer to (4).

NOTE: the literature review informing these guidelines excluded patients with a likely survival of > 2 years (including patients with early stage dementia).

From: *Clinical practice guidelines for communicating prognosis and end-of-life issues with adults in the advanced stages of a life-limiting illness, and their caregivers.* Josephine M Clayton, Karen M Hancock, Phyllis N Butow, Martin HN Tattersall, and David C Currow, MJA • Volume 186 Number 12 • 18 June 2007 • Copyright Medical Journal of Australia
• Reproduced with permission.

Advanced Care Planning discussions

When having Advanced Care Planning discussions it is recommended that health professionals consider the general principles outlined by the PREPARED acronym outlined in Table 21.1. In particular it is very important to first find out the person's understanding of their situation and preferences for information. Any new information about prognosis or end of life issues should be tailored to the person's understanding and preferences. Not all patients want to take part in detailed ACP discussions, and may prefer to defer decisions about their end of life care to their family or to their doctor. However, it is not possible to make assumptions about individuals information needs or preferences for involvement in decision-making based on their cultural background or demographic information. Hence, this needs to be sensitively explored with the individual. ACP discussions should be offered but not forced.

The most important component of Advanced Care Planning discussions is an exploration of the person's understanding, values, goals, and priorities in the context of their prognosis or health situation. Helpful questions for eliciting this information are shown in Box 21.3. Involvement of key family members or other trusted person(s) (whom the patient wishes to be involved in decisions

Box 21.3 Examples of questions for eliciting patient's understanding, values, goals, and priorities during Advanced Care Planning discussions

- What is your understanding of your health situation and what is likely to happen in the future?
- Do you have any thoughts or feelings about where things are going with your illness/health?
- What is most important to you now? What aspects of your life do you most value and enjoy?
- What are your goals over the next few weeks or months?
- When you look at the future what do you hope for?
- Do you have any thoughts about how you would like to be cared for in the future?
- What aspects of care are important to you for the future?
- Is there anything that you worry about happening? What would you NOT want to happen to you in terms of your care?
- How would you want decisions regarding your medical treatment to be made if you were too unwell to make them for yourself?
- Who would you want to have making these decisions?
- Is there a specific person (family member/friend or caregiver) that you would like to be involved in discussions about your care if you were unable to make decisions for yourself?
- Are there any situations where you would regard life prolonging treatments to be overly burdensome and prefer them to be stopped or withheld?
- If your condition gets worse where would you most like to be cared for?
- Do you have any special wishes or preferences or other comments?

about their care) has been shown to improve the effectiveness of ACP (9,10). Hence the 'P' for PREPARED in Table 21.1 is very important for ACP discussions—in particular finding out from the patient who they would like to be present when the discussion takes place. It can be helpful to explain to the person the importance of involving their proxy decision-makers in the discussion where appropriate. Further recommendations from the guidelines regarding ACP discussions are shown in Table 21.3.

Discussion about 'no cardiopulmonary resuscitation (CPR) orders'

In Australia is it routine for CPR to be commenced in acute care settings unless is it clearly documented in the medical records otherwise.

CPR discussions are a subset of ACP discussions, but an area that doctors often feel uncomfortable about. Partly because it can feel awkward discussing an intervention that could be considered irrelevant or futile, for patients who are expected to die from an advanced life limiting illness. There is also fear among health professionals that by raising this topic that patients may feel abandoned or loose hope.

Table 21.3 Recommendations from guidelines for Advanced Care Planning discussions

Recommendation	Useful phrases (where applicable)	Evidence Level
Describe simply and clearly what advance care planning is. Give a rationale for why having these conversations can be helpful for families and the healthcare team. ♦ Explain the mechanisms available for advance care planning within the patient's State or jurisdiction.	*"Have you thought about the type of medical care you would like to have if you ever became too sick to speak for yourself? That is the purpose of advance care planning, to ensure that you are cared for the way you would want to be, even in times when communication may be impossible." (11)* *"Do you know who would make decisions about your medical treatment if you were unable to make them for yourself?" "Is this the right person?"* *"Have you spoken to the person who will make decisions for you?" "Would you like to include them in these discussions, so they know what is happening and what might happen in future?"* *"Some people have thought about what they want and document their wishes in what is called an Advance Care Directive. Do you have an ACD? Would you like to complete one? I could get you some more information if you like (or refer you to someone who could explore this further with you)".* *"It's often easier to talk through tough decisions when there isn't a crisis." (12)* *"Have you talked to anyone about your wishes, if you become too unwell to make decisions for yourself, about potentially life prolonging treatment? Have you talked to your family or general medical practitioner about what you want?"*	CG DS
Involve the potential proxy decision maker in the discussions and planning in order that they understand the patient's wishes.	*"Sometimes people with your type of illness do lose the ability to make decisions (or communicate their wishes) as the illness progresses. Who would make decisions for you if you were unable to do this for yourself?* If the person can identify a substitute decision-maker *"Would you like to talk this through with them?"* *"Would you like me to assist you with this?"*	DS

(Continued)

Table 21.3 (contd) Recommendations from guidelines for Advanced Care Planning discussions

Recommendation	Useful phrases (where applicable)	Evidence Level
Develop an understanding of the patient's values and help them to work out their goals and priorities related to their remaining life and treatment of their illness, and document patient preferences.	"Each person has personal goals and values that influence their decision when discussing advance care planning. I would like to find out your goals regarding your health and your health care and the things you most value in life. For some people the goal may be to prolong life, for others relief of suffering, optimising quality of life, and others a comfortable and peaceful death. I suggest we go through examples of possible situations that may arise to help you decide your goals of care"	DS CG EO
♦ Consider using clinical scenarios to structure the discussion.		
♦ Document specific details such as timing/circumstances in which to cease blood tests, antibiotics, deactivation of implantable defibrillators, and no attempt at CPR. Consider referring to one of four potential levels of care (1–4), depending on the patient's condition at the time:		
1 comfort care only;		
2 limited care (includes comfort care)–use of antibiotics and intravenous medications where appropriate, but no surgery or other more invasive measures;		
3 surgical care–surgery and palliative chemotherapy where appropriate, but no ventilation or resuscitation except during and after surgery;		
4 intensive care–includes all possible treatments, including invasive measures, to maintain life (may not be appropriate to offer this level of care for this patient population).		
Emphasise that advance care planning is an ongoing process that will need to be reviewed and updated on a periodic basis, as the patient's wishes may change over time, particularly with major health changes.	"These are discussions we may need to revisit if there are changes in the course of your illness"	CG
Ensure that other HPs who are involved with the patient's care are aware of the patient's wishes. If an advance directive or formal medical power of attorney is completed make sure its existence is known by all treating HPs and it is available when the patient's place of care is being changed (e.g. from home or nursing home to hospital, during ambulance transfers).		CG

DS = Descriptive studies, CG = consensus guidelines, EO = published expert opinion - for full reference list refer to (4).

From: *Clinical practice guidelines for communicating prognosis and end-of-life issues with adults in the advanced stages of a life-limiting illness, and their caregivers.* Josephine M Clayton, Karen M Hancock, Phyllis N Butow, Martin HN Tattersall, and David C Currow, MJA • Volume 186 Number 12 • 18 June 2007 • Copyright Medical Journal of Australia • Reproduced with permission.

The topic of whether or not it is necessary to discuss CPR orders with dying patients was the section of the guidelines that proved the most difficult to reach consensus on within the expert advisory panel. Increasingly in Australia there is an expectation that 'no CPR orders' are discussed with the patient and/or their family if the patient is incompetent. The writing committee for the guidelines were hoping to provide some guidance about situations where is not necessary to specifically discuss 'no CPR orders' with dying patients and/or their families prior to documentation. Legal and expert ethical advice was sought. The final recommendations that were agreed by all members of the expert advisory group and writing committee for the guidelines (4) are shown in Box 21.4. In brief, the guidelines state that it is generally recommended that Health Professionals discuss 'no CPR orders' with patients (if they are competent) and their families prior to documenting 'no CPR orders' in the medical records. There are some situations where it may be appropriate to not discuss CPR orders prior to documentation. For example, when the patient and family prefers not to discuss end of life care and requests that the doctor make decisions relating to the patient's healthcare.

Box 21.4 Summary of recommendations regarding whether or not it is necessary to discuss 'No CPR orders prior to documentation' from guidelines

There is no common law requirement in Australia to attempt treatment, even life-prolonging treatment, which is judged to be of insufficient therapeutic benefit ('clinically futile') or is overly-burdensome. However, the use of the terms clinical/medical futility is also controversial: as it has been argued that such terms are not capable of objective definition and may give rise to disputes between the treatment team and the patient's family. There is little research evidence to guide policies about whether it is desirable to discuss 'no CPR' orders with dying patients prior to documentation.

Decisions about whether to offer or provide CPR should be made on an individual basis on the grounds of likely benefit versus likely burden. Nevertheless, in situations where it is clear that the patient is dying from a progressive far-advanced life-limiting illness and the clinician has decided that CPR is not to be performed on the basis of clinical futility (i.e. negligible chance of survival with or without CPR and burdens of CPR far outweigh the benefits) then it should not be presented to patients or their caregivers as if it were an appropriate treatment option. This does not mean that it should not be discussed (such discussions may still be an important part of terminal care), but mostly in these circumstances patients and/or families should not be asked to make a decision regarding CPR.

Specific discussions about CPR are recommended prior to documenting 'no CPR' orders in the following circumstances:

a When the illness trajectory is uncertain (i.e. CPR may not be clinically futile, for example a patient at an earlier stage of their illness and/or if a potentially reversible complication of treatment occurs)

b In response to a patient/caregiver request or question about CPR

c When the patient has made it clear that he or she wishes to be informed of all decisions made about their medical care

> **Box 21.4 Summary of recommendations regarding whether or not it is necessary to discuss 'No CPR orders prior to documentation' from guidelines** (*continued*)
>
> There are other circumstances where the responsible clinician may decide that it is not appropriate to have a specific discussion about CPR with a dying patient and/or their family, prior to documenting a 'no CPR' order in the medical record, including:
>
> a the patient is aware that they are dying and has already expressed a wish for care that is aimed at their comfort rather than prolonging life;
>
> b the patient prefers not to discuss end of life care and requests that the doctor and/or caregiver make any decisions relating to their healthcare;
>
> c the patient is clearly in the terminal phase of a progressive life-limiting illness and the doctor thinks that the harm of the discussion may outweigh the benefits.
>
> However, not discussing 'no CPR' orders with patients/caregivers in this latter circumstance may be open to contest and requires very careful consideration.
>
> From: *Clinical practice guidelines for communicating prognosis and end-of-life issues with adults in the advanced stages of a life-limiting illness, and their caregivers.* Josephine M Clayton, Karen M Hancock, Phyllis N Butow, Martin HN Tattersall, and David C Currow, **MJA** • Volume 186 Number 12 • 18 June 2007 • Copyright Medical Journal of Australia • Reproduced with permission.

Since publication of these communication guidelines (4) the New South Wales Department of Health have published a very helpful policy document regarding 'Decisions relating to No Cardio-Pulmonary Resuscitation (CPR) Orders' (13). They provide clear guidance about situations where it is possible to withhold CPR without explicit discussion with the patient or family, namely in the following circumstances:

◆ The patient (or family/person responsible) does not wish to discuss CPR. A decision is then devolved to the senior treating doctor

◆ The patient is aware that they are dying and has already expressed a desire for palliative care

◆ The health care facility does not provide CPR as a matter of course, consistent with the values and practices relevant to their patient population, such as hospices, and this has been made clear to the patient and their family during the course of admission, or when the facility assumes care

◆ The patient has had a long therapeutic relationship with another doctor than the attending doctor, and prior discussions have made the patient's views regarding resuscitation known.

Nevertheless it is still recommended in general that discussions regarding preferences for care, including CPR, should be offered to patients and their families or the family alone if the patient is incompetent even where the treating doctors believe that CPR will offer negligible clinical benefit. This is because patients and families may expect CPR based on exposure to the media, and overestimate its success rate, and underestimate the burden. This may lead to conflicts/concerns if CPR is not explicitly discussed. Furthermore patients may wish to be involved in such discussions. The goal of such a discussion 'is not to offer all treatments amongst which the patient, family, or 'person responsible' must choose, but rather to clarify prognosis and define appropriate and agreed treatment options for this patient at this time' (13).

Table 21.4 gives recommendations for communication about CPR should the clinician decide that such a discussion is appropriate. The principles outlined in the PREPARED statement in Table 21.2, and for Advanced Care Planning discussions in Table 21.3, are also very important for discussions about 'no CPR orders'. In particular it is important to explore the person's understanding, goals, and values prior to having a specific discussion regarding CPR orders (see Box 21.3). Where the person has an advanced life limiting illness and CPR is judged to have negligible benefits, it is advisable for health professionals to give clear recommendations regarding care during the dying process (i.e. rather than simply asking the patient whether or not they wish to have CPR). It can be very helpful to anchor these recommendations around the patient's own goals, where feasible.

Table 21.4 Recommendations for discussions about 'No CPR orders'

Recommendation	Useful phrases (where applicable)	Evidence Level
'No CPR' orders should not be discussed in isolation, but rather in the context of a general discussion about prognosis, the patient's values/ expectations and the goals of care.		CG
Check the patient and/or caregiver's understanding of CPR.	"Are you familiar with CPR? "What is your understanding of CPR?" "Do you know what CPR means?"	CG
Give a simple explanation of CPR making it clear that it was designed for previously well people with acute cardiopulmonary events. It is may not be not necessary to give a detailed description of CPR unless the patient/ caregiver requests clarification.	"Cardiopulmonary resuscitation or CPR is given when a person's heart stops beating or breathing stops. It is used to keep people alive temporarily until they can receive emergency treatment in hospital or until an ambulance arrives" If more detail required: "The chest is pumped and air is blown into the lungs to try and get the person's heart and breathing started again. In a hospital setting (or if ambulance called) it will also involve needles in a vein, tubes down the throat and potentially an electric shock to the chest"	RGP
Explain that when a person has a cardiac or respiratory arrest in an acute care facility or during ambulance transfers (e.g. between care settings) it is standard procedure for cardiopulmonary resuscitation to be attempted unless it is documented otherwise (i.e. 'no CPR' order in place).	"If an ambulance is called, the ambulance officers cannot diagnose; their primary role is to keep someone alive long enough to get to an emergency department. (14) It is standard policy for ambulance officers to start CPR in response to a cardiac arrest unless it is documented otherwise."	CG
Avoid describing CPR as "doing everything" as this can be easily misinterpreted (e.g. the implication of not doing CPR is that it means "doing nothing").	"We will continue to do everything that is possible to ensure your comfort"	CG

(Continued)

Table 21.4 (contd) Recommendations for discussions about 'No CPR orders'

Recommendation	Useful phrases (where applicable)	Evidence Level
When the clinician judges CPR to have no therapeutic benefit, explain that in your judgment CPR would have no chance of changing the course of their illness.	"I think we need to focus on making sure you are as comfortable and as active as possible. There are no invasive measures that are going to change the course of the illness now and we need to focus clearly on your comfort" "Our aim is to focus on your comfort. No measures are going to change the course of your cancer"	CG
♦ Consider reinforcing this by explaining that most people think CPR in hospitalised patients is successful. However the success rate of CPR in previously healthy people is low. The outcome of CPR in people with a serious illness is universally poor.	"Given the severity of your illness CPR has almost no chance of being effective (15). It might also mean that you cannot be with your family when you are close to death. I would recommend that we do not attempt it in your case but I can reassure you, that we will continue all treatments that are potentially effective for your comfort. What do you think about that?" "Allowing death to come naturally, and making sure that you are as comfortable and supported as possible is our goal when that time comes. Trying to reverse that process and prolong life with CPR at that time is almost certainly going to fail and we would not recommend we try and do so. Is that in keeping with your thoughts and wishes?"	CG DS
Where appropriate, explain that the patient's death is inevitable and that the aim is to ensure that their death is as comfortable as possible.	"Not giving CPR does not mean that we are giving up on you! On the contrary we will continue to be extremely active and supportive in our care for you. It simply means that when death does eventually come, our focus will be on keeping you comfortable and supported rather than prolonging the dying period"	DS
If CPR is judged to be clinically futile do not ask the patient/caregiver "what do you want done" when the patient dies; as this creates an inappropriate burden of choice when there is no choice to be made.	"Allowing death to come unhindered and naturally, and making sure that you are as comfortable and supported as possible is our goal when that time comes. From what we have already spoken about this would seem in keeping with your wishes—is this so?"	EO
Emphasise active support throughout the dying process and explain that all potentially effective treatments can still be given even if they have a "No CPR" order.	'Putting in place a 'No CPR' order does not mean that we will abandon doing everything we can for (patient's name)'s comfort and functioning. While some of the treatments have made small differences, it seems clear at this point that (patient's name) will probably not recover. Certainly more (chemotherapy/aggressive treatment) can't make him better at this point. We need to help him in ways that we know can make a difference for the better. We need to ensure that he doesn't suffer unnecessarily and that he is allowed to die in peace and comfort. Here's what I am proposing to do; we'll watch him carefully and make sure we do everything necessary to make him comfortable. When he dies we'll respond with humanity and kindness and not with futile measures involving machines and drugs. How do you feel about this?"(16) "CPR would not be helpful. It would not prevent the patient's death but may prolong their dying and cause more suffering"	CG

Table 21.4 *(contd)* Recommendations for discussions about 'No CPR orders'

Recommendation	Useful phrases (where applicable)	Evidence Level
The order should be clearly documented and state whether or not it has been discussed with the patient and/or their caregiver (and if discussed with a caregiver(s) their name(s)). Document that the focus should be on providing good palliative care, and specifically that "CPR should not be attempted".		CG
◆ Where a decision has been made not to involve the patient or their surrogate in decisions regarding "No CPR orders", an explanation should be recorded regarding the rationale for this.		
◆ "No CPR" orders should include a statement of the patient's underlying condition/prognosis justifying it, and the involvement of other HPs in the decision making process/discussion where applicable.		
◆ Check with your hospital or facility policy about any other requirements for documenting CPR orders.		

DS = Descriptive studies, CG = existing consensus guidelines, EO = published expert opinion, RPG = recommended good practice based on the clinical and consumer consensus opinion of the Australian and New Zealand Expert Advisory Group. For full reference list refer to (10)

From: *Clinical practice guidelines for communicating prognosis and end-of-life issues with adults in the advanced stages of a life-limiting illness, and their caregivers* .Josephine M Clayton, Karen M Hancock, Phyllis N Butow, Martin HN Tattersall and David C Currow, MJA • Volume 186 Number 12 • 18 June 2007 • Copyright Medical Journal of Australia • Reproduced with permission.

Dissemination of the guidelines

The guidelines were published in June 2007 as a supplement in the Medical Journal of Australia. They can be downloaded for free from the MJA Clinical Guidelines website:

http://www.mja.com.au/public/issues/186_12_180607/cla11246_fm.html

The guidelines were launched by the CEO of the Australian National Health and Medical Research Council (NHMRC) and the Parliamentary Secretary to the Australian Commonwealth Minister for Health and Ageing at Parliament House in Canberra in June 2007.

The guidelines were disseminated widely by the NHMRC plus the endorsing organizations' newsletters and websites (see Table 21.3).

Recent developments and future directions

Uptake of these guidelines has the potential to lead to improved outcomes for dying patients and their families. Guidelines in isolation are not enough to achieve this. However, these guidelines provide an important foundation for communication skills training modules for health professionals regarding end of life discussions. Communication skills training modules based on the content of these guidelines have been developed. A brief individualized module has been developed for junior medical staff in hospital settings regarding discussion of EOL issues and 'no CPR orders'. This module is currently being evaluated. A brief version of this communication module is also being developed for oncologists and trainees.

In addition, a more extensive module for advanced trainees in palliative medicine has been developed based on the content of these guidelines. The module was developed by a working party for the Australasian Chapter of Palliative Medicine/Royal Australasian College of Physicians, in collaboration with a US group called oncotalk *http://depts.washington.edu/oncotalk*. Completion of this module will soon become a compulsory requirement for training in palliative medicine in Australia and New Zealand. It is hoped that the module could be later adapted for other specialty groups and trainees.

Other recent developments regarding ACP in Australia include Palliative Care Australia's training resources and guidelines for health professionals regarding a 'Palliative Approach in Residential Aged Care' *http://agedcare.palliativecare.org.au*, including specific resources for Advanced Care Planning in this setting *http://agedcare.palliativecare.org.au/Default.aspx?tabid=1178* In addition, as outlined in Chapter 20, communication training modules for ACP discussions have been developed by the Respecting Patient Choices Programme at the Austin Hospital, Melbourne *http://www.respectingpatientchoices.org.au*. Online training has been developed by Respecting Patient Choices® and made widely available on the Royal Australasian College of General Practice website *http://www.racgp.org.au/guidelines/advancecareplans*. Update of this training by General Practitioners has the potential to greatly enhance ACP update. Further research is needed to examine the effect of such training and ACP discussions on patient outcomes.

Provision of a clear and simple template for documenting advanced planning discussions, which could be recognized in various States in Australia and across care settings including by paramedics, would be very helpful. However, reaching a consensus on the content of the documentation across various jurisdictions would no doubt be challenging.

Acknowledgements

I would like to thank the other members of the writing committee for the clinical practice guidelines described in this chapter: Karen Hancock, Phyllis Butow, Martin Tattersall, and David Currow. I would also like to thank the other members of the Australian and New Zealand Expert Advisory Group panel: Jonathan Adler, Sanchia Aranda, Kirsten Auret, Fran Boyle, Annette Britton, Katherine Clark, Richard Chye, Patricia Davidson, Jan Maree Davis, Afaf Girgis, Sara Graham, Janet Hardy, Kate Introna, John Kearsley, Ian Kerridge, Linda Kristjanson, Peter Martin, Amanda McBride, Anne Meller, Geoffrey Mitchell, Alison Moore, Beverley Noble, Ian Olver, Sharon Parker, Matthew Peters, Peter Saul, Professor Cameron, Lyn Swinburne, Bernadette Tobin, Kathryn Tuckwell, and Patsy Yates.

Development of the Clinical practice guidelines described in this chapter was supported by a Strategic Palliative Care Research Grant from the Australian National Health and Medical Research Council. The Chief Investigator on the project (and author of this chapter) was supported by a Cancer Institute NSW Clinical Research Fellowship.

Further resources

ACP in Australia:
The full version of the clinical practice guidelines that are described in this chapter contain many other

examples of sample phrases. The guidelines can be downloaded for free from: http://www.mja.com.au/public/issues/186_12_180607/cla11246_fm.html

An Australian palliative care website called Caresearch has sections for patients, families, and health professionals regarding Advanced Care Planning http://www.caresearch.com.au

Relevant New South Wales Health Guidelines: Using advanced directives: http://www.health.nsw.gov.au/policies/gl/2005/pdf/GL2005_056.pdf

End-of-Life Care and Decision-Making–Guidelines: http://www.health.nsw.gov.au/policies/gl/2005/pdf/GL2005_057.pdf

CPR: Decisions Relating to 'no cardiopulmonary resuscitation orders' http://www.health.nsw.gov.au/policies/gl/2008/pdf/GL2008_018.pdf

The Royal Australasian College of General Practitioners website has an excellent section on Advanced Care Planning: http://www.racgp.org.au/guidelines/advancecareplans

Respecting Patient Choices Program described in Chapter 20 http://www.respectingpatientchoices.org.au

The Benevolent Society has useful information for older Australians about Advanced Care Planning http://www.bensoc.org.au/director/whatwedo/olderpeople/planningyourfuture

References

1 Steinhauser KE, Christakis NA, Clipp EC et al. (2004). Factors considered important at the end of life by patients, family, physicians, other care providers. *JAMA: Journal of American Medical Association*, **284**:2476–82.

2 Gysels M, Richardson A, and Higginson I (2004). Communication training for health professionals who care for patients with cancer: a systematic review of effectiveness. *Support Care Cancer*, **12**:692–700.

3 Baile W, Lenzi R, Parker A et al. (2002). Oncologists' attitudes toward and practices in giving bad news: an exploratory study. *Journal of Clinical Oncology*, **20**:2189–96.

4 Clayton JM, Hancock KM, Butow PN, Tattersall MHN, and Currow DC (2007). Clinical practice guidelines for communicating prognosis and end-of-life issues with adults in the advanced stages of a life-limiting illness, and their caregivers. *Medical Journal of Australia*, **186**(12):S77–108.

5 Biegler P, Stewart C, Savulescu J, and Skene L (2000). Determining the validity of advance directives. *The Medical Journal of Australia*, **172**:545–48.

6 Parker S, Clayton JM, Hancock K, et al. (2006). Communication of prognosis and issues surrounding end of life (EOL) in adults in the advanced stages of a life-limiting illness: A systematic review. NHMRC Clinical Trials Centre, University of Sydney, available online at http://www.ctc.usyd.edu.au/research/publications/ctc-articles-2006.htm

7 National Health and Medical Research Council (1999). *A guide to the development, implementation and evaluation of clinical practice guidelines*. Canberra, Commonwealth of Australia.

8 Raine R, Sanderson C, and Black N (2005). Developing clinical guidelines: a challenge to current methods. *BMJ*, **331**:631–33.

9 Hammes B and Rooney B (1998). Death and end-of-life planning in one Midwestern community. *Archives of Internal Medicine*, **158**:383–90.

10 Prendergast T (2001). Advance care planning: Pitfalls, progress, promise. *Critical Care Medicine*, **29**:N34–39.

11 Emanuel LL, von Gunten CF, and Ferris FD (eds) (1999). Advance care planning. In: *The Education for Physicians on End-of-life Care (EPEC) curriculum*, The Robert Wood Johnson Foundation, Chicago.

12 Roter DL, Larson S, Fischer GS et al. (2000). Experts practice what they preach: A descriptive study of best and normative practices in end-of-life discussions. *Archives of Internal Medicine*, **160**:11–25.

13 New South Wales Department of Health Decisions relating to No Cardio-Pulmonary Resuscitation (CPR) Orders http://www.health.nsw.gov.au/policies/gl/2008/pdf/GL2008_018.pdf

14 Demoratz MJ (2005). Advance directives: getting patients to complete them before they need them. *Case Manager*, **16**:61–63.

15 Quill TE (2000). Perspectives on care at the close of life. Initiating end-of-life discussions with seriously ill patients: addressing the 'elephant in the room'. *JAMA: Journal of American Medical Association*, **284**:2502–2507.

16 Dugan DO and Gluck EH (2004). Discussing life-sustaining treatments: an overview and communications guide for primary care physicians. *Comprehensive Therapy*, **30**:25–36.

Chapter 22

Living and dying in style: Australia—an example of ACP in action

Eric Fairbank

Think ahead. Act now

Logo to promote Advance Care Planning from the Department of Human Services, Victoria, Australia

This chapter includes:

♦ An example of ACP from Victoria, the Living and Dying in Style project

♦ The Respecting Patient Choices® Program from Austin Health, Melbourne, Victoria.

♦ The Respecting Patient Choices® training programme

♦ Impact of the Living and Dying style projects and guidelines for the future.

Key Points:

♦ Dying can be hard work

♦ There are conversations that everybody needs to have, and nobody wants to start

♦ Advance Care Planning provides a framework to overcome this difficulty

♦ The Respecting Patient Choices® Program is an efficient method of Advance Care Planning

♦ Such preparation for end of life care contributes to living and dying in style.

Case study 1

Mr JB was a 75 year old man suffering from metastatic bowel cancer. His request was that no treatment be given that would prolong the dying phase of his illness. His family was not only scattered geographically, but also in their attitudes to the future management of his progressing illness.

Using the Advance Care Planning framework, he was able to initiate conversations within his family, and document his wishes with particular regard to resuscitation, and life prolonging treatments.

As a result he was able to die peacefully. He was surrounded by his family who were able to come together without conflict, respecting his wishes spelt out in advance.

Living and dying in style

'Living and Dying in Style' is the title of a project based in a rural part of southern Australia (a small city called Warrnambool, South West Victoria, with a population of 32 000) which aims to promote Advance Care Planning in both palliative care programmes and residential aged care facilities (care homes/nursing homes). These facilities are also situated in some of the smaller towns dotted throughout the region, which covers an area of 26,300 sq Km with a total population of just under 125,000 people (1).

Dying is hard work. It can be a struggle to do it well as the person confronts the multitude of physical, psychological, social, and spiritual problems. To still be yourself, while facing a life threatening illness, requires courage. There are necessary preparations to be made.

As patients and their families face the end of life, there are also challenges for health professionals, requiring courage and skill. Discussions about end of life issues are often sensitive and emotional, so for some, waiting for the 'right moment' seemed a reasonable thing to do. But opportunities were missed. People died unprepared.

Courageous therapeutic relationships with patients and their families need to be part of routine day-to-day care, and made easy by some sort of framework that means potentially difficult conversations are not postponed. No longer should it be that each is waiting for the other to raise an awkward topic.

Advance Care Planning can provide this framework, so that discussions about end of life issues can be started easily, without initially even mentioning the dreadful 'dying' word, to enable a more open and realistic discussion about future plans.

The respect for autonomy and providing a sense of control, preventing inappropriate aggressive medical treatments at the end of life with the completion of correct documentation, relieving the burden on families, and avoiding potential conflict are all worthy by-products of this process.

But the primary aim will always be having conversations about things that matter, about hopes and fears, strengthening relationships, beliefs and values, and creating a legacy—whatever it takes to be living and dying in style!

Advance Care Planning (ACP)

Advance Care Planning is a process involving conversations with people to help them make, and preferably document, decisions concerning their future health care; and also to appoint someone else to make sure those decisions are respected in case they are unable to speak for themselves. In Victoria this is done under the authority of The Medical Treatment Act Victoria 1988 which clarifies the right of an informed, competent adult to refuse unwanted medical treatment.

In spite of this legal avenue, ACP did not become established as a routine because there was no integrated system for its use, no-one was specifically trained in the process and any plans that were completed were often not readily available at times of crisis (probably tucked away in solicitors' filing cabinets).

However the failure that surrounded ACP in Australia was turned around by the Respecting Patient Choices® Program (2).

The Respecting Patient Choices (RPC) program

This programme is based on the Respecting Choices™ program from the Gundersen Lutheran Medical Foundation in La Crosse, Wisconsin, USA (3). Respecting Choices™ was the only bright light in ACP that Austin Health, Melbourne could find anywhere in the world. With modification of language and some system changes suitable for Australia, Austin Health was granted a licence to pilot what they called the Respecting Patient Choices® program.

The success of this pilot in 2002 led to RPC being introduced to other hospitals, palliative care programmes, and residential aged care facilities across Australia. South West Victoria's Living and Dying in Style project between 2003 and 2006 was the first to use RPC after Austin Health.

The nitty gritty of RPC

Conversations are the nitty gritty of the RPC programme. Preferably these will lead to documentation that ensures a person's choices for future health care are known, and consequently respected.

Under the RPC programme in common with that of the UK and other countries (2) an Advance Care Plan may consist of three specific things:

- ◆ A Statement of Choices. Although not legally binding in Victoria, but recognized in common law, this document provides written evidence of a person's wishes for future treatments, with specific options for resuscitation and life prolonging treatments recorded. The preferred site of care, important beliefs that may impact on care, and reassurance that palliative care to alleviate suffering will always be offered are also included on this form.

- ◆ A Refusal of Treatment Certificate. This is a legally binding document that allows a person to refuse a particular treatment, or treatment in general, for a current medical condition. It does not apply to new medical conditions that may arise in the future. A legally appointed agent may complete a certificate on behalf of their donor. (In practice very few of these are done, as consensus between patients, families, and their health care providers is usually achieved with discussions surrounding the Statement of Choices document.)

- ◆ An Enduring Power of Attorney (Medical Treatment). This is a legal document that records the appointment of a person (the agent) who is given the authority to make medical decisions on behalf of the donor, if the latter is unable to speak for themselves. A back-up alternative agent may also be appointed if desired. Contact details of the agent(s), documents that have been completed, and the whereabouts of the original and copies are all recorded on the reverse side of this document.

An important feature of the system is the so-called 'green sleeve'. This a special plastic pocket which is filed at the front of the medical history containing copies of the completed documents, along with a discussion record of conversations held, and those who participated.

While the person retains the original documents, copies are made available for agents, other family members, doctors, solicitors, and any other relevant hospitals. People are advised to have their documents readily available at home should they need to call an ambulance.

The RPC training course

Traditionally this has been a two-day course of face-to-face tuition. Another option is now being made available that involves web-based learning modules of the basics, followed by one day of tuition, concentrating particularly on communication skills.

The majority of those training to be ACP consultants are nurses, some counsellors, pastoral carers, and a few doctors. While up to 30 people are taken for each course, smaller groups work better.

The first day begins with an overview of ACP from a TV report. A brief history is then outlined, followed by use of a DVD prepared by RCP: 'Advance Care Planning for all Australians'. This leads into small group discussion about the pros and cons of ACP.

The legal considerations relevant to ACP in Victoria are discussed, including the various powers of attorney that exist, followed by the introduction of the Enduring Power of Attorney

(Medical Treatment) concept. Hands-on practice at filling in this document usually demonstrates how creative some people can be when given a form to complete!

Various ways of beginning the ACP process are discussed, with a demonstration of the 'five minute introduction' that may be used 'to get the ball rolling.'

Assessing mental capacity is an important topic, using conversation to determine a person's ability to understand, process information, and communicate decisions, rather than the more formal tools that have their own drawbacks.

Role-plays are never popular. Doing this in pairs rather than threes (i.e. dispense with the observer) seems to be more productive, and grudgingly agreed to be a good way of learning.

The second day begins with a discussion of ethics, including respect for the principle of autonomy, the crucial role of intent, and the principle of double effect.

Exploring resuscitation and life prolonging treatments, with the help of DVD material made by the RPC programme, highlights sometimes controversial issues such as nutrition and hydration, and withdrawing treatments. Discussion difficulties (see later) are an important hurdle to overcome. Techniques to use in conversations are then put into practice with more role-plays.

Case study 2

Boris, an 83 year old Ukrainian man, was admitted to the hospital palliative care unit two weeks after he and his English speaking daughter were introduced to ACP. When staff asked his daughter about her father's wishes for end of life care, she stated quite clearly that he would not wish to live if dependent on artificial feeding or if he was unable to interact in a meaningful way with family. She believed that he was approaching the end of his life, having nursed her mother with terminal care at home. Boris was given pain management and comfort care. He wanted to spend his birthday at home, but was too unwell and his birthday party was held at the hospital palliative care unit with his family. He received the Ukrainian right of 'anointing the sick' and died peacefully in the hospital palliative care unit. His family were nearby and returned to his bedside immediately.

Key learning: When ACP is raised and information provided, patients and their families have an opportunity to reflect upon this and discuss it between themselves, even if the discussion is followed up by other health professionals.

Case study 3

MJ was a 36 year old man who was living at home with is wife. He suffered a progressive form of Becker Muscular Dystrophy that left him wheelchair bound from the age of 13 and on nocturnal ventilation. He also had an enlarged heart. When he was first introduced to ACP he was keen to continue with aggressive interventions such as tube feeding into the stomach (percutaneous endoscopic gastrostomy or PEG tube) and mechanical ventilation via a tracheostomy. During his last hospital admission, however, he witnessed two cardiac arrests which prompted him to request ACP. He had several conversations with a Respecting Patient Choices® facilitator, leading to the appointment of a surrogate decision-maker and a documented Advance Care Plan. In this plan he stated that he would not wish to be resuscitated, nor would he like to have a permanent tracheostomy. He did proceed with the insertion of a PEG tube to assist with nutrition. MJ was discharged home with his wife and community support up until his death. He had no further admissions.

Key Learning: Patients' preferences for medical intervention change with experience and disease progression. As a consequence, Advance Care Plan documentation needs to also change. Discussions with trained facilitators about end of life preferences also need to be ongoing and involve the patient's doctors to address any of their current or future medical concerns. Family must be kept aware of any changes in the patient's wishes.

(Respecting Patient Choices, 2006, Final evaluation of the community implementation of the Respecting Patient Choices Program, Austin Health, Melbourne Victoria.)

Using the RPC system within their organization, integrating ACP into quality programmes, and promoting it in the workplace and the community brings the day to a conclusion—except for the presentation of badges, certificates, and posters! More details of the Respecting Patient Choices Program are in Box 22.1.

Box 22.1 Respecting Patient Choices. Contributed by William Silvester

Respecting Patient Choices®: a model of Advance Care Planning that has four major elements: organizational system changes; Advance Care Planning education and training; implementation of Advance Care Planning; and quality improvement. The model requires support from the organization's executive, management, and staff in order to facilitate the culture change necessary for the adoption of new work plans and systems and a change in clinical practice to facilitate Advance Care Planning. System changes include the correct and prominent filing of patients'/residents' Advance Care Plans and the transfer of these important documents between facilities (including between hospitals and aged care facilities). It is unacceptable for a patient/resident to have completed Advance Care Planning and recorded what sort of treatment that they do, or do not, want, only to have these wishes ignored simply because the Advance Care Plan is 'lost in the system'.

Some of the initiatives of the Respecting Patient Choices® program are:

- Training non-medical staff to undertake this important communication with patients and their families.

- Training general practice nurses to do Advance Care Planning in collaboration with their general practitioners, as part of the 75+ health assessment.

- Establishing Respecting Patient Choices® sites in every state and territory in Australia.

- Conducting a successful trial of Advance Care Planning in residential aged care facilities and in community palliative care.

- Conducting a successful randomized, controlled trial of Advance Care Planning in patients aged 80 and over (British Medical Journal—in press).

- Collaborating with the Australian General Practice Network and the Royal Australian College of General Practitioners to implement Advance Care Planning in GP surgeries throughout Australia.

- Working with Aged Care Standards and Accreditation Agency to scope the implementation of Advance Care Planning in aged care facilities across Australia.

- Establishing a website *www.respectingpatientchoices.org.au* which receives thousands of enquiries.

The Respecting Patient Choices® model of Advance Care Planning was introduced to 17 residential aged care facilities in 2004/2005. This highly successful pilot project was shown to improve quality of end of life care of aged care residents; resident and family satisfaction; and significantly reduce the likelihood of residents being transferred to hospital to die (Respecting Patient Choices, 2006).

In 2008 the Austin Health Respecting Patient Choices® program completed a randomized controlled trial demonstrating that Advance Care Planning in the elderly improves quality of care, patient and family satisfaction with care, the quality of end of life care and a reduction in the incidence of depression, anxiety, and post-traumatic stress in the surviving relatives of patients who die.

Discussion difficulties

Dying is still a taboo subject. Even amongst health professionals; and even when the death rate is one per person.

The Living and Dying in Style logo is a man in a top hat, with a big smile, enjoying a night out on the town, doing it in style. Or so I thought. One nurse didn't like him—she saw him as a cheerful undertaker! Imagine the difficulties she was going to have with conversations that inevitably lead to talking about dying.

Beginning the conversation is the hardest bit. Given the permission and the right atmosphere most people want to talk about these things. A protocol suggested by Respecting Choices begins by asking a simple question, underlining the fact that this a question asked of everybody:

'Have you appointed anyone to have Medical Enduring Power of Attorney?'

So begins a conversation explaining about Advance Care Planning in a way that is not threatening, that is about respecting wishes, leading onto a person's beliefs, values, healing versus curing, and so on.

The most important tool for these conversations is a chair. Sitting down with the person (preferably with their carer in support), unhurried, in a place that is quiet and private, and using lay expressions without euphemisms make up essential starting points.

Patients, doctors, and nurses all want to hope for the best (4); but hoping for the best while preparing for potential death need not be mutually exclusive. Some patients want to discuss their concerns about dying, others should—if they are likely to die sooner rather than later. Useful phrases and triggers are included in Box 22.2.

Health professionals do not need to fully share a patient's hopes or fears to respect, learn about, and respond to them. Hoping and preparing at the same time minimizes the weakness of each strategy on its own with a combination of optimism (let's hope) and realism (let's prepare).

Useful lessons

The framework of Advance Care Planning can be used to provide the kind of care that maintains dignity, provides autonomy and choice for all individuals, while acting with respect and compassion as end of life plans are made.

The Respecting Patient Choices program, developed by Austin Health, Melbourne from the Respecting Choices program in La Crosse, Wisconsin is an efficient system for ACP.

Box 22.2 Useful phrases might be

- 'It's a good plan to hope for the best, but at the same time to make some decisions in case things don't go as well as we hope'.
- 'Would you like to talk about your concerns if things do not go as we hope?'
- 'Preparing for the worst does not mean giving up—it means arranging the best medical care for you, no matter what happens'
- 'It's important that doctors and nurses and your family know how you want to be treated in the future. There may be some treatments you would like and others you don't want at all'.

Open questions are always useful for continuing conversations: (5)

- 'What worries you most about… (e.g. what may happen)?'
- 'As you think about the future… what is most important to you?

Advance Care Planning does take time. Its successful implementation requires that it be given priority in daily practice, otherwise the length of time taken will be used as an excuse to delay conversations about end of life issues. Rather than completing plans in one go, a series of shorter conversations may be more appropriate. The time taken is also time well spent, avoiding the potential for future crises at inconvenient times.

Any agency introducing ACP needs support from their executive team for any policy changes, with written agreements to minimize the impact of senior staff turnover. Every agency also needs a 'clinical leader' to promote the cause, support ACP consultants, and to generally raise awareness amongst health professionals, health care agencies, the legal profession, and the community.

There were misconceptions in all these groups needing explanations that reassured people that ACP was part of routine care, that ACP consultants were not aware of serious prognostic information that had not been discussed previously, that there was no plan to deny people treatment, and that it had nothing to do with euthanasia.

Specific funding is needed to acknowledge the time, knowledge and skills required to fill this role.

The impact of living and dying in style

Everything gets evaluated these days—both quantitatively and qualitatively to assess impact and areas for further improvement.

Evaluation included the training course, the utilisation of ACP in different agencies in different parts of the region; the effect on the patient and family; and a survey of local general practitioners; as well as feedback from the ACP consultants themselves.

Suffice to say that the overall impact was positive:

- The training programme was judged to have met its objectives by most.
- Utilisation across the region did vary, depending on executive support at each agency, stability of staff, and individual enthusiasm of ACP consultants.
- There were many comments about improved communication, a feeling of relief, a better sense of control, and having everything in order.
- The awareness of general practitioners was raised and, very pleasingly, they said that they would respect the wishes of patients expressed in a plan.
- ACP consultants felt they were improving care, involving families better, helping people prepare for the future and, when the time comes, giving them a better opportunity to die with dignity.
- Difficulties reported were the time taken in an already busy schedule, that some people felt it was either not necessary or too confronting, and a few were overwhelmed by the paper work.

Given the positive response to the Living and Dying in Style project, sustainability became the next issue, so that ACP is not only an accepted practice in palliative care and aged care, but also in other areas of inpatient and community care.

The future

Progress in ACP has been such that the Victorian Government is now drafting policy with five guiding principles being considered for its implementation: see Box 22.3 (6).

'To implement sustainable ACP, supportive systems and workforce capacity must exist between health services and other relevant services in the broader community.'

A lot has been achieved, but there is still plenty to do!

Box 22.3 ACP: a policy for Health Services; Victoria Government, Melbourne, Victoria

1 ACP is person-centred i.e. individual, flexible, voluntary, and recognized as being valid

2 ACP is founded on the best available evidence

3 All Victorians have access to ACP and to information about their rights under laws that are relevant to ACP

4 ACP is integrated across the health care system, and provided in a coordinated way

5 Health services take responsibility for assisting people with ACP.

Conclusion

The use of Advance Care Planning as a framework helps to provide the kind of day-to-day palliative and aged care that maintains dignity, provides autonomy and choice for all individuals and their families, while acting with respect and compassion as end of life plans are made.

Acknowledgement

This chapter would not be complete without acknowledging the significant contribution of my colleague Mabel Mitchell RN, BAppSci, MSc to the Living and Dying in Style project. In particular, the brief mention on evaluation of the project does not do justice to her efforts in this regard, nor are the many hours she spent travelling to support over 200 newly graduated ACP consultants across the region recorded.

Further resources

Materials of the Respecting Patient Choices® Program, and further information may be obtained from the website: www.respectingpatientchoices.org

References

1 Mitchell M, Fairbank E (2006). *Living and Dying in Style Final Report*. South Western Regional Palliative Care Program, Warrnambool, Victoria.

2 Lee MJ, Heland M, Romios P, Naksook C, and Silvester W (2003). Respecting Patient Choices: advance care planning to improve patient care at Austin Health. *Health Issues*, **77**:23–26.

3 Hammes BJ and Rooney BC (1998). Death and end-of-life planning in one mid-western community. *Archives of Internal Medicine*, **158**:383–90.

4 Back A (2003). Hope for the Best, Prepare for the Worst. *Annals of Internal Medicine*, **138**;(5):439–42.

5 Clayton JM, Hancock KM, Butow PN, Tattersall MHN, and Currow DC (2007). Clinical practice guidelines for communicating prognosis and end-of-life issues with adults in the advanced stages of a life-limiting illness, and their caregivers. *Medical Journal of Australia*, **186**(12):S77–S108.

6 Roberts G et al. (2008). *ACP: a policy for health services*. Department of Human Services, Victorian Government, Melbourne, Victoria.

Section 5

Practicalities and getting going

Chapter 23

Communication skills and Advance Care Planning

Jackie Beavan, Carolyn Fowler, and Sarah Russell

'The problem with communication . . . is the illusion that it has been accomplished.'
George Bernard Shaw

This chapter includes:
- Clarification of communication skills and Advance Care Planning
- Evidence for the value of effective communication in Advance Care Planning
- Key communication skills with useful examples of opening gambits
- Examples of blocking behaviours
- Models of communication and suggestions for implementation
- Workforce issues: recommendations for further education and training.

Key points
- Communicating about end of life care is challenging but essential
- Defining communication and communication skills can be a complex business
- There is plenty of evidence to suggest that effective communication is a key element in allowing patients to decide how they are cared for at the end of life
- Specific communication skills and models can be instrumental in encouraging patients to share concerns, ideas, and expectations, while some communication behaviours can inhibit patient disclosure
- A systematic approach to developing a workforce skilled in end of life communication is achievable and desirable

Introduction

Talking with anyone about how they would like to be cared for at the end of their lives is rarely going to be an easy task. However, being aware of the communication skills that can help and developing these skills can make this task less daunting and more rewarding for both the health professional and the patient.

Defining communication

Good communication forms a key part of the interaction between the patient and health care professional in providing psychological support, information-giving with regard to treatments, medication, and rehabilitation, and for encouraging and facilitating difficult conversations and decisions towards the end of life (1). The early work of Glaser and Strauss (2) highlighted the importance of communication in serious illness or terminal care. Communication is not just concerned with explaining and supporting treatment decisions but also with accompanying the individual along their illness experience journey. Communication about end of life issues is central to decision-making in life-threatening illness (3).

Before proceeding any further, though, it is important to define what we mean here by 'communication' amongst the multiplicity of definitions that abound. In simple terms, 'Communication involves the reciprocal process in which messages are sent and received between two or more people.' (4) Some definitions include modes of communication, such as Brooks and Heath (5) who see communication as 'the process by which information, meanings and feelings are shared by persons through the exchange of verbal and non-verbal messages'. Groogan (6) asserts that communication is 'not something that people do to one another, but rather it is a process in which they create a relationship by interacting with each other'. Effective communication in healthcare has been defined as being 'an open two way communication in which patients are informed about the nature of their disease and treatment and are encouraged to express their anxieties and emotions' (7). If definitions of communication vary so much, it is not surprising that there are differences in defining the skills required to do it effectively. Chant et al. (8) observe that there is inconsistency as to exactly what constitutes a communication skill. They suggest that communication involves the process of message transmission itself and the mode of transmission used, in terms of which senses and sensory outputs are involved. Clusters of these 'sensory outputs' form communication skills, which themselves can be grouped to form communication strategies. Small wonder that those who write about communication skills tend to list examples, rather than strive for a definition! However, it is generally accepted that there are attitudes, behaviours, and traits that support effective communication skills (Table 23.1).

The evidence base for the importance of communication in Advance Care Planning

A review of the literature reveals complexity in terms of health professional, patient, and family agendas, but provides clear evidence for the importance of effective communication (see Table 23.2). Studies suggest that advance directives (now called advance decisions to refuse treatment) are ineffective without the accompanying communication skills and trust-building processes (11).

Table 23.1 Key communication attitudes, behaviours, and traits

Empathy	The ability to understand a person's experiences and feelings accurately including demonstrating that understanding (9).
Genuineness	The ability to be yourself despite your professional role (9).
Respect	The ability to accept the patient as he or she is (9).
Unconditional positive regard	The ability to take a non-judgemental approach (10).
Reflexivity	Immediate, dynamic, and continuing self awareness and reflection (10).

Table 23.2 The value of communication in Advance Care Planning

Barnes et al. 2007 (17)	This study of 22 palliative care and oncology patients, relatives and user group members showed that, although some patients welcome the opportunity to discuss end of life care, others may not feel ready or able to do so. The timing of a discussion is likely to influence its acceptability and effect. The person initiating discussion should be skilled in responding to the cues of the patient, and should enable the patient to close the topic down at the end of the discussion, in order to avoid dwelling too much on the end of life. Advance Care Planning should take place over a number of meetings, and be conducted by an appropriately trained professional with sufficient time to talk through the issues raised, and with the knowledge and skills to answer questions, tailor the discussion to the individual, and avoid destroying hope.
Clayton et al. 2007 (15)	This was a systematic review of studies of adults with advanced progressive life-limiting illness with less than two years to live and/or the caregivers (including bereaved relatives) of such patients and qualified health care professionals. The authors concluded that avoidance can lead to poorer patient satisfaction and psychological morbidity. If information provision is not honest and detailed, patients may perceive that health care professionals are withholding potentially frightening information. Although many health care professionals believe introducing the topic will unnecessarily upset the patient and dispel any hope, evidence suggests that patients can engage in such discussions with minimal stress and maintain a sense of hope even when the prognosis is poor. In addition, awareness of prognosis is associated with greater satisfaction with care and lower depression levels in patients.
Prendergast 2001 (11)	This review of studies assessing the effectiveness of advance directives finds that they have no effect on outcomes. In contrast, it highlights one successful programme that focuses on the patient and their family and treats end of life discussions as an ongoing process, requiring effective communication skills, the building of trust over time, and working within the patient's most important relationships.
Schickedanz et al. 2008 (18)	One hundred and forty-three English and Spanish speakers aged 50 and older (mean 61) enrolled in an advance directive preference study in San Francisco County. Six barrier themes emerged: perceiving ACP as irrelevant (84%), personal barriers (53%), relationship concerns (46%), information needs (36%), health encounter time constraints (29%), and problems with advance directives (29%). Understanding ACP barriers may help clinicians prioritize and address them and may also provide a framework for tailoring interventions to improve ACP engagement.
Seymour et al. 2004 (12)	This was a study of 32 older people or their representatives who belonged to six diverse community groups in Sheffield, UK, which used focus groups to explore older people's views about advance statements and the role these might play in end of life care decisions. Trust between doctor and patient built up over time, and was perceived to be important in creating an environment in which the communication necessary to underpin ACP could take place. It concludes that, rather than emphasizing the completion of advance statements, it may be preferable to conceptualize ACP as a process of discussion and review between clinicians, patients, and families.
Sudore et al. 2008 (13)	This descriptive study measured self-reported ACP contemplation, discussions with family, friends, and clinicians, and documentation six months after subjects were exposed to two advance directives. It concluded that the ACP paradigm should be broadened to include contemplation and discussions and that one of the most important targets for ACP interventions may be promoting discussions with family and friends.
Wenrich et al. 2001 (14)	A study of 137 cancer and chronically and terminally ill patients' views on patient-physician communication identified key areas. These included the physician talking honestly and straightforwardly, being willing to talk about dying, giving bad news in a sensitive way, listening to patients, encouraging questions, and being sensitive to timing of such discussions.

Seymour et al. (12) also found that, in patients from a range of ethnic backgrounds, trust-building through ongoing discussion was more important than completing advance statements and Sudore et al. (13) recommended that facilitating discussion between family and friends was a key element in Advance Care Planning (ACP). Other studies have shown that patients value honesty, clarity, and sensitivity in their doctors when they discuss end of life issues (14); and that avoidance of honest and detailed discussion may lead to poorer patient satisfaction and increased psychological distress (15). There is evidence that ACP may be a series of discussions rather than just one event and that some of those discussions will be exploratory conversations rather than decision-making ones (e.g. to decide and agree an advance decision to refuse treatment) (12).

The evidence also tells us that health care professionals need to be aware of their own competency and confidence in communicating at the end of life (16). Barnes et al. (17) found variations in the readiness of patients to engage in end of life conversations and emphasized that health professionals should be skilled in judging the timing of such discussions. The ability of health professionals in recognizing barriers to discussing Advance Care Planning was also seen as vital by Schickedanz et al. (18). Wenrich et al. (14) describe the importance of emotional support and identify key elements of communication, as being 'compassion, responsiveness to emotional needs, maintaining hope and a positive attitude, providing comfort (through touch) and personalization (treating the whole person and not just the disease), making the patient feel unique and special, and considering the patient's social situation'.

Points to consider when talking about Advance Care Planning

There is a considerable body of evidence, then, that effective and skilled communication is perceived by patients as being beneficial when discussing their care towards the end of life. The discussions that take place can vary greatly from patient to patient and a range of considerations may need to be taken into account:

a. **The point in the process at which the discussion takes place**

   A first attempt to introduce end of life issues may be very different from later discussions when earlier concerns and wishes are reviewed and perhaps confirmed or amended.

b. **The content of the conversation**

   Topics discussed may range from consideration of preferences and wishes or general concerns to Advance Decisions to Refuse Treatment or preferred place of care or death. There may be an emphasis on practicalities such as 'Just in Case Boxes' (anticipatory prescribing), managing possible death anxiety associated with having the conversation, or even bereavement care for relatives after death. Some topics may require referral to other professionals.

c. **The context and circumstances of the conversation**

   The discussion may have been instigated by admission to a nursing home or hospital, or take place at a pivotal point in a person's physical illness and treatment plan or personal life.

d. **Proactive to crisis Advance Care Planning conversations**

   The discussion that follows a patient being identified as likely to die in the next year* where both patient and health professional have time to build rapport and trust will be very different from the crisis conversation carried out late on a Friday afternoon before a bank holiday, where urgent practical issues need to be considered.

   * This may be after an affirmative response by a health professional to the Gold Standards Framework surprise question: 'Would you be surprised if this person died in the next 6 months or so?' (19)

e. **Cultural sensitivity**

   Cultural factors, including ethnicity, religion, gender, and sexual orientation, may influence how a person wants to be cared for at the end of life and how they wish to negotiate this.

The health professional may need to acknowledge their uncertainty and respectfully enquire how best to meet the patient's needs.

f. **Confidence and competence of different staff groups**

Some practitioners may work in end of life care all the time and feel confident to facilitate and implement these conversations while others who deal infrequently in end of life care may need support.

As can be seen, one Advance Care Planning discussion may be very different from the next, being affected by the stage of the patient's illness, recent life events, the stage in the ACP process, cultural factors, and the skills and experience of the health professional.

Key communication skills

Once it has been established that it may be appropriate to initiate a discussion about end of life issues (taking into account all of the aspects mentioned in the previous section) the judicious use of effective communication skills is essential in starting this process. The initial aim of the Advance Care Planning discussion is to create an environment in which the patient feels comfortable to disclose what is really in their mind about the future. Maguire et al. (20) and Maguire and Pitceathly (21), describe certain behaviours (key communication skills) that may help patients disclose their concerns and express their feelings. They also identify ways in which health professionals can effectively block these disclosures (see Table 23.3).

Table 23.3 Facilitating behaviours

Open directive questions	These can be used very effectively at the start of any conversation about Advance Care Planning to find out patients' understanding of their situation and how ready they are to discuss how they wish to be cared for in the future. They are open in that they allow the patient to give us information in their own way, but directive in that they focus on one aspect of the patient's experience.	Examples: 'Can you tell me how things have been for you over the past few weeks?' 'What have you been told so far about your illness?'
Questions with a psychological focus	Much of what a patient discusses might be about physical aspects such as pain, fatigue or clinical procedures, but focusing only on these may lead the patient to believe that discussion of emotional and psychological aspects is not appropriate. However, it is important to find out how they feel about the often momentous events that are occurring in their life at this time.	Examples: 'How do you feel about going into the hospice for a couple of weeks?' 'When the doctor told you that your illness is terminal, what thoughts were going through your mind?'
Questions which explore answers to psychological questions	The initial response to a psychological question may be brief, even consisting of one word, and this requires some clarification if we are to understand what is meant.	Examples: 'You say you are frightened about going into the hospice. What is it exactly that frightens you about this?' 'So you felt angry when the doctor told you. Can you tell me more about this?'

(Continued)

Table 23.3 (*continued*) Facilitating behaviours

Empathic statements	We can never really know what another person is going through, but we can signal that we care and that we are eager to understand. This can be done in several ways. We can acknowledge that their situation is difficult; we can reflect what we see or sometimes we can stay silent for a while to allow someone to talk.	Examples: *'This is clearly a very worrying time for you.'* *'From what you have said, this has been a very difficult decision to make.'*
Screening questions	Finding out whether there are any concerns that have not been mentioned yet is important, because health professionals sometimes offer advice before patients have managed to present all of their key complaints (22) Screening questions ('what else' questions) can help here.	Examples *'You have mentioned some concerns already—is there anything else that is worrying you?'* *'What else is on your mind?'*
Summarizing	In a conversation about ACP we might receive a good deal of information from the patient. It is useful to summarize at intervals and at the end of a conversation, just to check that what we understand is what the patient actually meant and that we have picked up all the important points. It also shows the patient that we have been listening.	Examples: *'So you're going to discuss lasting power of attorney with your family and let us know your decision.'* *'You've told me that you would like to stay at home as long as possible, but when you can no longer look after yourself, you would like to go into a nursing home.'*

A word about cues

Sometimes, a patient may say something or behave in a way that suggests that they are experiencing feelings that have not been discussed yet—this is often a cue that is useful to pick up and explore. Del Piccolo et al. (23) defined a cue as being: 'a verbal or non verbal hint which suggests an underlying unpleasant emotion and would need a clarification from the health provider'.

Cues include words or phrases that hint at emotions that have been left unarticulated, repeated mentions of specific issues that suggest concerns, or non-verbal behaviours such as crying, sighing, frowning, or fidgeting.

Blocks to effective communication

There are also communication behaviours that can act as blocks to patient disclosure. These were identified as follows:

Closed questions

While closed questions (those that can be answered with 'yes' or 'no') certainly have their place in clinical encounters, using only closed questions gives little opportunity for patients to explain their ideas, concerns, and expectations in their own words.

Leading questions

Leading questions tend to include the expected answer in some way, for example, 'You've got on very well at the day hospice, haven't you?' This can discourage patients from giving an honest response.

A focus on physical aspects

Like closed questions, questions with a physical focus are an essential part of many consultations and assessments. However, staying with the physical side can be an effective way of avoiding discussing more sensitive issues—for the patient and the health professional!

Premature advice or reassurance

When a patient introduces a problem, it can be tempting to go into advice or reassurance mode before that problem has been fully explored. Although this may seem to be what the patient wants, it effectively closes down any further discussion of the problem and significant information may be suppressed. Furthermore, premature reassurance may give false hope.

Explaining away distress as normal

It may seem helpful to respond to a patient's fears, for example, about going into a nursing home by saying something like, 'Everyone feels like that when they give up their home'. However, this can lead to the patient feeling that their concerns have been dismissed and prevent them from explaining further.

'Jollying' patients along

Encouraging patients to 'look on the bright side' or to 'keep positive' may be counter-productive if it stops them from discussing their concerns.

Switching the topic

When we feel uncomfortable discussing emotional issues, we might change the subject as an avoiding strategy. We can do this in various ways.

Switching person

Patient: My husband is worried about me being at home.
HCP: What do you think about it?

Switching time frame

Patient: I felt really down yesterday.
HCP: But how do you feel this morning?

Removing the emotion

Patient: The pain makes me feel so helpless.
HCP: Have you been taking the painkillers?

When we do this, we are ignoring important cues and making it very difficult for the patient to have their issues addressed.

Training can help health professionals to recognize when they are blocking a patient's concerns and to avoid blocking behaviours. Similarly, it can help them to be more confident in using facilitating behaviours (21,24,25) Models of interacting with patients, for example when breaking bad news or discussing end of life issues, can also help by incorporating key communication skills into a framework.

Models of communication

There are several models that can be used to help structure important and sensitive conversations with patients. Four of these models are of particular value, although only two of these were designed specifically for end of life discussions. SPIKES (26) was originally intended as a protocol for breaking bad news, but can be usefully adapted for Advance Care Planning discussions. Calgary-Cambridge (27) is a more generic model for structuring a medical consultation, but again contains elements that can be applied to an end of life setting. PREPARED (15) and SAGE and THYME (28) were both developed to help health practitioners deal with the challenging task of discussing with patients how they would like to be cared for as their life draws to a close.

There are certain elements that appear in all of these models, for example, they all emphasize the importance of obtaining the patient's perspective and the value of empathy. In addition, they all include the need to summarize at the end of the discussion. Three out of four place great importance on preparation for the meeting, including privacy and the opportunity to include significant others. SPIKES and PREPARED both recommend caution in checking exactly what and how much a patient wishes to know and to discuss; recognizing that some patients may be more reticent than others. SAGE and THYME focuses heavily on questions to ask the patient, while PREPARED also includes the needs of care-givers. Of course, none of these models should be used in a rigid manner, but should be adapted to meet the needs of the particular patient. Table 23.4 demonstrates some of the commonalities and differences between the four models.

Table 23.4 Models that can lend structure to Advance Care Planning discussions

SPIKES	PREPARED	SAGE & THYME	CALGARY-CAMBRIDGE
Setting: Includes privacy, involving significant others, listening mode and body language	**Prepare for the discussion:** Check patient's diagnosis and results; Privacy; Significant others	**Setting:** Create privacy and choose right time to discuss emotions and concerns	**Initiating the session:** Establish initial rapport; Identify reason for consultation with open questions; Listen without interrupting; Confirm and screen for further problems; Negotiate agenda
	Relate to the person: Develop rapport and show empathy		
Perception: The 'before you tell, ask' principle; You should glean a fairly accurate picture of the patient's perception of their medical condition	**Elicit patient and caregiver preferences:** Clarify aim of meeting; Elicit patient's understanding and expectations	**Ask:** Specific questions about feelings **Gather:** Make a list of things the patient tells you **Empathy:** See below **Talk:** Ask if patient has anyone they can talk to **Help:** Have they been helped in the past? **You:** 'What do you think would help?' **Me:** 'Would you like me to do anything?'	**Gathering information:** Explore patient's problems; Open to closed questions; Listen attentively; Facilitate patient responses; Pick up cues; Clarify unclear statements; Summarize periodically; Use clear questions; Establish and sequence of events; Explore patient's ideas, concerns, expectations, and feelings

SPIKES	PREPARED	SAGE & THYME	CALGARY-CAMBRIDGE
Invitation: Check how much patient wants to know about diagnosis and treatment; Obtaining overt permission respects the patient's right to know (or not to know).	**Provide information:** Offer to discuss issues, giving patient option not to discuss it		
			Providing structure: Summarize appropriately; Signpost; Use logical sequence; Keep to time
			Building relationship: Appropriate non-verbal behaviour; Develop rapport, use empathy, provide support; Involve patient
Knowledge: Give information at patient's pace using the same language as them; 'Chunk and check'.	**Provide information:** Give information at patient's pace, using clear language; Explain uncertainty; Consider caregiver's and family's information needs		**Explanation and planning:** Correct amount and type of information; Aid recall and understanding; Shared understanding; Shared decision-making
Empathy: Listen for, identify, acknowledge and validate emotions	**Acknowledge emotions and concerns:** Explore, acknowledge and respond to fears, concerns and emotions	**Empathy:** Use silence, give space, reflect patient's feelings	
	(Foster) Realistic hope: Be honest, offering appropriate reassurance, but not false hope		

(Continued)

Table 23.4 (*continued*) Models that can lend structure to Advance Care Planning discussions

SPIKES	PREPARED	SAGE & THYME	CALGARY-CAMBRIDGE
	Encourage questions and further discussions: Check understanding; Emphasise discussion can be ongoing		
Strategy and Summary: Summarize discussion, give chance for questions or concerns; Clarify next steps	**Document:** Write summary of discussion; Contact other relevant health care providers	**End:** Reflect, acknowledge and conclude meeting, emphasizing main points	**Closing and planning:** Forward planning; Summary; Final check

Case studies

Awareness and understanding of communication skills are extremely useful and models which show how to combine these skills (as outlined above) can also enhance confidence in health professionals who become involved in ACP. However, knowing about these skills and models is not enough—being able to use them in response to individual patient needs is most important. The case studies that follow are designed to give you an opportunity to consider what skills might be most useful in specific situations.

Case study 1

Josie has had lung cancer for three years. She and her husband have two teenage children and have chosen not to involve health care professionals in discussions about ongoing care or emotional/psychological support. At clinic on a Friday afternoon she was told the disease was progressing and that there was no more treatment on offer. She and her husband were devastated and appeared extremely shocked by the news. There had been no Advance Care Planning started and the consultant decided to ask her where she wanted to die. Both Josie and her husband were shocked by this question and very angry at the bluntness of the question.

You are the GP who sees Josie and her husband directly after they have seen the consultant. They are still very angry and upset.

How might you proceed with Advance Care Planning in this situation?

You might have considered the following:

♦ Checking whether you are the right person to have this conversation—if not who is?

♦ Establishing the patients understanding of the news they have heard.

♦ Acknowledging how difficult it was to receive bad news.

♦ Acknowledging the anger and distress they are feeling.

♦ Letting them set the pace—it is the patient's agenda.

- Asking if they are ready to discuss how Josie would like to be cared for and if they aren't, making it clear that the door is open for when they are ready.

- Chunking and checking their understanding of any information you give.
  Which communication skills do you think would be particularly important here?
  You might have thought of:

- Open directive questions e.g. *What have you been told by your consultant so far?*

- Questions with a psychological focus e.g. *How has this left you feeling?*

- Empathic statements e.g. *This is obviously a very difficult time for you.*

- Summarizing e.g. *So the shock of receiving this news has left you unable to discuss your care at the moment, but you are aware that you can contact me when you feel more prepared.*

Case study 2

Mrs Jones has been living in a care home for the past three years. She talks openly about her palliative diagnosis and jokes about living on borrowed time. You, as a nurse at the care home, ask if she has everything in order, and she says the GP knows everything. You do not explore this at the time and then feel awkward about bringing it up again.

How might you proceed with Advance Care Planning in this situation?
You might have considered the following:

- Advance Care Planning has started and is an ongoing process—this information can be built on when you next have an opportunity to talk together.

- Clarifying what you meant by 'having everything in order' and checking what the patient understood by this.

- Being honest and admitting that you are not aware of Mrs Jones's wishes about her future care.

- Explaining that knowing more would help you and others in the team caring for her.

- Asking whether Mrs Jones would prefer to just discuss her future care with her GP and if this is the case, whether she would mind you talking to the GP so that the care team is also aware of her wishes.

- Making it clear that you are happy to talk about these issues at any time.
  Which communication skills do you think would be particularly important here?
  You might have thought of:

- Open directive questions e.g. *So how do you see things unfolding over the next few weeks/months?*

- Picking up cues e.g. *Living on borrowed time? What makes you say that?*
  When you say the GP knows everything, what do you mean?

- Questions with a psychological focus e.g. *You seem to be able to talk openly about your diagnosis—how do you feel about it?*
  How do you feel about discussing how you'd like to be cared for with me?

- Screening questions e.g. *What concerns do you have that we haven't talked about yet?*

- Educated guesses e.g. *You seem to be saying that everything is sorted with your GP—I wonder if you feel uncomfortable talking about this with me?*

Case study 3

Mr Singh is a 60 year old Sikh gentleman with advanced heart failure. You are the district nurse visiting him and you are concerned at how quickly he is deteriorating and the fact that you do not know what his wishes are about what happens in the time he has left. He speaks some English, but you do not always understand each other. You decide to try and talk to him about this. You find it difficult to approach the subject and start by talking about the hospice. Mr Singh becomes very angry and tells you not to mention that word again. You have now lost your confidence but know you have to continue visiting.

How might you proceed with Advance Care Planning in this situation?

You might have considered the following:

◆ Advance Care Planning has started, the patient may not wish to talk about it and this is his choice.

◆ Apologising for any distress caused by mentioning the hospice.

◆ Acknowledging his anger.

◆ Exploring the possibility of involving a professional interpreter (although he speaks some English, many people who are ill would prefer to communicate in their first language).

◆ Gently probing the source of his anger about hospice care.

◆ Establishing the patient's understanding of his disease and what it might mean for him.

◆ Respectfully enquiring if there is anything that it might help to know about his faith that would help you and the team care for him.

◆ Working towards building a trusting and honest relationship.

◆ The issues of risk-taking for professional and patient.

◆ The continuous process of informed consent.

◆ The patient's agenda, establishing his wishes/preferences.

Which communication skills do you think would be particularly important here?

You might have thought of:

◆ Open directive questions e.g. *How do you think things are going for you at the moment?*

◆ Questions with a psychological focus e.g. *How are you feeling about the future?*

◆ Empathic statements e.g. *I can see that this is difficult for you.*

◆ Educated guesses e.g. *You seemed so angry when I last visited—I guess you're very worried about what the future holds.*

The way forward: developing the workforce

This chapter has so far identified the relevance and importance of communication skills in Advance Care Planning. It has also explored the behaviours, knowledge, and attributes required

Table 23.5 Work Force Groups

Group Definition	Minimum Skill and Knowledge Level
Group A—Staff working in specialist palliative care and hospices who essentially spend the whole of their working lives dealing with end of life care.	These to include communication skills, assessment, Advance Care Planning and symptom management as they relate to end of life care.
Group B—Staff who frequently deal with end of life care as part of their role.	These to include communication skills, assessment, Advance Care Planning and symptom management as they relate to end of life care. This group has the greatest potential training need.
Group C—Staff working as specialists or generalists within other services who infrequently have to deal with end of life care.	This group must have a good basic grounding in the principles and practice of end of life care and be enabled to seek expert advice or information.

Reproduced from (29) with permission.

to use these skills effectively. The challenge is to embed these skills into practice and develop a confident workforce to practise these skills. Therefore there are two aspects to education, firstly that the workforce have the knowledge and skills and secondly that they have the confidence to use them.

The end of life workforce identified by the End of Life Strategy 2008 (29) has three broad groups (Table 23.5).

Senior health care professionals in cancer and palliative care have for some time been able to access an advanced communication skills training course, now called Connected (30). This course will now be rolled out to senior professionals working in end of life care. Groups A and B will benefit from this programme, but there is still a need to establish a robust training programme of intermediate and basic communication skills for other group B staff and Group C.

Evaluations of programmes of education around ACP highlighted the relevance of experiential learning in the form of guided role play using actors (31). Fry et al. (32) consider that 'experiential learning is based on the notion that understanding is not a fixed or unchangeable element of thought but is formed and reformed through experience'. Our own values and beliefs will be brought to the learning but it is likely that learning will only be achieved if reflection is embedded, a concept supported by Kolb's Learning Cycle (33). This is significant as it informs the way we continue to deliver communication skills training for all workforce groups, not just senior professionals. It also establishes the need for education as a continuous process rather than a one-off event. Therefore, workplace mentors may be useful in evaluating practice through observation and reflection of individuals and facilitating the confidence to use new skills.

A competency and principles framework for health and social care workers working with adults in end of life care has been developed as a collaborative approach by the Department of Health, National End of Life Programme, Skills for Health and Skills for Care 2009 (34). Advance Care Planning and communication are two of the five main competencies. These will inform and direct design and delivery of educational programmes. However, to ensure a change of practice, the competences mentioned will need to be adopted into workplace learning, so that individuals can practise the skills they have acquired and reflect on their practice. Practising the skills with guidance from a competent practitioner and reflecting on practice are essential in establishing a skilled and confident workforce able to facilitate Advance Care Planning.

In considering education for ACP, communication is paramount but other knowledge and skills are required. Understanding the process of ACP, the terminology, and legal aspects is crucial. Table 23.6 below identifies a competency framework for understanding educational needs.

It is also relevant to consider education of the public and a public awareness coalition has been created and led by the National Council for Palliative Care in partnership with the Department of Health (35). Its aim is to change attitudes and behaviours in society in relation to death and dying.

Table 23.6 Education Model for Delivering Advance Care Planning to End of Life Work Force Groups in Health and Social Care

Level of Education	Content	Audience
Level 4	Complex Advance Care Planning, discussions and documentation of statement of wishes and preferences	EoL workforce A and B Educators Specialist key worker
	Advance Decisions	
	Sign post to Medical/Legal Consultants/experts	
	Advanced Communication Skills Training	

(Continued)

Table 23.6 (*continued*) Education Model for Delivering Advance Care Planning to End of Life Work Force Groups in Health and Social Care

Level of Education	Content	Audience	
Level 3	Documentation of statement of wishes and preferences	EoL workforce A and B	National End of Life Competencies
		Generalist key worker	
	Intermediate Communication Skills		
Level 2	Understanding the process	EoL workforce B and C	
	Facilitation of process and ACP discussions		
	Sign posting to appropriate professional		
	Introductory Communication Skills		
Level 1	Awareness raising of what ACP is.	EoL workforce C	
	Purpose of ACP	Management	
	Impact of ACP	The public	
		Patients and carers	
		User groups	

Each level will build on the previous level (31).

Conclusion

The importance of Advance Care Planning is being increasingly recognized in modern healthcare systems. Similarly, communication skills, viewed with some suspicion until fairly recently, are now considered by many as belonging with other core clinical skills. The growing body of evidence supporting the benefits, both for patients and health professionals, of combining ACP with effective communication skills provides a powerful impetus to develop appropriate education and training for all health professionals for whom end of life care is an issue. Getting this right is essential for all of us as human beings.

References

1   Russell S and Knowles V (2009). Palliative Care in Chronic Obstructive Pulmonary Disease in Stevens E, Jackson S, and Milligan (eds), *Palliative Nursing Across the Spectrum of Care*, p. 126. Wiley-Blackwell, Oxford.

2   Glaser B and Strauss A (1968). *Time for Dying*. Aldine, New York.

3   Norton SA and Bowers BJ (2001). Working towards consensus: providers' strategies to shift patients from curative to palliative treatment choices. *Research in Nursing andHealth*, 24(4):258–69.

4   Balzer-Riley J (2004). *Communication in Nursing*, 6. Mosby, Missouri.

5   Brooks W, Heath R (1985). *Speech Communication*, 7th edn. Madison, Oxford.

6   Groogan S (1999). Setting the scene. In Long A (ed) *Interaction for Practice in Community Nursing*. Macmillan, London.

7   Wilkinson S (1991). Factors which influence how nurses communicate with patients with cancer. *Journal of Advanced Nursing*, 16:677–88.

8   Chant S, Jenkinson T, Randle J, and Russell G (2002). Communication Skills: some problems in nursing education and practice. *Journal of Clinical Nursing*, 11:12–21.

9 Coulehan JL and Block MR (2006). *The Medical Interview: Mastering Skills for Clinical Practice*. 5th edn. FA Davies Co, Philadelphia.

10 Finlay L and Gough B (2003). *Reflexivity: A Practical Guide for Researchers in Health and Social Sciences*. Blackwell Publishing, Oxford.

11 Prendergast TJ (2001). Advance care planning: pitfalls, progress, promise. *Critical Care Medicine*, **29**(2):SupplN34–9.

12 Seymour J, Gott M, Bellamy G, Ahmedzai SH, and Clark D (2004). Planning for the end of life: the views of older people about advance care statements. *Social Science and Medicine*, **59**(1):57–68.

13 Sudore RL, Schickedanz AD, Landefeld CS, et al. (2008). Engagement in multiple steps of the advance care planning process: a descriptive study of diverse older adults. *Journal of American Geriatrics Society*, **56**(6):1006–13.

14 Wenrich MD, Curtis JR, Shannon SE, Carline JD, Ambrozy DM, and Ramsey PG (2001). Communicating with dying patients within the spectrum of medical care from terminal diagnosis to death. *Archives of Internal Medicine*, **161**(6):868–74.

15 Clayton JM, Hancock KM, Butow PN, Tattersall MH, and Currow DC (2007). Clinical practice guidelines for communicating prognosis and end-of-life issues with adults in the advanced stages of a life-limiting illness, and their caregivers. The *Medical Journal of Australia*, **186**(12):S77, S79, S83–S108.

16 Russell S and Russell R (2007). Challenges in end of life communication in COPD. *Breathe*, **4**(2): 133–39.

17 Barnes K, Jones L, Tookman A, and King M (2007). Acceptability of an advance care planning interview schedule: a focus group study. *Palliative Medicine*, **21**(1):23–8.

18 Schickedanz AD, Schillinger D, Landefeld CS, Knight SJ, Williams BA, and Sudore RL (2009). A Clinical Framework for Improving the Advance Care Planning Process: Start with Patients Self Identified Barriers. *Journal of American Geriatrics Society*, **57**(1):31–9.

19 Thomas K and Free A. GSF Prognostic Indicator Guidance http://www.goldstandardsframework.nhs.uk/Resources/Gold%20Standards%20Framework/PIG_Paper_Final_revised_v5_Sept08.pdf

20 Maguire P, Faulkner A, Booth K, Elliot C, and Hillier V (1996). Helping cancer patients disclose their concerns. *European Journal of Cancer*,**32**A(1):78–81.

21 Maguire P (2002). Key Communication Skills and how to acquire them. *BMJ*, **325**:697–700.

22 Roter D and Frankel R (1992). Quantitative and qualitative approaches to evaluation of the medical dialogue. *Social Science and Medicine*, **34**:1097–1103.

23 Del Piccolo L, Goss C, and Bergvik S (2006). The fourth meeting of the Verona Network on Sequence Analysis: Consensus finding on the appropriateness of provider responses to patient cues and concerns, *Patient Education and Counseling*, **61**:473–75.

24 Fallowfield L, Jenkins V, Farewell V, Saul J, Duffy A, and Eves R (2002). Efficacy of a Cancer Research UK communication skills training model for oncologists: a randomised controlled trial. *Lancet*, **359**:650–56.

25 Wilkinson SM, Perry R, Linsell L, Blanchard K, and Roberts A (2006). A randomised controlled trial to evaluate the effectiveness of a three day communication skills training programme for palliative care nurses. *Palliative* Medicine, **20**(2):139.

26 Baile WF, Buckman R, Lenzi R, Glober G, Beale EA, and Kudelka AP (2000). SPIKES—a six-step protocol for delivering bad news: application to the patient with cancer. *Oncologist*, **5**:302–311.

27 Silverman JD, Kurtz SM, and Draper J (1998). *Skills for Communicating with Patients*. Radcliffe Medical Press, Oxford.

28 Connolly M and Duck A (2008). Communication skills in end-stage respiratory disease: managing distressed patients and breaking bad news, *Breathe*, **5**(2):147–54.

29 Department of Health (2008). *End of Life Care Strategy*. Department of Health, London.

30 Connected website http://www.connected.nhs.uk

31 Russell S and Fowler C (2009). *Report on: Pilot Advance Care Planning Workshops in Mount Vernon Cancer Network* - February to May 2009. V3. Mount Vernon Cancer Network, Internal Report.

32 Fry H, Ketteridge S, and Marshall S (2003). *A Handbook for Teaching and Learning in Higher Education*. Routledge Falmer, Oxon.

33 Kolb, D A (1984). *Experiential Learning*. Prentice-Hall, Englewood Cliffs, New Jersey.

34 Department of Health (2009). Common Core competences and principles for health and social care workers working with adults at the end of life. Department of Health, London http://www.endoflifecareforadults.nhs.uk

35 National Council for Palliative Care (2009). Help us to promote living and dying well. http://www.ncpc.org.uk/download/Coalition/CoalitionNewsletter01.pdf

Chapter 24

Working with local commissioners to deliver Advanced Care Planning

Jennifer Stothard

Commissioning is the process of specifying, securing and monitoring services to meet people's needs at a strategic level (1).

This chapter includes:

◆ The role of the commissioner

◆ Commissioning of end of life care services

◆ Commissioning to deliver Advanced Care Planning (ACP)

◆ Engaging commissioners to support delivery of ACP

◆ Challenges for delivery.

Key points

◆ Commissioners have a duty to ensure efficient and effective use of finite resources to deliver the best possible outcomes for the local community

◆ Commissioners (as well as providers) must culture quality, innovation, and productivity to better deliver these outcomes

◆ Health and Social Care stakeholders and their communities need to work in strategic partnerships and with transparency and probity

◆ ACP as part the end of life care has become a strategic and clinical priority especially in care homes or specific pathways e.g. cancer, dementia, long term conditions

---

Throughout the previous chapters you will have read the evidence to support the use of Advanced Care Planning for patients nearing the end of their life, examples of successful introduction of ACP in both health and social care sectors and examples of international best practice relating to ACP.

This chapter will focus on how to achieve engagement with local commissioners to ensure support for the introduction and sustained use of ACP within the local community. To achieve this the role of the commissioner will be discussed both in terms of general commissioning and in terms of commissioning end of life care services, potential outcome measures will be suggested; in particular how the use of ACP can enable service providers to deliver against these outcome measures, and finally issues regarding the delivery of effective commissioning of end of life care services will be discussed.

The role of the commissioner

Commissioners have a duty to ensure efficient and effective use of finite resources to deliver the best possible outcomes for the local community. Within the healthcare setting the statutory responsibility of PCT's in relation to commissioning can be defined as 'to determine local health needs and determine what services are to be provided to meet those needs, having regard to the resources available to them' (2).

The role of the commissioner can best be described through the implementation of a number of separate functions that when undertaken together form the process of commissioning, these can be summarized within the structure of a commissioning cycle (Fig. 24.1).

The commissioner's role is to assess the needs of the population and review the evidence to determine which interventions have been proven to be effective in meeting those needs. Prioritization must be undertaken both in terms of the needs of the population and the potential services to be provided, based on which will provide the greatest benefit in the most cost effective way, and which meet the strategic aims of the commissioner and local community. The prioritized services to be delivered must be defined within a service specification and then procured through the agreement of contractual terms and conditions or service level agreements (SLA) ensuring value for money is achieved. Upon agreement of the contract or SLA the performance of the provider in delivering the service is monitored by the commissioner against the key performance indicators and outcomes, as agreed within the contract terms, to ensure effective delivery of services. Delivery of the specified outcomes should ensure the needs of the population are met; however, this should be regularly monitored due to the changing needs of the population and potential changes in service delivery.

The many and varied roles of the commissioner have been described within *World Class Commissioning* guidance published in 2007 by the Department of Health. The guidance describes the 11 key competencies as a prerequisite to ensure effective commissioning within the health service. By undertaking the processes as detailed within the guidance commissioning organizations can ensure they are effective in undertaking their duties for the local heath community.

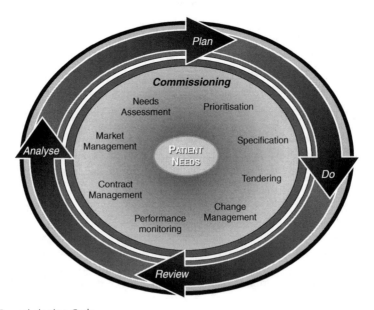

Fig. 24.1 Commissioning Cycle.

Commissioning end of life care services

In terms of end of life care services the aim of the commissioner is to work with providers of services to ensure that all patients at the end of life have access to consistent high quality, responsive care in all settings. An example of a generic service specification for the provision of end of life care services is provided within the document *Information for Commissioning End of Life Care* published by National End of Life Care Programme, 2008.

End of life care services are complex and ensuring the numerous services are in synergy is one of the greatest challenges for the commissioner. Commissioners must ensure there is a whole system approach to the delivery of end of life care services to ensure efficient and effective use of resources. As no two patients' needs or journeys are identical the challenge for commissioners is to ensure that the multitude of providers deliver consistent high quality responsive services which are adaptable to meet patient needs. To achieve this, the commissioner may use a number of different market management techniques including the provision of integrated care and prime contractor models, however, of vital importance is to ensure coordination is achieved between providers to enable efficient use of capacity and resources.

Commissioning to deliver ACP

Evidence shows that the most prominent issue within healthcare complaints made relating to palliative care is that patients and families were not given sufficient or timely information to enable them to make informed choices regarding the care they received (3). This evidence shows a requirement for commissioners to specify that information is provided to ensure that patients and carers feel sufficiently informed to make decisions regarding the care they wish to receive as their health declines. The implementation of Advanced Care Planning should empower patients and families to detail their needs and preferences in concise documentation which can be used to inform all services who provide care.

Commissioners must work with key stakeholders to agree the documentation to be used and then specify within contracts and SLAs that all providers must take account of the information contained within the Advanced Care Plan when delivering care. It is vital to ensure that all providers acknowledge the same documentation and consult this when creating patient care plans.

The Advanced Care Plan needs to be owned, coordinated, and updated regularly. Commissioners should work with key stakeholders to agree which provider will lead the discussion of ACP with patients and carers; this should then be reflected within service specifications and contract documentation. Service specifications for all providers should include the requirement to consult and utilize information provided within the Advanced Care Plan to ensure that the care provided for patients wherever possible meets the patient's needs and preferences.

Commissioners should include within the specification for end of life care services specific key performance indicators relating to the use of Advanced Care Plans which can be quantifiably measured at frequent intervals. Examples of potential key performance indicators relating to the use of Advanced Care Plans are included in Table 24.1. These key performance indicators should be supported by annual audits of key information sources to determine the quality of the service provided.

Delivery of the preferred place of care within the Advanced Care Plan should be considered as a key outcome measure for commissioning of end of life care services. However, measurement of this outcome must take into account that patients preferences may change as their health deteriorates; the wishes of families and carers may change; and the health needs of the patient may not enable the preferred place of care to be realized.

Table 24.1 Examples of key performance indicators relating to the provision of Advanced Care Planning to be included in the service specification

- ◆ % of patients offered ACP discussion
- ◆ % of patients at end of life with ACP documentation
- ◆ User satisfaction (patient/family/carers)
- ◆ Number of staff trained in use of ACP
- ◆ Number of staff trained in advanced communication skills

Case study detailing action undertaken in Derbyshire County to facilitate the use of ACP by service providers

To embed widespread use of ACP within the community, commissioners (both health and social care) established a project group with service providers. The aim of the project was to facilitate preference discussions with patients nearing the end of life and to assist in the planning of these wishes. A stakeholder consultation highlighted the need for a local overarching document which would be used to capture a patient's wishes and preferences and can be consulted by all service providers without replacing any of the care plan documentation required for use within each service provider. The overarching document facilitates the discussion with patients around planning for their care. More detailed discussions regarding advanced decisions to refuse treatment or lasting power of attorney are captured on other national documentation following discussions with appropriately trained staff.

To ensure the sustained use of the ACP tools within the community contractual terms have been agreed with the key service providers. In relation to primary care providers this will be incorporated in a locally enhanced service contract relating to end of life care. Reference has been made with regards to the use of ACP within the specification documents which include the training and competency level expected for the different staffing groups involved in providing end of life care; specific training required for the delivery of ACP; and information to be provided to commissioners on a regular basis. Following consultation with all other service providers involved in providing end of life care contractual terms will be agreed which detail the requirement to consult all ACP documents when creating a patient care plan.

Engaging commissioners to support delivery of ACP

In England there are many national strategic drivers which promote the improvement of end of life care as a priority for the local community these include the *National end of life care strategy* (2008), *High quality care for all* (2008) and the *Cancer reform strategy* (2007) all published by the Department of Health. However, one of the greatest drivers for every local community must be that the quality of end of life care provided should be seen as a marker for how we care for people within our society.

To deliver Advanced Care Planning in the end of life care setting may require additional competencies and capacity from service providers, which may represent a need for additional resources. To ensure investment for providing ACP is prioritized over other population needs the commissioner must be convinced of the importance of ACP in delivering the required outcomes. Examples of potential outcome measures for end of life care services are provided in Table 24.2; along with a description of how the use of ACP can help the provider deliver against these outcomes.

The information contained within the Advanced Care Plan can be used by commissioners to determine the expected level of demand for services, the service specification, and the structure of

Table 24.2 Examples of end of life care outcome measures and how the use of Advanced Care Planning can help providers deliver against the measures

End of life care outcome measure	Advanced Care Plan link
Number of deaths achieved in the place of choice	The Advanced Care Plan should be used to document the patient's preferences regarding place of care. This can be shared with all care providers to ensure services can be proactively planned to meet the patient's preferences
Number of deaths achieved at home	Information contained within the Advanced Care Plan can be audited to determine whether the patients preferences were met
User / carer satisfaction	Provision of Advanced Care Plans will improve user and carer satisfaction through ensuring patients and carers have the opportunity to determine the services they are provided
Individualized care	By understanding and documenting patient's preferences service providers can aim to provide care that meets patient's needs and preferences.

the supply model. It can also be used to support review of services and redesign of the patient journey or pathway. It is acknowledged that the introduction of ACP in the delivery of end of life care services does not reliably reduce healthcare costs (4); however, it is expected that cost shifts can be achieved by reducing the number of terminal hospitalizations and unplanned admissions in the last few months of life, and reinvesting the resource in community services to provide planned care (5).

Challenges for delivery

Management of change is never easy in a complex system and whole system redesign often requires a shift in organizational culture. Commissioners have a significant responsibility, as do providers, to instigate quality improvements and manage any changes required sensitively and effectively to ensure that providers are not destabilized and patients continue to receive the services they need.

One of the main challenges for commissioners in enabling delivery of patients' preferences is in terms of contracting sufficient resources to be available flexibly to meet the patients' needs and choices. To enable this it is stated that commissioners must ensure that there is a range of safe, effective, and accessible local services delivered by appropriately qualified healthcare professionals (6).

An argument against the use of Advanced Care Planning could be that it raises patient's and carer's expectations that all their preferences with regards to end of life care can be fulfilled; when in reality this may not be achievable for a variety of reasons, including declining health status requiring more intensive support, increased carer needs, or lack of service availability. Due to all the benefits derived from the use of Advanced Care Plans for end of life care the challenge for the commissioner is to ensure that providers make every reasonable effort to ensure care is provided in accordance with the preferences as stated within the Advanced Care Plan.

Conclusion

Whilst the role of the commissioner is not vital in delivering Advanced Care Planning for patients and carers, the engagement of the commissioner is key to ensuring that ACP is seen as a local priority and therefore is prioritized to gain investment to enable effective delivery. Gaining the support of commissioners will enable clinicians to successfully embed the use of ACP through securing resources within contractual terms.

The information captured within Advanced Care Plans is invaluable to commissioners to support strategic planning both in terms of the specification of the service requirement and to quantify expected level of demand.

Effective use of Advance Care Plans will ensure that providers of services deliver against the end of life care outcome measures to meet the needs of the population.

Further resources

Information for Commissioning End of Life Care (National End of Life Care Programme, 2008) www.end-oflifecare.nhs.uk

National end of life care strategy (Department of Health, 2008) www.dh.gov.uk/en/Publicationsandstatistics/Publications/PublicationsPolicyAndGuidance/DH_086277 (Accessed 28 June 2010)

World Class Commissioning (Department of Health, 2008) www.dh.gov.uk

End of Life care (National Audit Office, 2008) www.nao.org.uk

NICE guidance on supportive and palliative care for cancer patients (National Institute for Health and Clinical Excellence, 2004)www.nice.org.uk

End of Life care—a commissioning perspective (National Council for Palliative Care, 2007) www.ncpc.org.uk

References

1   Social Services Inspectorate/Audit Commission (2003). *Making Ends Meet.*

2   Department of Health (2008). *World Class Commissioning–The role of the Primary Care Trust board in world class commissioning.*

3   Healthcare Commission (2008). *Spotlight on complaints–A report on second-stage complaints about the NHS in England.*

4   Royal college of Physicians (2009). *Advanced Care Planning–Concise Guidance to Good Practice,* London.

5   Shiner A and Stothard J (2007). Shifting End of Life Care Back into the Community. *Journal of Integrated Care,* **15**(4)28–35.

6   Curry T (2005). Royal College of Nursing–Real Choice in the Health Service *The Real Choice Debate.* London.

Appendix 1

Useful websites and resources

Mental Capacity Act 2005: Information booklets
Current information is available from:
   http://www.justice.gov.uk/guidance/mental-capacity.htm
   http://www.opsi.gov.uk/acts/acts2005/ukpga_20050009_en_1
Mental Capacity Act: Code of Practice (2007):
   http://www.publicguardian.gov.uk/mca/code-of-practice.htm

Royal College of Physicians: National Guidelines Advance Care Planning: Concise
guidance to good practice, number 12. An excellent guidance document produced by the Royal
College of Physicians on the benefits and uses of ACP in England
   http://www.rcplondon.ac.uk/clinical-standards/organisation/Guidelines/concise-guidelines/
Pages/Advanced-Care-Planning.aspx

Advance Care Planning: A Guide for Health and Social Care Staff
http://eolc.cbcl.co.uk/eolc/files/F2023-EoLC-ACP_guide_for_staff-Aug2008.pdf
   Guidance on key issues and challenges of incorporating ACP into routine patient care, key
principles and definitions of ACP and related terms, and how ACP links to the Mental Capacity
Act.

Advance Decisions to Refuse Treatment: A Guide for Health and Social Care Staff
http://eolc.cbcl.co.uk/eolc/files/NHS-EoLC_ADRT_Sep2008.pdf
   A guide to help health and social care professionals understand and implement the new law
relating to advance decisions to refuse treatment, as contained in the Mental Capacity Act 2005.

Advance Decisions to Refuse Treatment
This approved website contains valuable resources for both patients and professionals on Advance
Decisions and many related end of life care issues: www.adrtnhs.co.uk
   ADRT decisions check list: http://www.adrtnhs.co.uk/pdf/Advance_Decisions_Checklist.pdf

My Advance Decisions to Refuse Treatment Form
ADRT example proforma: http://www.adrtnhs.co.uk/pdf/EoLC_appendix1.pdf
   People and professionals might use this example or develop it to meet their own individual or
local needs. There are other examples but care is required to ensure that they comply with the
legal requirements.

Decisions relating to cardiopulmonary resuscitation:
A joint statement from the British Medical Association, the Resuscitation Council (UK),
   and the Royal College of Nursing www.resus.org.uk/pages/dnar.pdf

Clinical Decisions Algorithm
The process for making clinical decisions in serious medical conditions in patients over 18 years.
In Regnard C, Hockley J, Dean M. (2008) *A guide to Symptom Relief in Palliative Care*. Radcliffe
Publishing, 6th ed.

Differences between general care planning and decisions made in advance (PDF)

http://www.endoflifecareforadults.nhs.uk/assets/downloads/differences_between_acp_and_adrt.pdf

A guide to show differences between ACP and ADRT published March 2010

Planning for your future care: a guide (PDF)

http://www.endoflifecareforadults.nhs.uk/assets/downloads/pubs_Planning_for_your_future_care.pdf

A simple and easy to understand guide for patients making Advance Care Plans for their future. It may prove relevant to family members and informal carers.

Gold Standards Framework

http://www.goldstandardsframework.nhs.uk/AdvanceCarePlanning

General guidance and information on the use of Advance Care Planning as part of the Gold Standards Framework programmes in end of life care, primary care, care homes, acute hospitals, and other settings. GSF helps to identify which patients may be in the final year or so of life, using the Prognostic Indicator Guidance Paper (Appendix 2) and thereby to trigger the ACP discussion. Examples of an ACP tool the 'Thinking Ahead' paper that is frequently used in care homes is included.

http://www.goldstandardsframework.nhs.uk/Resources/Gold%20Standards%20Framework/138%20GSF%20PIG%20Vol%204%20No%201.pdf

The National Council for Palliative Care

www.ncpc.org.uk/publications

- The Mental Capacity Act in Practice
- Good Decision Making: The Mental Capacity Act and End of Life Care

Liverpool Care Pathway for the Final days

http://www.mcpcil.org.uk/liverpool-care-pathway/

Preferred Priorities of Care

http://www.endoflifecare.nhs.uk/eolc/ppc.htm

Some examples from other countries (others included in the relevant chapters):

Australian: Respecting0 Patient Choices

An extensive ACP programme run in many settings in Australia, based at Austin Hospital, Melbourne www.respectingpatientchoices.org.au

USA

Literature Review on advance directives. Wilkinson AM, Wenger N, Shugarman LR. (2007). Available at: http://aspe.hhs.gov/daltcp/reports/2007/advdirlr.pdf

'Respecting Choices Advance Care Planning Facilitators Manual,' Gundersen Lutheran Programs for Improving End-of-Life Care, Gundersen Lutheran Medical Foundation, 2000. http://www.gundluth.org/eolprograms

Canada

Advance Care Planning: 'Let's Talk'

  http://www.fraserhealth.ca/HealthInfo/AdvanceCarePlanning/Default.htm

  Living Lessons® is an information and resource program developed through a partnership between the GlaxoSmithKline Foundation and the Canadian Hospice Palliative Care Association. More information may be found at http://www.living-lessons.org.

Appendix 2

Aids to communication

SATNAV: See Chapter 12 (Holman 2009)

Summarize	A good place to start is to summarize the resident's history. It may be that the conversation is being initiated following repeated hospital admissions or in the light of deteriorating health or new diagnosis of a life limiting illness or early dementia.
Aim	Get to the point. It can often feel uncomfortable to get to the point and use words that have a definite understanding. Phases like 'the reason I am having this conversation is to...' can help to direct the conversation.
Test the water	It is important to know the effect that the conversation is having on the person, be it the resident or the family. It is therefore helpful to 'test the water' and check how appropriate it is to continue. For example to ask the question at this point 'Are you happy for us to continue with this discussion?' can help to gauge the appropriateness of continuing.
Navigate a way forward	It is not uncommon that a resident or family member may not know how to proceed from this point. It is therefore helpful to be able to guide them, for example to suggest 'What you might want to do/consider is...' Or 'perhaps what might be helpful at this stage is...'
Add further information	It is important to be able to help residents and families make informed decisions. Therefore at this point it can be helpful to offer supporting information. It may be about suggesting other services that may be available or other sources of information that might help. It could include information about treatment.
Vocal reassurance	Each conversation should end with significant vocal reassurance. It should be remembered that many people do not remember everything that is said and may indeed only remember the 'good news'. As uncomfortable as these conversations may become, how a person is left feeling may be more important than what has been said.

PREPARED: Key recommendations for discussions about ACP and end of life issues (see Chapter 21)

* From: 'Clinical practice guidelines for communicating prognosis and end-of-life issues with adults in the advanced stages of a life-limiting illness, and their caregivers'. Josephine M Clayton, Karen M Hancock, Phyllis N Butow, Martin HN Tattersall and David C Currow, **MJA** • Volume 186 Number 12 • 18 June 2007 • Copyright Medical Journal of Australia • Reproduced with permission.

P	**Prepare for the discussion**, where possible:
	◆ Confirm pathological diagnosis and investigation results before initiating discussion.
	◆ Try to ensure privacy and uninterrupted time for discussion.
	◆ Negotiate who should be present during the discussion.
R	**Relate to the person:**
	◆ Develop rapport.
	◆ Show empathy, care and compassion during the entire consultation.
E	**Elicit patient and caregiver preferences:**
	◆ Identify the reason for this consultation and elicit the patient's expectations.
	◆ Clarify the patient's or caregiver's understanding of their situation, and establish how much detail and what they want to know.
	◆ Consider cultural and contextual factors influencing information preferences.
P	**Provide information** tailored to the individual needs of both patients and their families:
	◆ Offer to discuss what to expect, in a sensitive manner, giving the patient the option not to discuss it.
	◆ Pace information to the patient's information preferences, understanding and circumstances.
	◆ Use clear, jargon-free, understandable language.
	◆ Explain the uncertainty, limitations and unreliability of prognostic and end-of-life information.
	◆ Avoid being too exact with timeframes unless in the last few days.
	◆ Consider the caregiver's distinct information needs, which may require a separate meeting with the caregiver (provided the patient, if mentally competent, gives consent).
	◆ Try to ensure consistency of information and approach provided to different family members and the patient and from different clinical team members.
A	**Acknowledge emotions & concerns:**
	◆ Explore and acknowledge the patient's and caregiver's fears and concerns and their emotional reaction to the discussion.
	◆ Respond to the patient's or caregiver's distress regarding the discussion, where applicable.
R	(foster) **Realistic hope** (e.g. peaceful death, support):
	◆ Be honest without being blunt or giving more detailed information than desired by the patient.
	◆ Do not give misleading or false information to try to positively influence a patient's hope.
	◆ Reassure that support, treatments and resources are available to control pain and other symptoms, but avoid premature reassurance.
	◆ Explore and facilitate realistic goals and wishes, and ways of coping on a day-to-day basis, where appropriate.

E **Encourage questions** and further discussions:

♦ Encourage questions and information clarification; be prepared to repeat explanations.

♦ Check understanding of what has been discussed and if the information provided meets the patient's and caregiver's needs.

♦ Leave the door open for topics to be discussed again in the future.

D **Document:**

♦ Write a summary of what has been discussed in the medical record.

♦ Speak or write to other key health care providers involved in the patient's care. As a minimum, this should include the patient's general practitioner.

Appendix 3

Guidance and useful ACP tools

Excerpts from Royal College of Physicians Concise Guidelines on Advance Care Planning

Reproduced from: Royal College of Physicians, National Council for Palliative Care, British Society of Rehabilitation Medicine, British Geriatrics Society, Alzheimer's Society, Royal College of Nursing, Royal College of Psychiatrists, Help the Aged, Royal College of General Practitioners. *Advance care planning*. Concise Guidance to Good Practice series, No 12. London: RCP, 2009 with permission. Available here: http://www.rcplondon.ac.uk/pubs/contents/9c95f6ea-c57e-4-db8-bd98-fc12ba31c8fe.pdf

---

Box A3.1 Tips for a successful ACP discussion

- The individual needs to be ready for the discussion – it cannot be forced.
- Discussions usually need to take place on more than one occasion (over days, weeks, months) and should not be completed on a single visit in most circumstances.
- Discussions take time and effort and cannot be completed as a simple checklist exercise.
- Discussions should take place in comfortable, unhurried surroundings; time is a key factor.
- It is important that capacity is maximized by ensuring the treatment of any transient condition affecting communication and optimising sensory function (e.g. by obtaining the patient's hearing aid).
- A step-by-step approach should be used.
- Discussions should be characterised by truthfulness; respect; time; compassion and empathy.
- A tool to introduce the concept and guide the discussion may help professionals to address ACP with people (see Box A3.2).
- Information should be given using words the person understands.
- Clarify any ambiguous terms used by your patient, for example: 'could you explain what you mean by not wanting any heroics?'
- Checking and reflecting in this way is a key part of effective communication.
- Individuals should be given sufficient information about their possible options and under what circumstances their plan would be activated. They need to understand what the consequences of their decision would be.
- The professional should look out for cues that the individual wishes to end the discussion.
- The professional should summarize and check understanding with the patient.

Box A3.1 Tips for a successful ACP discussion *(continued)*

- The discussion should be documented if the patient so wishes.
- Not all people will be able to document their wishes, but may well be able to nominate their preferred decision maker and discuss their long-term values, as these come to mind more readily than anticipating abstract situations.
- Audio-visual recordings might be helpful in providing the individual a record of the discussion.
- Plan for a review.

Box A3.2 Suggested content for an ACP document

A document is not a requirement of ACP, unless the patient specifically wishes to record an ADRT refusing life-sustaining treatment.

However, we reviewed a variety of ACP documents (see below); none is ideal. In practice a combination of documents are likely to be required:

- an administrative section with relevant contact numbers
- a tool to help people express their preferences, such as the Hammersmith Expression of Healthcare Preferences
- an MCA-compliant ADRT (if the individual wishes this), which should help direct care and a reference to any LPA.

Accompanying notes should be clear, concise, and unambiguous. It should, however, be emphasized that ACP is more about discussion and communication than the forms, although documentation is important, especially for ADRTs.

ACP documents examined:

- Let Me Decide Molloy DW MV. *Let Me Decide*, 2nd ed. Hamilton, OntarioMcMaster University Press, 1990.
- The Medical Directive Emanuel LL EE. The Medical Directive: a new comprehensive advance care document. *JAMA.* 1989;**22**(261):3288–93.
- Dignity in Dying (www.dignityindying.org.uk/livingwills)
- Alzheimer's Society living will (www.alzheimers.org.uk/site/scripts/documents_info.php?documentID=143)
- Hammersmith Expression of Healthcare Preferences137
- Thinking Ahead – ACP planning discussion (www.goldstandardsframework.nhs.uk/advanced_care.php)
- Advanced Clinical management plan (Minnie Kidd House)
- Care Home Support Team – health care choices form
- Physician Orders for Life Sustaining Treatment (POLST) (www.ohsu.edu/polst)
- Lawpack Advance Medical Decision (www.lawpack.co.uk/Family/product859.asp)
- ADRT.nhs.uk (www.adrtnhs.co.uk/pages/links.htm)
- Preferred Priorities of Care (www.endoflifecareforadults.nhs.uk/eolc/ppc.htm)

If the patient **does not** have an impairment or disturbance of mind or brain, assume the patient has capacity

If an impairment is present, is this sufficient to cause a lack of capacity?
The patient's capacity for this decision can be assessed as follows:
   1. Can they understand the information?
      NB. this must be imparted in a way the patient can understand
   2. Can they retain the information?
      NB. This only needs to be long enough to use and weigh the information
   3. Can they use and weigh up that information?
      NB. They must be able to show that they are able to consider the benefits and burdens of the alternatives to the proposed treatment
   4. Can they communicate the decision?
      NB. The carers must try every method possible to enable this
The result of each step of this assessment should be documented, ideally byquoting the patient.

Does the person have capacity for this decision?	Ask the patient. NB. An eccentric or unwise decision does not imply a lack of capacity

Is there an Advance Decision to Refuse Treatment (ADRT) and/or A Lasting Power of Attorney for Personal Welfare (LPA-PW)	• **If the ADRT is the most recent decision:** - check that the circumstances of the ADRT match the current circumstances and that the ADRT is valid and applicable, ie. if it specifies treatments to be refused even if life is at risk, is signed and witnessed This ADRT then overrides any previous ADRT or LPA appointment - follow the decision(s) stated in the ADRT • **If the appointment of a LPA(PW) is the most recent decision:** - seek verification by viewing the signed LPA document and its accompanying third party certificate - check that the LPA document is signed and includes the authority to decide on life sustaining treatment This LPA(H&W) then overrides any previous ADRT or LPA appointment - fully inform the LPA(PW) of the clinical facts - ask the LPA(PW) for their decision NB. there may be more than one LPA

Is the patient without anyone whom is appropriate to consult about their best interests?	• In an emergency, act in the patient's best interests (see below). • For certain serious medical decisions, it is necessary to involve an Independent Mental Capacity Advocate (IMCA) who are available locally

• The person legally responsible for the patient (often the GP or consultant) makes a decision as below.
• **The person assessing the patient's best interests must**
   1. Make sure not to make any judgements using the professionals' view of the patient's quality of life.
   2. Consider all the relevant circumstances and options without discrimination
   3. Not be motivated by a desire to bring about the patient's death
   4. Consult with family, partner or representatives as to whether the patient previously had expressed any opinions or wishes about their future care.
   5. Consult with the clinical team caring for the patient. If necessary ask for an opinion from a specialist with knowledge of the patient's condition.
   6. Consider any beliefs and values likely to influence the patient if they had capacity
   7. Consider any other factors the patient would consider if they were able to do so.
   8. Consider the patient's feelings.

If there unresolved conflicts, consider involving
- the local ethics committee
- the Court of Protection

Fig. A3.1 Guidance on the process for making clinical decisions in serious medical conditions in patients over 18 years.

V9 © 2008. Regnard C, Hockley J, Dean M. A Guide to Symptom Relief in Palliative Care, Radcliffe Publishing, 6th ed.
Reproduced with permission from C Regnard.

Extract from preferred priorities of care document

For full document and other details see
http://eolc.cbcl.co.uk/eolc/files/F2110-Preferred_Priorities_for_Care_V2_Dec2007.pdf

Your preferences and priorities
Version 2 December 2007 Review date December 2009

In relation to your health, what has been happening to you?

What are your preferences and priorities for your future care?

Where would you like to be cared for in the future?

Signature   **Date**

Please record any changes to your preferences and priorities here
(Please sign and date any changes)

Further information
You can use this page to make a note of any further information you need or questions you might
want to ask your professional carers (like your doctor, nurse or social worker).

Excerpt from ACP developed by St Christopher's Hospice Feb 2010

> Copies of the ACP booklet are available through St Christopher's bookshop and can be
> ordered by contacting d.brady@stchristophers.org.uk

Your personal preferences and choices

1 Where would you like to be cared for if you are no longer able to care for yourself?
   - First preference
   - Second preference
2 Bearing in mind that your circumstances may change, where would you prefer to be cared for
   when you are dying? e.g. home, care home, hospital, or hospice
   - First preference
   - Second preference
3 Who knows you well and understands what is important to you?
4 Who do you view as your next of kin?
5 Who or what supports you when things are difficult?
6 Do you have a particular faith or belief system that is important to you?
7 Would you like to talk to anyone about it?
   YES ☐   NO ☐   If YES, who?
8 What concerns you most about your health, now and for the future?

9 Are there discussions with family and/or friends you feel would be helpful?
Would you like anyone to help you with this?

YES ☐   NO ☐   If YES, who?

10 Have you made a will?

YES ☐   NO ☐

- If YES, where is it held?
- If NO, would you like to discuss how to make a will?

11 Does anyone have Lasting Power of Attorney (Property and Affairs) for you?
See page 9

YES ☐   NO☐

- If YES, please add their full contact details to page 11
- If NO, would you like to discuss this? YES NO

12 Do you want to be buried or cremated?

BURIED ☐   CREMATED☐

13 Do you have any arrangements in place?

YES ☐   NO☐

If YES, please provide details

14 If it were possible, would you wish to donate any of your organs?

YES ☐   NO☐

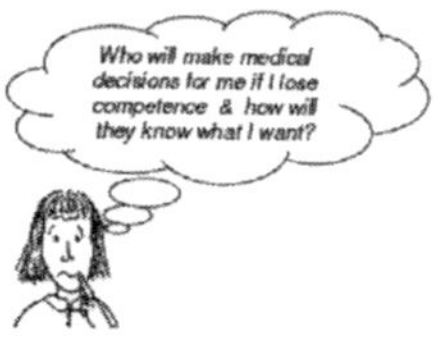

Who will make medical decisions for me if I lose competence & how will they know what I want?	**Advance Care Planning in 3-Steps**		
	Advance	A	Appoint an Agent
	Care	C	Chat and Communicate
	Planning	P	Put it on Paper

Talking to your patients about Advance Care Planning

A Appoint an Agent	**C Chat and Communicate**	**P Put it on Paper**
It is important to remember that the competent patient can: • Consent to or refuse treatment for themself • Legally appoint an Enduring Power of Attorney - Medical Treatment to consent to or refuse treatment on their behalf if / when incompetent to make these decisions for themself • Nominate their Person Responsible in writing	Encourage and facilitate patients and families / friends to talk about: • Things I value are.... • Future situations that I would find unacceptable in relation to my health are.... • Specific treatments that I would NOT want considered for me are.... • This is who I would like to be involved in decisions....	Advise your patient that if there is something they feel strongly about they can write it down and give a copy of their documents to the relevant people. Advance Care Planning documents can include: • Handwritten letter • Statement of Choices / Preferences • Refusal of Treatment Certificate

'ACP in 3-Steps' © Northern Health 2009

NH Advance Care Planning Program
9495 3235 or acp@nh.org.au

Fig. A3.2 Copyright Northern Health (Melbourne, Australia). Reproduced with permission.

Example proforma for ADRT

NHS End of Life Care – Advance decisions to refuse treatment
http://www.adrtnhs.co.uk/pdf/EoLC_appendix1.pdf

My Advance Decision to Refuse Treatment

My Name	Any distinguishing features in the event of unconsciousness
Address	Date of Birth
	Telephone Number

What is this document is for?

This advance decision to refuse treatment has been written by me to state in advance which treatments I don't want in the future. These are my decisions about my healthcare, in the event that I have lost mental capacity and can not consent to or refuse treatment. This advance decision replaces any previous advance decision I have made.

Advice to the reader

I have written this document to identify my advance decision. I would expect any health care professionals reading this document in the event I have lost capacity to check that my advance decision is valid and applicable, in the circumstances that exist at the time.

Please check

Please do not assume I have lost capacity before any actions are taken. I might need help and time to communicate.

If I have lost capacity please check the validity and applicability of this advance decision.

This advance decision becomes legally binding and must be followed if professionals are satisfied it is valid and applicable. Please help to share this information with people who are involved in my treatment and care and need to know about this.

Please also check if I have made any other statements about my preferences or decisions that might be relevant to my advance decision.

This advance decision does not refuse the offer and or provision of basic care, support and comfort.

My Name

My advance decision to refuse treatment

I wish to refuse the following specific treatments:	*In these circumstances:*

(Please note that refusal of life sustaining treatments must include the statement this decision applies 'even if my life is at risk')

My Signature	**Date of Signature**
(or nominated person)	
Witness	Witness Signature
Name	Telephone
Address	Date

Person to be contacted to discuss my wishes:

Name	**Relationship**
Address	**Telephone**

I have discussed this with (e.g. name of Healthcare Professional)

Profession / Job Title

Contact Details

Date

I give permission for this document to be discussed with my relatives / carers

Yes   **NO**   (please circle one)

My General Practitioner is: (name)

Address

Telephone Number

Optional Review   ·   Date/Time

Comment

Maker's Signature   Witness Signature

The following list identifies which people have a copy and have been told about this Advance Decision to Refuse Treatment (and their contact details)

Name	Relationship	Telephone number

Advance Decisions Check List

Always assume the person has capacity to consent to or refuse treatment. Please maximise the person's capacity and facilitate communication.

QUESTION	Answer Yes/No	GUIDANCE
Does the person have capacity to give consent to or refuse treatment him or herself, with appropriate support where necessary		**YES:** the person has capacity to make the decision him or herself. The advance decision is not applicable. Ask what s/he wants to do **NO:** Continue with check list

IS THE ADVANCE DECISION VALID

	QUESTION	Answer Yes/No	GUIDANCE
1	Has the person withdrawn the advance decision? (this can be done verbally or in writing)		**YES:** This is not a valid advance decision. Make sure that you have identified and recorded the evidence that the person withdrew the advance decision. **NO:** Continue with the checklist
2	Since making the advance decision, has the person created a lasting power of attorney (LPA) giving anybody else the authority to refuse or consent to the treatment in question?		**YES:** This is not a valid advance decision. The donee(s) of the LPA must give consent to or refuse the treatment. The LPA decision must be in the person's best interests. **NO:** Continue with the checklist

3	Are there reasonable grounds for believing that circumstances exist which the person did not anticipate at the time of making the advance decision and which would have affected his/her decision had s/he anticipated them?	**YES:** If such reasonable grounds exist, this will not be an applicable advance decision. It is important to identify the grounds, discuss this with anybody close to the person, and identify why they would have affected his/her decision had s/he anticipated them, and record your reasoning. **NO:** Continue with the checklist
4	Has the person done anything that is clearly inconsistent with the advance decision remaining his/her fixed decision?	**YES:** This is not a valid advance decision. It is important to identify what the person has done, discuss this with anybody close to the person, explain why this is inconsistent with the advance decision remaining his/her fixed decision, and record your reasons. **NO:** The advance decision is valid Continue with the checklist.

IS THE ADVANCE DECISION APPLICABLE

5	(a) Does the advance decision **specify** which treatment the person wishes to refuse?* (b) Is the treatment in question that specified in the advance decision?	**YES to both (a) and (b):** Continue with the checklist **NO:** This is not an applicable advance decision
6	If the advance decision has specified circumstances in which it is to apply (see question 3 above), do **all** of those circumstances exist at the time that the decision whether to refuse treatment needs to be made? *(N.B. It is possible for a person to decide that the advance decision should apply in **all** circumstances)*	**YES:** Continue with the checklist **NO:** This is not an applicable advance decision

LIFE SUSTAINING TREATMENT

8	Is the decision both valid and applicable according to the criteria set out above?	**YES:** Continue with the check list **NO:** This is not a binding advance decision to refuse the specified life sustaining treatment

9	In your opinion is the treatment in question necessary to sustain the person's life?	**YES:** Continue with the checklist **NO:** This is a binding advance decision to refuse the specified non-life-sustaining treatment. It must be respected and followed.
10	Does the advance decision contain a statement that it is to apply even if the person's life is at risk?	**YES:** Continue with the checklist **NO:** This is not a binding advance decision to refuse the specified life-sustaining treatment.
11	Is the advance decision: In writing AND Signed by the person making it or by somebody else on his behalf and at his direction AND Signed by a witness?	**YES TO ALL:** This is a binding advance decision to refuse the specified life-sustaining treatment. It must be respected and followed. **NO TO ANY:** This is not a binding advance decision to refuse the specified life-sustaining treatment.

Gold Standards Framework prognostic indicator guidance paper

available at

http://www.goldstandardsframework.nhs.uk/Resources/Gold%20Standards%20Framework/PIG_Paper_Final_revised_v5_Sept08.pdf.

Index

Printed and bound by CPI Group (UK) Ltd, Croydon, CR0 4YY